Register Now for Online Access to Your Book!

SPRINGER PUBLISHING
CONNECT™

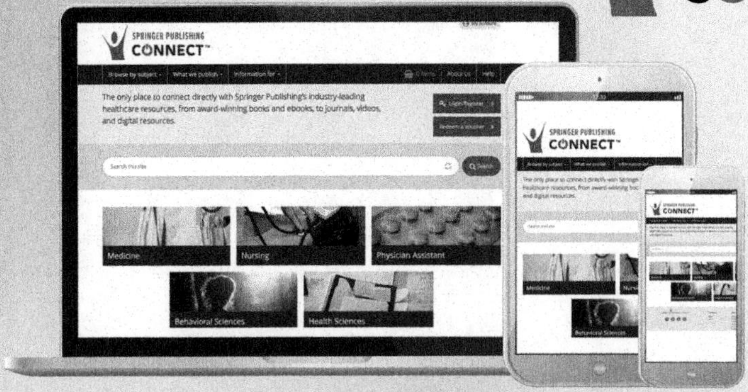

Your print purchase of *Guidelines for Nurse Practitioners in Ambulatory Obstetric Settings, Third Edition,* **includes online access to the contents of your book**—increasing accessibility, portability, and searchability!

Access today at:

http://connect.springerpub.com/content/book/978-0-8261-4854-4
or scan the QR code at the right with your smartphone. Log in or register, then click "Redeem a voucher" and use the code below.

NMYMXNL9

Scan here for quick access.

Having trouble redeeming a voucher code?
Go to https://connect.springerpub.com/redeeming-voucher-code

If you are experiencing problems accessing the digital component of this product, please contact our customer service department at cs@springerpub.com

The online access with your print purchase is available at the publisher's discretion and may be removed at any time without notice.

Publisher's Note: New and used products purchased from third-party sellers are not guaranteed for quality, authenticity, or access to any included digital components.

SPRINGER PUBLISHING
View all our products at springerpub.com

Guidelines for Nurse Practitioners in Ambulatory Obstetric Settings

Kelly D. Rosenberger, DNP, APRN, CNM, WHNP-BC, FAANP, is a women's health nurse practitioner (NP) and certified nurse midwife with more than 25 years of experience providing high-quality, patient-centered OB/GYN care. Her clinical service initially began at the Cleveland Clinic Foundation in the 1990s, and she currently has a robust clinical practice at the University of Illinois Chicago (UIC) Mile Square L.P. Johnson FQHC in Rockford, Illinois. Dr. Rosenberger is also a Clinical Assistant Professor at UIC in the Department of Human Developmental Nursing Science in the College of Nursing and in the Department of Family and Community Medicine in the College of Medicine.

At UIC, Dr. Rosenberger taught the Clinical Skills course to medical students from 2007 to 2014 at the Rockford Campus. Dr. Rosenberger has also taught numerous advanced practice clinical and DNP courses for the College of Nursing in addition to precepting numerous NP and medical students since 1997. In 2016, Dr. Rosenberger was honored with the Preceptor of the Year Award. Dr. Rosenberger has served as a manuscript reviewer and guest editor as invited for her expertise in OB/GYN. She is well published and has numerous presentations on many topics.

Dr. Rosenberger has been a member of many professional organizations, including the American College of Nurse-Midwives and the American Association of Nurse Practitioners (AANP). In 2018, she received AANP's highest honor with induction as a Fellow. In 2021, Dr. Rosenberger received the I-TEAM Award from the UIC for her excellence in interprofessional clinical practice and development of teaching innovations with the National Center for Rural Health Professions.

Nancy J. Cibulka, PhD, WHNP, FNP-BC, FAANP, is a women's health and family nurse practitioner (NP) with extensive practice experience providing prenatal, postpartal, and well woman care to inner city women at Barnes-Jewish Hospital and at Washington University's OB/GYN clinic. She is also an Associate Professor in Nursing at Saint Louis University teaching in the DNP program. Dr. Cibulka's experience as an NP spans more than 40 years, including with the OB/GYN clinic (Barnes-Jewish Hospital), Health Resources Center (Saint Louis University free clinic), Vista Staffing Solutions (Milwaukee, Wisconsin), Take-Care Health Systems (St. Louis), Unity Corporate Health Services, and private practice Perinatal Group at Washington University School of Medicine (St. Louis) and Gratiot Community Hospital private practice (Alma, Michigan).

In addition to her current teaching position at Saint Louis University, Dr. Cibulka was an associate professor of nursing at Maryville University (St. Louis, Missouri) and an instructor at the University of Iowa College of Nursing. Dr. Cibulka has taught undergraduate courses in maternal–child nursing and taught advanced graduate clinical courses in advanced health assessment; care of the adolescent, adult, and older adult; care of childbearing and childrearing families; professional role development; and advanced clinical practicum. Additional clinical experience includes being an NP, Planned Parenthood of East Central Ohio; nurse consultant, Maternal & Child Health Bureau, Iowa Department of Public Health; and clinical consultant, March of Dimes Perinatal Project, Wisconsin Vocational Studies Center, University of Wisconsin. She has published articles in the *Journal of Obstetric, Gynecologic, & Neonatal Nursing; American Journal of Nursing; Journal of the Association of Nurses in AIDS Care; The Journal for Nurse Practitioners; Journal of Nursing Education;* and *Journal of the American Association of Nurse Practitioners*; among others. She has presented papers at national conferences, including the Association of Women's Health, Obstetric, and Neonatal Nurses; National Organization of Nurse Practitioner Faculties (NONPF); Midwest Nursing Research Society; Sigma Theta Tau International (STTI); and the annual evidence-based practice conferences. Honors and awards include the Research Abstract Award (American Association of Nurse Practitioners [AANP] in 2008), research poster (STTI in 2005), School of Health Professions Distinguished Faculty Award (2005), the scholarship/fellowship award (Abbott Labs in 2005), and the Maryville University President's Faculty Award for Exemplary Service for Scholarship (2005), among others. She is a member of the AANP and, in June 2012, she was inducted into the Fellows.

Mary Lee Barron, PhD, APRN, FNP-BC, FAANP, is an associate professor, School of Nursing, Southern Illinois University Edwardsville (SIUE). Additionally, she is the Director of Marquette Fertility Education, offering direct patient care services and research in natural family planning. Formerly, she taught at Saint Louis University in the FNP program and served as Director of the Master's and DNP Programs. With more than 40 years of nursing experience, her nurse practitioner (NP) clinical experience has focused on OB/GYN at the OB/GYN clinic (Barnes–Jewish Hospital) and affiliated with Washington University School of Medicine and Saint Louis University. She has taught the Marquette Method as a Natural Family Planning Instructor and has been trained by the Pope Paul VI Institute, Omaha, Nebraska, as a Medical Consultant and Fertility Care Practitioner. She also served in the U.S. Naval Reserve, where she advanced to the rank of Lieutenant Commander.

At SIUE, Dr. Barron teaches graduate Advanced Management of Women's Health with Practicum, Nursing Research, Theory-Guided Practice, and Emerging Roles in Advanced Nursing Practice. She has published 23 peer-reviewed articles in a variety of journals. Dr. Barron has authored the March of Dimes module on Antepartum Care and Laboratory Examination since 1998 and served as a visiting professor presenting "Born Too Soon" for the Los Angeles chapter. She has authored 10 book chapters and presents widely on topics related to the health benefits of breastfeeding, natural family planning, obesity and pregnancy, and hormone replacement therapy. Dr. Barron is the recipient of several awards, including March of Dimes Nurse of the Year (Advanced Practice) in 2017, Leadership Academy Fellow (American Association of Colleges of Nursing [AACN]), and Alpha Sigma Nu (Jesuit Honor Society). She is a member of the American Association of Nurse Practitioners (AANP) and in June 2014 she was inducted into the Fellows.

Additionally, she has held membership in Sigma Theta Tau International (STTI), Association of Women's Health, Obstetric, and Neonatal Nurses (AWHONN), National Organization of Nurse Practitioner Faculties (NONPF), and serves as a manuscript reviewer for a number of journals, including *Clinical Nursing Research, MCN: The American Journal of Maternal Child Nursing* and *Biological Research for Nursing*.

Guidelines for Nurse Practitioners in Ambulatory Obstetric Settings

Third Edition

Kelly D. Rosenberger, DNP, APRN, CNM, WHNP-BC, FAANP

Nancy J. Cibulka, PhD, WHNP, FNP-BC, FAANP

Mary Lee Barron, PhD, APRN, FNP-BC, FAANP

SPRINGER PUBLISHING

First Springer Publishing edition 2013; subsequent edition 2017

Springer Publishing Company, LLC
11 West 42nd Street, New York, NY 10036
www.springerpub.com
connect.springerpub.com/

Acquisitions Editor: Rachel X. Landes
Compositor: diacriTech

ISBN: 978-0-8261-4845-2
ebook ISBN: 978-0-8261-4854-4
DOI: 10.1891/9780826148544

22 23 25 25 / 5 4 3 2 1

Library of Congress Control Number: 2021922673

Printed in the United States of America.

Contents

IV. Guidelines for Management of Selected Complications of Pregnancy

Appendices

Contributors

Karen Cotler, DNP, FNP-BC, FAANP
Dr. Cotler is a faculty member of the University of Illinois Chicago (UIC) College of Nursing, where she teaches and directs the FNP program. She also has a robust FNP clinical practice caring for individuals with HIV. Dr. Cotler contributed to Chapter 20.

Anna J. Fischer Colby, BFA, MS, MPP
Anna Colby is a senior research associate at Public Policy Associates (PPA) in Lansing, Michigan. She has extensive experience in public policy, development, research, and evaluation in food systems, healthcare, education, and other areas. Prior to joining PPA in 2019, Ms. Colby worked as a policy advocate for California Food Policy Advocates (CFPA) and was assistant director of the Tomas Rivera Policy Institute (TRPI) of the University of Southern California. Ms. Colby contributed the graphics in Figure 2.1 and created Table 19.1.

Lisa Hickman, BSN, RNC-OB
Ms. Hickman is a current student of Dr. Rosenberger in the NMW/WHNP Program at the University of Illinois Chicago (UIC) College of Nursing. She is a certified OB RN with many years of labor and delivery experience. She contributed to Chapter 2.

Michael P. Rosenberger, BSc, MPH
Mr. Rosenberger is currently completing his third year as a medical student. With a bachelor's in chemistry, a master's in public health, and interest in endocrinology, he has presented on several topics related to women's healthcare. He contributed to Chapters 10 and 23.

Amy M. Seibert, DNP, WHNP-BC
Dr. Seibert is a former student of Dr. Rosenberger's and has published with Dr. Rosenberger on OB/GYN topics, such as asymptomatic GBS bacteriuria. She has a robust clinical practice as a WHNP-BC at the Midwest Center for Women's Healthcare. She contributed to Chapters 12, 13, and 24.

Janet Thorlton, PhD, MS, RN, CNE
Dr. Thorlton is a faculty member of the University of Illinois Chicago (UIC) College of Nursing, where she teaches DNP students and conducts a program of research surrounding consumer use of performance enhancing ingredients contained in dietary supplements and energy drinks. She contributed to Chapter 3.

Preface

The third edition of *Guidelines for Nurse Practitioners in Ambulatory Obstetric Settings* is designed for nurse practitioners, nurse midwives, clinical nurse specialists, physician assistants, students in these areas, and other health professionals who provide prenatal and postpartum care in outpatient settings. The initial decision to write this book was prompted by our mutual desire to incorporate more than 100 years of combined practice experience caring for women and newborns with the best evidence currently available to positively impact pregnancy outcomes. Since the first edition was published, practice knowledge has changed in many areas, and we were aware of the importance of updating the information. The extensive revisions in this edition reflect new guidelines for practice endorsed by professional organizations and/or the government. Each chapter has been updated with new references and contains new management strategies. Throughout history, quality care before, during, and after childbirth has played an important role in reducing maternal and fetal death, preventing birth defects, and decreasing the incidence of other preventable health problems. Healthcare providers have a remarkable opportunity to provide health education, assessment, and early problem identification and management during the preconception and childbearing years. To help achieve these goals, the third edition of this book presents the best available practice evidence for providing preconception, prenatal, and postpartum care in one easy-to-use publication.

This book is organized into four sections. Part I, "Guidelines for Preparation for Pregnancy," comprehensively covers preconception counseling and care, as well as the latest guidelines on screening for genetic disorders before and during pregnancy. Part II, "Guidelines for Routine Prenatal and Postpartum Care," provides a wealth of information on key assessments, including laboratory and ultrasound diagnostics for the initial prenatal visit and for subsequent visits. Management of uncomplicated pregnancies and the discomforts that commonly occur are addressed, along with safe medication use and antenatal surveillance recommendations. The continuum of obstetric care does not end with the delivery of the infant; thus, in-depth recommendations are provided for postpartum care in the ambulatory setting. Topics such as general care and health promotion, early parenting issues, breastfeeding for success, and assessment and management of selected postpartum complications are offered, so that the clinician can guide patients as they make the transition from childbearing to parenting. Throughout the book, we have presented topics using a problem-based schema that highlights history, physical examination, laboratory and diagnostic testing, differential diagnosis, management, indications for consultation and/or referral, and follow-up care. This format is particularly evident in Parts III and IV, "Guidelines for Management of Common Problems of Pregnancy" and "Guidelines for Management of Selected Complications of Pregnancy." Several unique topics are included in these sections to address the complex and evolving nature of prenatal care in the 21st century. For example, the latest trends in preterm labor prevention, disaster planning, managing exposure to the Zika virus, obesity, dermatoses, and HIV in pregnancy are important contemporary topics that we have included because they are highly relevant to today's clinicians.

The third edition has two new chapters to reflect emerging issues and other pertinent practice concerns based on our conversations with students and ambulatory obstetric providers. The new chapters cover the following areas:

- Thyroid Disorders in Pregnancy and Postpartum
- COVID-19 During Pregnancy and Postpartum

Other special features and updates include:

- A greatly expanded section on the array of choices for noninvasive prenatal testing for aneuploidy in the genetics chapter
- New information from the Food and Drug Administration on drug labeling to assist healthcare providers to assess benefits and risks in pregnant and nursing mothers
- Updated tables and content on medications commonly prescribed during pregnancy
- The addition of information on the contraction stress test, maximum vertical pocket (of amniotic fluid), and further clarification of Doppler velocimetry in the antenatal fetal surveillance chapter
- Updated imaging recommendations for assessing postpartum hemorrhage, updated antibiotic choices for sexually transmitted infections (STIs) and postpartum endometritis management, and updates for assessing and managing postpartum depression, along with links to the Association of Women's Health, Obstetric, and Neonatal Nurses position statement and the American College of Obstetricians and Gynecologists (ACOG) Depression Resource Center
- Recommendations from four professional and/or governmental organizations on screening for anemia in pregnancy
- Updated information on risks and management of influenza and COVID-19 during pregnancy and the latest recommendations for influenza and COVID-19 vaccination for pregnant and lactating individuals
- New nomenclature and diagnostic criteria for hypertensive disorders of pregnancy as well as recommendations for prevention with low-dose aspirin for those individuals at risk are detailed in the chapter on hypertensive disorders in pregnancy
- The latest in ongoing knowledge development on prevention of preterm birth, use of progesterone, and ACOG guidelines on use and timing of antenatal corticosteroids, tocolytics, and magnesium sulfate to reduce complications of prematurity in the neonate
- A link to the free March of Dimes Preterm Labor Assessment Tool Kit can be found in the preterm labor chapter
- An explanation of the fourth-generation HIV test can be found in the chapter on HIV-1 and pregnancy, along with very important information on prescribing preexposure prophylaxis (PrEP) to pregnant and lactating individuals at high risk of HIV infection (i.e., having an HIV-infected partner)
- Online resources and government websites for patients and providers have been updated throughout with two new appendices added covering Telehealth Resources and Best Practice Guides as well as LGBTQIA+ Resources.

We hope that clinicians who care for low- to moderate-risk pregnant individuals will continue to find this book to be helpful and user friendly. It is designed for easy reference in a busy clinical practice setting. Numerous website addresses are listed throughout the text and in the appendices for quick access to additional complex information, credible resources, and free patient education materials. The bibliographies are extensive for each topic and very current, reflecting the latest literature on evidence-based practice.

As seasoned educators, we also designed this book to assist faculty who provide content on ambulatory obstetric care within their curricula. It is difficult to find a text that provides the depth and breadth of material needed by students who seek to develop competency in ambulatory obstetrics; this book will fulfill their educational needs. In addition, we have been quite thorough in specifying appropriate assessments, possible differential diagnoses, and indications for referral. This presentation style will help students and beginning clinicians develop their critical thinking skills and identify scope-of-practice parameters.

We welcome comments from all providers, educators, and students. It is our hope that this book will continue to provide comprehensive up-to-date guidelines for high-quality ambulatory obstetric care and will nourish practice development from student or novice to expert clinician.

Kelly D. Rosenberger
Nancy J. Cibulka
Mary Lee Barron

I. Guidelines for Preparation for Pregnancy

I. Preconception Counseling and Care

MARY LEE BARRON | KELLY D. ROSENBERGER

A. BACKGROUND

The purpose of preconception care is to deliver risk screening, health promotion, and effective interventions as part of routine healthcare. Preconception healthcare is essential because the lifestyle behaviors and exposures that occur before prenatal care is initiated may affect fetal development and subsequent maternal and perinatal outcomes.

1. **Goal 1**: Improve the knowledge, attitudes, and behaviors of people related to preconception health.
2. **Goal 2**: Ensure that all individuals of childbearing age in the United States receive preconception care services (i.e., evidence-based risk screening, health promotion, and interventions) that will enable them to enter pregnancy in optimal health.
3. **Goal 3**: Reduce risks indicated by a previous adverse pregnancy outcome through interventions during the inter-conception period.
4. **Goal 4**: Reduce health disparities in adverse pregnancy outcomes.

To accomplish these goals, the Centers for Disease Control and Prevention (CDC; Johnson et al., 2006) developed 10 recommendations for improving preconception and inter-conception care as part of a strategic plan to improve the health of individuals, their children, and their families.

B. RECOMMENDATIONS TO IMPROVE HEALTH

1. **Individual Responsibility Across the Life Span**: Every person and couple should be encouraged to have a reproductive life plan.
2. **Consumer Awareness**: Increase public awareness about the importance of preconception health behaviors and preconception care services by using information and tools appropriate across various ages; promote literacy, including health literacy, in all cultural/linguistic contexts.
3. **Preventive Visits**: As part of primary care visits, provide risk assessment and educational and health-promotion counseling to all people of childbearing age to reduce reproductive risks and improve pregnancy outcomes.
4. **Interventions for Identified Risks**: Increase the proportion of people who receive interventions as follow-up to preconception risk screening, focusing on high-priority interventions (i.e., those with evidence of effectiveness and greatest potential impact).
5. **Inter-conception Care**: Use the inter-conception period to provide additional intensive interventions for people who have had a previous pregnancy that ended in an adverse outcome (e.g., infant death, fetal loss, birth defects, low birth weight, or preterm birth).

6. Prepregnancy Checkup: Offer, as a component of maternity care, one prepregnancy visit for couples and persons planning pregnancy.

7. Health Insurance Coverage for People With Low Incomes: Increase public and private health insurance coverage for people with low incomes to improve access to preventive health, preconception, and inter-conception care.

8. Public Health Programs and Strategies: Integrate components of preconception health into existing local public health and related programs, including emphasis on inter-conception interventions for people with previous adverse outcomes.

9. Research: Increase the evidence base and promote the use of the evidence to improve preconception health.

10. Monitoring Improvements: Maximize public health surveillance and related research mechanisms to monitor preconception health.

The most updated CDC recommendations can be found on the Planning for Pregnancy website at: www.cdc.gov/preconception/planning.html Additionally, the National Preconception Health and Health Care Initiative clinical workgroup note achievement of these nine targets indicate quality preconception care: absence of tobacco use, absence of uncontrolled depression, absence of sexually transmitted infections, teratogen avoidance, healthy weight (body mass index [BMI] >18 and <30 kg/m$^{2)}$, folic acid use 3 months or more before conception, optimal glycemic control, planned pregnancy, and first prenatal visit before 12 weeks gestational age.

C. HISTORY

Nurse practitioners (NPs) provide healthcare for patients before, during, and in between pregnancies in a variety of settings. The care NPs provide seats them at the forefront to assess for, and address, known risk factors for maternal complications prior to pregnancy and tailor a care plan for each patient's individual needs to mitigate risks and foster the best patient outcomes. Preconception risk assessment includes the same history taking that is done at a prenatal visit (see Chapter 3) because the goals are the same—healthy people and optimal birth outcomes. Ideally, the partner should also be included in a preconception visit. The difference is in the timing of behavior changes to ensure a healthy pregnancy, that is, correcting behaviors to attain the best possible health and avoiding unnecessary risks. Specifically, is there identification of any medical conditions or medication use in either parent, genetic disorders, high-risk exposures (e.g., tobacco, drug, and alcohol use), and environmental hazards (e.g., firearms, toxins, chemicals, including pesticides, gases, and foods)? In addition, the NP is able to review past menstrual, gestational, and pregnancy histories, as well as family, vaccination, surgical, social, and mental health histories. The NP should assess the couple's plans for conceiving and the level of their fertility literacy. *Fertility literacy* is defined as the degree to which people understand fertility information. For men, this would include the effect of modifiable lifestyle factors on male fertility (Barron, 2013a). For women, this would include knowledge of the normal events (i.e., including signs of ovulation) and characteristics of the menstrual cycle, as well as modifiable lifestyle factors that affect those characteristics (Barron, 2013b).

D. PHYSICAL EXAMINATION

1. Baseline height, weight, BMI, and vital signs
2. General physical examination, including the mouth, thyroid, heart, lungs, breasts, abdomen, and pelvic area
3. Comprehensive examination based on medical history

E. LABORATORY AND DIAGNOSTIC TESTING

1. Pap smear as indicated
2. Baseline studies to consider:
   a. Blood type and Rh
   b. Complete blood count (CBC)
   c. Urinalysis
   d. Sexually transmitted disease (STD) screening:
      i. HIV
      ii. Herpes
      iii. Rapid plasma reagin (RPR) or venereal disease reaction level (VDRL) for syphilis
      iv. Gonorrhea
      v. Chlamydia
      vi. Wet mount for bacterial vaginosis
      vii. Trichomoniasis
   e. Possible checks:
      i. Hemoglobin electrophoresis to determine carrier of sickle cell disease or trait or other hemoglobinopathy
      ii. Hepatitis B, C antibody
      iii. Varicella titer
      iv. Rubella titer
      v. Tuberculosis (purified protein derivative [PPD] skin test)
      vi. Toxoplasmosis
      vii. Cytomegalovirus
      viii. Thyroid panel (if indicated)
      ix. Zika (if in endemic area)
      x. Hemoglobin A1c (if >45 years old, obese, or having gestational diabetes mellitus [GDM] history)
      xi. Lead level (if at risk for exposure, often found in low-income housing areas)
      xii. Serum phenylalanine level (if suspected)

F. PATIENT EDUCATION

1. Review menstrual cycle events, including observation of cervical mucus, so the patient can identify the fertile window. Recommend charting of cycles. There are many menstrual-cycle-tracking apps available for smartphones and other electronic devices. However, most apps base identification of ovulation on a 28-day cycle.
   a. Review what to expect regarding menstrual cycle variability posthormonal contraception. Immediately after discontinuing oral contraceptive (OC) use, almost 60% of first cycles after discontinuation are ovulatory. The cycle length may be prolonged until the ninth cycle. Cycle disturbance and insufficient luteal phases are more frequent in the first six cycles after discontinuation.
   b. Following depot medroxyprogesterone acetate (DMPA), the mean time of returning fertility is 260 days.
   c. Following the removal of etonogestrel (Implanon or Nexplanon), 88% of patients regained fertility within 3 months of removal.
2. Review the effects of stress on cycle length.
   a. Stress may shorten a cycle, delay ovulation, or lengthen the cycle depending on the nature of the stress and its acute or chronic duration.
3. Review sleep hygiene and effects of nighttime ambient light exposure.
   a. Light at night (in the sleeping environment) may alter menstrual cycle parameters (length, phases, and cervical mucus secretion), especially in

vulnerable people. The sleeping area should be maximally darkened; avoid the use of blue or green alarm clock lights and do not use night lights.

4. Encourage achievement of normal body weight and a healthy gut microbiome (both partners).

a. History of bariatric surgery: In a recent retrospective cohort study (January 1, 1980 to May 30, 2013) examining the risk of perinatal complications ($N = 10{,}296$), individuals who were within 2 years of bariatric surgery had greater risk for prematurity, neonatal intensive care unit admission, and small-for-gestational-age status than those who waited longer to conceive. These findings could inform a decision on the optimal timing between surgery and conception (Parent et al., 2017). Newer research has found high maternal BMI during pregnancy is associated with several physical, cognitive, and mental health problems in offspring across the life span (Norr et al., 2020).

b. Healthy maternal gut microbiome is essential for metabolism, fetal neurologic system maturation, and overall well-being (Edwards et al., 2017). The human gut microbiome begins developing before birth in a systematic fashion and may be affected by factors such as the maternal oral microbiome, type of delivery, maternal diet, and environmental exposures (Brown et al., 2013). Disruptions of the gut microbiome during early development from major illness, stress, and/or high-dose broad-spectrum antibiotics may lead to increased risk of maternal and/or fetal disorders, chronic disease, and mental disorders later in life (Borre et al., 2014). Without a healthy microbiome, bacteria cross the gut into the general circulation increasing systemic inflammation (Power et al., 2014). This increased intestinal permeability is linked with inflammatory disorders such as obesity, insulin resistance, and type 2 diabetes (Mokkala et al., 2016). Additionally, the typical Western diet consists of excessive processed foods, dietary fat, and sugars, leading to excess weight gain and a dysbiotic gut (Dunlop et al., 2015; Morrison & Regnault, 2016). Diet and lifestyle habits are modifiable factors that affect the brain–gut axis and the long-term health of pregnant individuals and infants. NPs can promote a healthy gut in patients considering pregnancy or currently pregnant by counseling to follow a diet with 70 to 90 g low-fat organic protein daily, unsaturated fatty acids, whole grains, high fiber, low processed sugars and diary probiotics or other cultured foods containing *L. acidophilus, B. lactis, and L. rhamnosus*, and encouraging omega-3 intake.

5. Review the "Fertility Diet" (recommended to enhance fertility and overall health). From 2007 to 2018, Chavarro et al. published a number of articles regarding diet and fertility and the book *The Fertility Diet* (2007). Their research focused on modifiable risk factors of people who became pregnant versus those who did not, using data from a large retrospective study (Nurses' Health Study II, 1991–1999). Additional work has demonstrated adherence to healthy diets, such as the Mediterranean Diet that includes fish, poultry, whole grains, fruits, and vegetables, are related to improved fertility in women and improved semen quality in men (Gaskins & Chavarro, 2018). Because polycystic ovarian syndrome (PCOS) and anovulation are significant causes of infertility, some of the recommendations focus on this population. For example, the recommendation to drink whole milk or consume a full-fat dairy product is based on the fact that skim milk has a more stimulant effect on insulin growth factor-1, leading to more insulin resistance, which is linked to the pathogenesis of PCOS (Table 1.1).

TABLE 1.1 DIETARY RECOMMENDATIONS TO SUPPORT FERTILITY HEALTH

WOMEN	MEN
Take a daily multivitamin (containing folic acid 400 mcg, iron, and zinc)	Take a daily multivitamin (containing folic acid, zinc, and selenium)
Saturated fat ≤8% of daily intake	Saturated fat ≤7% of daily intake
Daily serving of a full-fat dairy food, such as whole milk, ice cream, or cheddar cheese	
Both	
Avoid transfats: Do not consume any product with partially hydrogenated vegetable oil; don't bake with shortening, don't eat fried foods (most commercial baked goods and "fast food") Replace unhealthy fats with healthy types, such as monounsaturated or polyunsaturated fats	
Eat healthy oils (coconut or olive), omega-3, and nuts (10%–15% of daily calories or 22–27 g)	
Drink water (plain, flavored, and sparkling) instead of sodas	
Eat popcorn instead of chips	
Slow the carbs (slowly digested, rich in fiber), focusing on quality and diversity: whole grains, whole-grain pasta, beans, vegetables, and whole uncooked fruit Avoid processed soy products Cut back on red meat and processed meats Get protein and iron from vegetables and nuts Reduce caffeine use to less than 800 mcg/d	

Source: Adapted from Chavarro and Willett (2007), Moyad (2012), and Gaskins and Chavarro (2018).

5. Women with phenylketonuria (PKU) should begin a low phenylalanine diet.
6. Reduce the risk of food-borne illness:
   a. Practice good personal hygiene (handwashing and care of kitchen utensils, cookware, and surfaces)
   b. Consume meats, fish, poultry, and eggs that are fully cooked
   c. Avoid unpasteurized dairy and fruit/vegetable products
   d. Wash fresh fruits and vegetables before eating (to reduce pesticide residues)
   e. Avoid raw sprouts (alfalfa, clover, radish, and mung bean)
   f. Avoid listeriosis by refraining from processed/deli meats, hot dogs, soft cheeses, smoked seafood, meat spreads, and pâté

G. FERTILITY HEALTH PROMOTION

1. Cease smoking, vaping, alcohol consumption, and use of illicit drugs
   a. Recognizing that 50% of pregnancies are unplanned, substance use is best addressed when included in preventative or primary care visits. Recognize that many individuals are unable to stop without support. A single screening question will provide insight regarding the patient's use. For example, "How many times in the past year have you had 4 or more drinks in a day?" (CDC, 2014). Phrasing the question regarding substance use as a "how many . . ." is a nonjudgmental way to approach the topic. There are other brief screening tools available at www.cdc.gov/ncbddd/fasd/documents/redalcohpreg.pdf.
   b. Evidence exists supporting a range of pharmacological and behavioral interventions as effective strategies for increasing smoking cessation in adults. Additionally, behavioral interventions may assist

pregnant individuals to stop smoking and vaping. Data on the effectiveness and safety of electronic cigarettes used in adults and pregnant individuals for smoking cessation is limited. Further studies are focusing on drug classification comparisons of different combinations among diverse populations on the safety and efficacy of electronic cigarettes (Patnode et al., 2021).

c. New evidence suggests a risk of small-for-gestational-age newborns may be increased during pregnancy in patients vaping. During pregnancy, patients reported utilizing vaping as a healthier alternative to smoking. However, there is a lack of data regarding the information on maternal and fetal outcomes after vaping during pregnancy. There is a need for further studies to evaluate the in utero and long-term effects of vaping during pregnancy (Nagpal et al., 2021). Thus, while there is emerging evidence, the authors do not recommend vaping as a behavioral intervention for smoking cessation at this time.

d. A recent posthoc analysis of a multicenter U.S. trial of individuals with a history of pregnancy loss found taking low-dose aspirin before conception may improve birth outcomes. The study involved 1,227 patients aged 18 to 40 years with one or two prior pregnancy losses randomly assigned to receive 81 mg daily aspirin or placebo while trying to conceive. If they became pregnant, the low-dose aspirin was continued through 36 weeks gestational age. In the posthoc analysis, the investigators assessed participants' adherence to the protocol using pill bottle weights. The results of the trial found compared with placebo, taking aspirin 5 days a week led to 8 more pregnancies, 15 more live births, and 6 fewer pregnancy losses for every 100 participants. Aspirin's effect on live births was greatest when individuals began taking it at least 4 days a week prior to conception and throughout their pregnancy (Slomski, 2021).

2. Review use of over-the-counter (OTC) and prescription medications. Consult with the primary care provider if any are teratogenic.

3. Encourage a daily vitamin supplement containing the following:

a. Folic acid 0.4 mg; individuals at risk for neural tube defects should increase to 4 mg/d

b. Vitamin D supplementation of 400 IU (10 mcg) daily is recommended and can be found in most prenatal vitamins

c. Calcium 1,200 to 1,500 mg/d

d. Iron is added to vitamin supplements if hemoglobin is less than 12 g/dL

4. Discuss beneficial effects of exercise, particularly on insulin levels; encourage the initiation of exercise if not already getting 20 to 30 minutes of aerobic exercise three times per week, for example, fast walking, swimming, and dancing.

5. Avoid emptying the cat litter box to reduce the risk of toxoplasmosis.

6. Avoid hot tubs and saunas (bringing body temperature above 101°F can damage the embryo).

7. For partners specifically:

a. Maintain scrotal temperature to promote sperm production by avoiding hot tubs, tight underwear, high temperature working conditions, and cycling wearing lycra pants.

b. Avoid long periods of sitting that could raise the scrotal temperature, for example, using a laptop on one's lap.

c. Avoid alcohol, marijuana, and reduce caffeine use to less than 800 mcg/d.

d. There is increasing evidence cell phones may be associated with decreased semen quality and infertility in men. Testicular tissues may be damaged by increased oxidative stress, heating, and radiation from cell phones. In men, cell phone radiation may result in decreased sperm volume, sperm concentration, sperm count, motility, and viability (El-Hamd & Aboeldahab, 2018). Thus, men should be encouraged to minimize the amount of time exposed to cell phone radiation and not to carry cell phones in their pants pockets.

8. Do not use lubricants, as these are often spermicidal (PreSeed is not spermicidal). PreSeed is a "fertility-friendly" isotonic formula specifically designed to meet the need for safe lubrication when trying to get pregnant. Common lubricants damage sperm because they are not isotonic and are the wrong pH, thus causing dehydration of sperm and decreased or absent motility. Some lubricants also contain sperm-toxic ingredients, such as glycerol (glycerin).

9. Avoid environmental toxins

a. See the CDC website for more information on toxic substances and preconception health (www.cdc.gov/preconception/men.html and www.cdc.gov/preconception/women.html)

b. In addition, the National Institute for Occupational Safety and Health supports a comprehensive website within the CDC. Not only does this site offer a list of workplace hazards, but it also lists programs in place to support employers and employees in evaluation of health hazards specific to the workplace (www.cdc.gov/niosh/hhe).

10. Ideally, education regarding relevant areas is discussed with the prospective parents. Preconception counseling does make a difference; it is associated with positive maternal health behaviors that increase the likelihood of a healthy individual, pregnancy, and infant.

H. REFERRAL/CONSULTATION

1. Genetic counseling, if indicated
2. Evaluation of prescription medication use as needed
3. Substance abuse counseling
4. Nutritional counseling if indicated
   - **a.** Obesity
   - **b.** Diabetes
   - **c.** Gestational diabetes with prior pregnancy
   - **d.** Vegan
   - **e.** Eating disorder history
   - **f.** Anyone at risk for nutritional deficiencies
5. Community/federal programs for financial assistance, if indicated
6. Domestic violence intervention

I. FOLLOW-UP

1. Refer for obstetric care if not provided at the facility

2. If conception does not occur within 1 year and the patient is younger than 35 years, or if conception does not occur within 6 months and the patient is older than 35 years, further evaluation is warranted.

Bibliography

American College of Obstetrics and Gynecologists. (2019). Committee opinion no. 762: Prepregnancy counseling. *Obstetrics & Gynecology, 133*, e78–e89. https://doi.org/10.1097/AOG.0000000000003013

American College of Obstetrics and Gynecologists and Society for Maternal Fetal Medicine. (2019). Obstetrical care consensus: Interpregnancy care. *Obstetrics & Gynecology, 133*(1), e51–e72. https://doi.org/10.1097/AOG.0000000000003025

Baker, F., & Driver, H. (2007). Circadian rhythms, sleep, and the menstrual cycle. *Sleep Medicine, 8*(6), 613–622. https://doi.org/10.1016/j.sleep.2006.09.011

Barron, M. L. (2007). Light exposure, melatonin secretion, and menstrual cycle parameters: An integrative review. *Biological Research for Nursing, 9*(1), 49–69. https://doi.org/10.1177/1099800407303337

Barron, M. L. (2013a). Fertility literacy for men in primary care settings. *Journal for Nurse Practitioners, 9*, 155–160. https://doi.org/10.1016/j.nurpra.2012.10.002

Barron, M. L. (2013b). Fertility literacy for women in primary care settings. *Journal for Nurse Practitioners, 9*, 161–166. https://doi.org/10.1016/j.nurpra.2012.11.001

Borre, Y. E., O'Keefe, G. W., Clarke, G., Stanton, C., Dinan, T. G., & Cryan, J. F. (2014). Microbiota and neurodevelopment windows: Implications for brain disorders. *Trends in Molecular Medicine, 20*, 509–518. https://doi.org/10.1016/j.molmed.2014.05.002

Brown, J., de Vos, W. M., DiStefano, P. S., Dore, J., Huttenhower, C., Knight, R., Lawley, T. D., Raes, J., & Turnbaugh, P. (2013). Translating the human microbiome. *Nature Biotechnology, 31*, 304–308. https://doi.org/10.1038/nbt.2543

Centers for Disease Control and Prevention. (2014). *Planning and implementing screening and brief intervention for risky alcohol use: A step-by-step guide for primary care practices*. National Center on Birth Defects and Developmental Disabilities.

Chavarro, J. E., Rich-Edwards, J., Rosner, B., & Willett, W. (2009). Caffeinated and alcoholic beverage intake in relation to ovulatory disorder infertility. *Epidemiology, 20*(3), 374–381. https://doi.org/10.1097/EDE.0b013e31819d68cc

Chavarro, J. E., & Willett, W. C. (2007). *The fertility diet*. McGraw-Hill.

Dunlop, A. L., Mulle, J. G., Ferranti, E. P., Edwards, S., Dunn, A. B., & Corwin, E. J. (2015). Maternal microbiome and pregnancy outcomes that impact infant health: A review. *Advances in Neonatal Care, 15*(6), 377–385. https://doi.org/10.1097/ANC.0000000000000218

Edwards, S. M., Cunningham, S. A., Dunlop, A. L., & Corwin, E. J. (2017). The maternal gut microbiome during pregnancy. *The American Journal of Maternal Child Nursing, 42*(6), 310–317. https://doi.org/10.1097/NMC.0000000000000372.

El-Hamd, M. A., & Aboeldahab, S. (2018). Cell phone and male infertility: An update. *Journal of Integrative Nephrology and Andrology, 5*, 1–5. https://doi.org/10.4103/jina.jina_34_17

Fantasia, H. C., Harris, A. L., & Fontenot, H. B. (2020). *Guidelines for nurse practitioners in gynecologic settings* (12th ed.). Springer Publishing Company.

Finer, L. B., & Zolna, M. R. (2011). Unintended pregnancy in the United States: Incidence and disparities, 2006. *Contraception, 84*(5), 478. https://doi.org/10.1016/j.contraception.2011.07.013

Frayne, D. J., Verbiest, S., Chelmow, D., Clarke, H., Dunlop, A., Hosmer, J., Menard, M. K., Moos, M. K., Ramos, D., Stuebe, A., & Zephyrin, L. (2016, May). Health care system measures to advance preconception wellness: Consensus recommendations of the clinical workgroup of the national preconception health and health care initiative. *Obstetrics & Gynecology, 127*(5), 863–872. https://doi.org/10.1097/AOG.0000000000001379

Fotherby, K., & Howard, G. (1986). Return of fertility in women discontinuing injectable contraceptives. *Journal of Obstetrics and Gynecology, 6*(Suppl. 2), S110–S115. https://doi.org/10.3109/01443618609081724

Frey, K., Navarro, S., Kotelchuck, M., & Lu, M. (2008). The clinical content of preconception care: Preconception care for men. *American Journal of Obstetrics & Gynecology, 199*(Suppl. 2), S389–S395. https://doi.org/10.1016/j.ajog.2008.10.024

Funk, S., Miller, M. M., Mishell, D. R., Archer, D. F., Poindexter, A., Schmidt, J., Zampaglione, E., & Implanon US Study Group. (2005). Safety and efficacy of Implanon, a single-rod implantable contraceptive containing etonogestrel. *Contraception, 71*, 319–326. https://doi.org/10.1016/j.contraception.2004.11.007

Gaskins, A. J., & Chavarro, J. E. (2018, April). Diet and fertility: A review. *American Journal of Obstetrics & Gynecology, 218*(4), 379–389. https://doi.org/10.1016/j.ajog.2017.08.010

Gnoth, C., Frank-Herrmann, P., Schmoll, A., Godehardt, E., & Freundl, G. (2002). Cycle characteristics after discontinuation of oral contraceptives. *Gynecological Endocrinology: The Official Journal of the International Society of Gynecological Endocrinology, 16*(4), 307–317. https://doi.org/10.1080/gye.16.4.307.317

Jensen, J. T., & Creinin, M. D. (2020). *Speroff & Darney's clinical guide to contraception* (6th ed.). Walters Kluwer.

Johnson, K., Posner, S., Biermann, J., Cordero, J. F., Atrash, H. K., Parker, C. S., Boulet, S., & Curtis, M. G. (2006). Recommendations to improve preconception health and health care—United States: A report of the CDC/ATSDR preconception care work group and the select panel on preconception care. *Morbidity & Mortality Weekly Report, 55*, 1–23. https://doi.org/10.1037/e506902006-001

Koskelo, R., Zaproudina, N., & Vuorikari, K. (2005). High scrotal temperatures and chairs in the pathophysiology of poor semen quality. *Pathophysiology, 11*(4), 221–224. https://doi.org/10.1016/j.pathophys.2005.02.006

Mokkala, K., Roytio, H., Munukka, E., Pietila, S., Ekblad, U., Ronnemna, T., Eerola, E., Laiho, A., & Laitinen, K. (2016). Gut microbiota richness and composition and dietary intake of overweight pregnant women related to serum zonulin concentration, a marker for intestinal permeability. *Journal of Nutrition, 146*, 1694–1700. https://doi.org/10.3945/jn.116.235358

Morrison, J. L., & Regnault, T. R. (2016). Nutrition in pregnancy: Optimizing maternal diet and fetal adaptations to altered nutrient supply. *Nutrients, 8*(6), 342–346. https://doi.org/10.3390/nu8060342

Moyad, M. (2012). The optimal male health diet and dietary supplement program. *Urologic Clinics of North America, 39*(1), 89–107. https://doi.org/10.1016/j.ucl.2011.09.006

Nagpal, T. S., Green, C. R., & Cook, J. L. (2021). Vaping during pregnancy: What are the potential health outcomes and perceptions pregnant women have? *JOGC, 43*(2), 219–226. https://doi.org/10.1016/j.jogc.2020.05.014

Nassan, F. L., Chavarro, J. E., & Tanrikut, C. (2018). Diet and men's fertility: Does diet affect sperm quality. *Fertility and Sterility, 110*(4), 570–577. https://doi.org/10.1016/j.fertnstert.2018.05.025

Nassaralla, C., Stanford, J., Daly, K., Schneider, M., Schliep, K., & Fehring, R. (2011). Characteristics of the menstrual cycle after discontinuation of oral contraceptives. *Journal of Women's Health, 20*(2), 169–177. https://doi.org/10.1089/jwh.2010.2001

National Association of Nurse Practitioners in Women's Health. (2016). *Prevention of alcohol-exposed pregnancies*. Author.

Norr, M. E., Hect, J. L., Lenniger, C. J., Van den Heeuvel, M., & Thomason, M. E. (2020). An examination of maternal prenatal BMI and human fetal brain development. *The Journal of Child Psychology and Psychiatry, 62*(4), 458–469. https://doi.org/10.1111/jcpp.13301

Parent, B., Martopullo, I., Weiss, N. S., Khandelwal, S., Fay, E. E., & Rowhani-Rahbar, A. (2017). Bariatric surgery in women of childbearing age, timing between an operation and birth, and associated perinatal complications. *JAMA Surgery, 152*(2), 1–8. https://doi.org/10.1001/jamasurg.2016.3621

Patnode, C. D., Henderson, J. T., Melnikow, J., Coppola, E. L., Durbin, S., & Thomas, P. (2021). *Interventions for tobacco cessation in adults, including pregnant women: An evidence update for the U.S. Preventative services task force*. Agency for Healthcare Research and Quality (US).

Power, S. E., O'Toole, P. W., Stanton, C., Ross, R. P., & Fitzgerald, G. F. (2014). Intestinal microbiota, diet and health. *British Journal of Nutrition, 111*, 387–402. https://doi.org/10.1017/S0007114513002560

Salas-Heutos, A., James, E. R., Aston, K. I., Jenkins, T. G., & Carrell, D. T. (2019). Diet and sperm quality: Nutrients, foods and dietary patterns. *Reproductive Biology, 19*, 219–224. https://doi.org/10.1016/j.repbio.2019.07.005

Slomski, A. (2021). With good adherence, daily aspirin may prevent pregnancy loss. *JAMA, 325*(12), 1135. https://doi.org/10.1001/jama.2021.1788

Williams, L., Zapata, L. B., D'Angelo, D. V., Harrison, L., & Morrow, B. (2011). Associations between preconception counseling and maternal behaviors before and during pregnancy. *Maternal Child Health Journal, 16*(9), 1854–1861. https://doi.org/10.1007/s10995-011-0932-4

Yu-Han, C., Chavarro, J. E., & Souter, I. (2018). Diet and female fertility: Doctor, what should I eat? *Fertility and Sterility, 110*(4), 560–569. https://doi.org/10.1016/j.fertnstert.2018.05.027

2. Screening for Genetic Disorders and Genetic Counseling—Preconception and Early Pregnancy

NANCY J. CIBULKA | LISA HICKMAN | KELLY D. ROSENBERGER

Genetics and Genetic Testing

Genetics refers to the study of a gene, gene sequence, and heredity in living organisms. The term *aneuploidy* refers to chromosome regions having extra or fewer copies than normal. Because each chromosome is made up of a very large number of genes, the loss or addition of chromosomal material significantly disrupts human development. A genetic test analyzes DNA, RNA, chromosomes, or specific metabolites to detect aneuploidy and heritable abnormalities. Birth defects are structural or functional abnormalities present at birth that cause physical or mental disability, which can lead to infant mortality. It is important to keep in mind that birth defects are known to occur in 3% to 5% of all newborns. In some cases, birth defects are caused by chromosomal abnormalities. In other cases, birth defects are caused by a combination of genetic and environmental factors, including exposure to teratogens during a critical stage of embryonic development. Most chromosomal abnormalities are not inherited but occur by chance before conception when an egg or sperm receives an abnormal amount of chromosomal material.

The prenatal care provider needs to determine whether pregnant individuals or those contemplating pregnancy are at risk for offspring with genetic abnormalities or birth defects, including those caused by environmental exposures. A carefully elicited medical, genetic, family, and personal history will give important information about potential genetic problems. All pregnant individuals and those considering a future pregnancy should be offered carrier screening for cystic fibrosis (CF), spinal muscular atrophy, and hemoglobinopathies (American College of Obstetricians and Gynecologists [ACOG], Committee on Genetics, 2017a). A referral to a genetic counselor is essential when patients are at risk for genetic problems.

All patients may wish to consider preconception and/or prenatal screening or diagnostic tests to determine risk to their offspring. *Screening tests*, such as blood and ultrasound examinations, do not indicate with certainty whether chromosomal abnormalities are present but give important information about individual risk. The purpose of genetic *diagnostic testing* is to determine whether a specific genetic disorder is present in the fetus; testing is available for some but not all genetic disorders. These diagnostic tests mostly require a sample of fetal DNA for analysis. *Carrier testing* can be performed to identify individuals who have a gene mutation for a disorder inherited in an autosomal recessive or X-linked pattern but do not have symptoms of a genetic condition. Carrier testing is offered to individuals who have family members with a genetic disorder, family members of known carriers, and those of an ethnic or racial group known to have a higher carrier rate for a particular condition. When both parents are carriers of an autosomal recessive disorder, there is a one-in-four chance in each pregnancy that the child will be born with the disorder (see Figure 2.1). *Diagnostic tests,* including analysis of preimplantation embryonic cells, chorionic villus sampling (CVS), and amniocentesis, provide 99.9% accuracy about chromosomal abnormalities; however, they carry a very small risk of miscarriage (ACOG, 2016a). Noninvasive prenatal testing (NIPT) for analysis of cell-free DNA from maternal plasma is now a widely available screening method; however, due to its limited ability for identification of chromosomal abnormalities, NIPT should not be considered a diagnostic tool (ACOG, Committee on Genetics and Society for Maternal–Fetal Medicine, 2015).

Preconception and prenatal genetic screening and testing are available for a variety of genetic conditions because they provide individuals and families with the option to avoid conception of an affected child, to consider pregnancy termination, to detect and treat a fetal condition in utero (rarely), or to prepare for the birth of a child with serious health problems. Screening tests should be offered with a full explanation as to why the test might be considered, what the test will or will not reveal, follow-up for positive screening results, what course of action or treatment might be considered, and all risks of undergoing testing, including emotional distress. No screening test is perfect, and both false-positive and false-negative results may occur. Some couples do not wish to pursue invasive diagnostic testing because of personal reasons, fear of miscarriage, or other issues. For these reasons, and if the test results would not change the plan for the pregnancy, patients may decline screening tests. Factors that influence an individual's decision-making about genetic screening include personal beliefs, sociocultural background, family context, and religious beliefs. Informed consent should be obtained prior to all testing. Because decisions of this nature can be extremely difficult for parents, referral to support networks or counseling must be available.

Ideally, genetic screening should be offered preconceptionally or, if not possible, during early pregnancy. If screening is positive for a genetic disorder, or if the health assessment and/or family history indicate risk for a genetic problem,

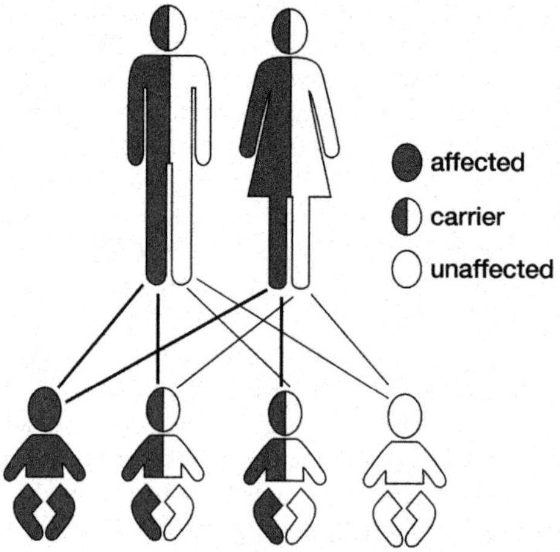

FIGURE 2.1 Examples of inheritance patterns for autosomal recessive disorders.

consider referral to a genetic counselor to discuss risks and additional screening opportunities. The goals of genetics counseling and screening are to calculate and communicate genetic risks for current and/or future pregnancies, confirm or rule out genetic conditions through specialized testing, and provide care and psychosocial support for the patient and family members when genetic disorders are diagnosed. Some couples may desire information about in vitro fertilization with preimplantation genetic diagnosis (PGD) or prenatal genetic diagnosis with CVS or amniocentesis. PGD has been used for the diagnosis of translocations and single-gene disorders, such as CF, X-linked disorders, and other inherited mutations. Genetics counselors can be located through the National Society of Genetic Counselors (NSGC) website at www.nsgc.org. Genetic testing is a rapidly evolving field, and clinicians will need to stay up to date with new information. Additional information for parents and healthcare providers can be found in Appendix A.

Initial History for Genetic Risk Factors

A. RELEVANT MEDICAL AND OBSTETRIC HISTORY

1. Age; increased risk for aneuploidy if the mother is 35 years of age or older

2. Mother has a known or suspected genetic disorder, birth defect, or chromosomal abnormality

3. Mother has a medical condition known or suspected to affect fetal development

4. Two or more prior pregnancy losses (a "red flag" for genetic defects)

5. Birth defects, learning problems, mental disability, or genetic disorders in previous children

6. Exposure to medications, especially any known to be teratogenic

7. Exposure to viral illness during pregnancy

B. FAMILY AND GENETIC HISTORY

1. Take a detailed, three-generational family history for both parents. The family history can be collected using a family history questionnaire or a pedigree. General questioning about more distant relatives can help to uncover possible X-linked disorders or autosomal dominant disorders with reduced penetrance.

2. Web-based tools are available for public use, such as the Surgeon General's Family Health History initiative at www.hhs.gov/familyhistory; March of Dimes: Your Family Health History at www.-marchofdimes.com/pregnancy/trying_healthhistory.html; and through the NSGC at www.nsgc.org

3. Family history should include any genetic disorders, birth defects, chromosomal abnormalities, learning problems, and chronic health conditions with age at diagnosis. If deceased, indicate the cause of death and age at death. Any positive responses should be followed up to obtain more detail.

4. Determine if the patient has a family history of adverse pregnancy outcomes such as miscarriage, preterm birth, preeclampsia, or abnormal newborn screening test results. A positive family history may increase the risk of poor pregnancy outcomes.

5. Determine if there is a close biological relationship between parents or grandparents. Consanguinity increases the risk for birth defects and genetic disorders.

6. The ethnic background of each grandparent should be given for the consideration of ethnic predisposition to certain genetic disorders.

7. If using the ACOG forms or other electronic medical record systems, the genetic screening section guides the interviewer to ask about family and personal history of thalassemia, neural tube defects (NTDs), congenital heart defects, Tay–Sachs and other neuromuscular syndromes, Down syndrome, sickle cell disease (SCD) or trait, hemophilia, muscular dystrophy, CF, Huntington's chorea, mental disability, autism, fragile X, and maternal metabolic disorder such as insulin-dependent diabetes or phenylketonuria (PKU).

8. Ask if the father of the baby has other children and if they are healthy or have any birth defects, learning disabilities, or health problems.

9. The information gathered by the history will help to determine if the patient is a candidate for carrier screening for genetic conditions.

C. PERSONAL HISTORY: SOCIAL AND ENVIRONMENTAL FACTORS

1. Exposure to known or suspected environmental teratogens
2. Exposure to radiation or biological hazards
3. Tobacco, alcohol, and/or substance abuse during pregnancy
4. Exposure to secondhand tobacco smoke

Prenatal Genetic Screening Tests

A. DOWN SYNDROME/ANEUPLOIDY SCREENING FOR TRISOMIES 13, 18, AND 21

1. Definition and background: Screening for aneuploidy identifies women whose fetuses are at increased risk for trisomy 21 (Down syndrome), 18, and 13. Chromosomal abnormalities are associated with severe birth defects, mental disability, miscarriage, and neonatal or infant demise.

2. ACOG recommends that all pregnant women be offered aneuploidy screening or diagnostic testing early in pregnancy, ideally at the first prenatal visit (ACOG, 2016a).

3. Screening tests for aneuploidy are available in all trimesters. Screening can provide a reasonably accurate risk estimate of individual Down syndrome risk.

4. Baseline risk is determined first by maternal age and history. The risk of aneuploidy increases with advancing age, but age should not be the only factor used to determine screening or diagnostic tests offered. Counseling is provided to inform the patient about specific risk of aneuploidy and to review the options for screening or diagnostic testing (including the option to decline) using a framework of shared decision-making.

5. First-trimester screening is generally performed between 10 and 13 6/7 weeks gestation. It includes a blood test for two markers, free beta-human chorionic gonadotropin (beta-HCG) or total human chorionic gonadotropin (HCG) and pregnancy-associated plasma protein A (PAPP-A), together with ultrasound for nuchal translucency (fluid collection at the back of the fetal neck). Accurate measurement of nuchal translucency is essential for risk assessment. The detection rate for Down syndrome is 82% to 87% (ACOG, 2020). If nuchal translucency alone is used without the blood test, the detection rate for Down syndrome is approximately 70%.

6. Second-trimester biochemical screening includes the triple, quad, or penta screen for markers in maternal serum. Risk of open NTD is calculated in addition to aneuploidy risk (see Section III.B). The triple screen tests for alpha-fetoprotein (AFP), free or total HCG, and unconjugated estriol; the detection rate of the triple screen for Down syndrome is approximately

70%. Inhibin A is added in the quadruple (or "quad" screen) to improve the detection rate of Down syndrome to approximately 80%. The penta screen adds invasive trophoblast antigen, but data are limited on whether the accuracy of the penta screen is improved compared to the quad screen. Choice of test often depends on institutional preference. A maternal blood sample should be drawn between 15 and 22 weeks gestation (optimally between 16 and 18 weeks). Risks for Down syndrome, trisomy 18, and NTDs are calculated based on the results.

7. Combining first- and second-trimester screening (i.e., integrated, sequential, or contingent screening) is another option. If biochemical testing is completed in the first trimester and then repeated at 15 to 22 weeks with nuchal translucency, the detection rate for Down syndrome is 95% to 96%; without nuchal translucency, it is around 88%. Blood work must be sent to the same laboratory for interpretation.

8. Screening by second-trimester ultrasound alone is not as predictive as combined screening. Fetuses with trisomy 13 or 18 usually have major structural anomalies that are readily visible on ultrasound, but findings for Down syndrome can be subtler. The major structural anomalies associated with Down syndrome include cardiac anomalies and duodenal atresia, which are usually identified on second- and third-trimester ultrasounds. However, there are several nonspecific "soft" markers for aneuploidy that are also common in unaffected fetuses (such as renal pelvis dilation, choroid plexus cyst, or an echogenic intracardiac focus). Thus, isolated findings of "soft" markers on ultrasound are not considered predictive for Down syndrome, but if other screening has not been performed, it should be offered.

9. NIPT that uses cell-free DNA from maternal plasma is another option for fetal aneuploidy. ACOG and the Society for Maternal–Fetal Medicine (SMFM) recommend NIPT as a screening option for individuals at increased risk of aneuploidy but not as first-line screening for low-risk individuals in the general population. Given the limitations of cell-free DNA screening performance and testing, conventional screening methods are the most appropriate choice for these individuals. Cell-free DNA testing is recommended as an option for pregnant individuals age 35 or older, those with a history of trisomy in a prior pregnancy, fetuses with findings suspicious for aneuploidy on ultrasound, and others at increased risk of aneuploidy.

10. NIPT screens for trisomy 13, 18, and 21 and reports sex chromosomes if requested. Other chromosomal abnormalities cannot be detected. NIPT can be performed as early as 9 or 10 weeks gestation and can continue until birth. Several laboratories offer NIPT and all tests have a high sensitivity and specificity for trisomies 18 and 21. The fetal fraction (amount of cell-free DNA in the maternal sample that is of fetal origin) is necessary for interpretation, and most laboratories require at least 4% for an accurate result. Fetal fraction may be low in pregnant individuals weighing more than 250 pounds and, more concerning, with an aneuploidy fetus; thus, if results are "indeterminate" or "uninterpretable" or "positive" (a "no call" test result), refer for genetic counseling and offer comprehensive ultrasound evaluation as well as diagnostic testing (ACOG, 2015). Results are available within 5 to 7 days (Palomaki et al., 2021).

11. Cell-free DNA testing is not recommended for women with multiple gestations and should not be used to screen for microdeletions. This test does not assess the risk of neural tube or ventral wall defects, so pregnant individuals should be offered maternal serum AFP (MSAFP) in addition to ultrasound evaluation in the second trimester.

12. Detection rates of aneuploidy screening vary from 64% to 99%, depending on the combination of tests performed (ACOG, 2020). Screening options are limited in multiple gestations.

13. Informed consent must be obtained prior to testing. Counseling should include the limitations of the screening tests, their advantages and disadvantages, and future options if test results are positive.

14. Patients need to understand that not all affected fetuses will be detected and that there will be some false-positive screens. Pregnant individuals also need to be advised that screening provides an individual risk assessment but is not diagnostic for Down syndrome and will not detect all chromosomal abnormalities.

15. If test results show an increased risk for aneuploidy and/or if the patient will be 35 years of age or older at delivery, refer for genetic counseling. Patient may desire definitive testing by CVS or amniocentesis.

- **a.** CVS is performed between 10 and 13 weeks gestation. Under continuous ultrasound guidance, a catheter inserted through the cervix or a needle through the abdomen removes a small amount of placental tissue.
- **b.** Amniocentesis is performed after 15 weeks. Under ultrasound visualization, a small amount of amniotic fluid is removed with a needle through the abdomen. Besides testing for Down syndrome, other chromosomal abnormalities, such as Turner syndrome and Klinefelter syndrome and microdeletion syndromes, can be detected.
- **c.** Risk of miscarriage is estimated to be 1 in 370 to 769 procedures for amniocentesis at 15 weeks and is similar for CVS (ACOG, 2016a).
- **d.** Prenatal diagnostic laboratory techniques using fetal samples are beyond the scope of this chapter. Information is available in Appendix A.

B. NEURAL TUBE DEFECTS

1. Definition and background: NTDs are congenital structural abnormalities of the brain and vertebral column resulting from incomplete closure of the neural tube during embryogenesis. The most commonly occurring NTDs are anencephaly and spina bifida. Anencephaly accounts for one half of the cases and is incompatible with life. Although the majority of infants with spina bifida survive, most live with some degree of disability. NTDs are the second most common major congenital malformation worldwide, second only to cardiac malformations.

2. The incidence of NTDs is highly variable and is affected by ethnic and geographic factors, and by whether folic acid supplementation and/or food fortification programs are widely available. The incidence of NTDs historically was cited as 1 in 1,000 pregnancies in the United States; however, by 2006, the incidence was about 0.3 per 1,000 births (Hochberg & Stone, 2016). Isolated NTDs are most likely the result of a combination of genetic predisposition and environmental influences. However, NTDs can also be one manifestation of a chromosomal syndrome.

3. Risk factors for NTD include individuals with a previously affected pregnancy, personal or family history of NTD, and those taking certain antiseizure medicines or other folate antagonists. Diabetes and obesity are also considered to be risk factors. Individuals at high risk of NTD should be referred directly to a genetic counselor. Early diagnosis of NTD provides patients with information that allows them to consider whether they wish to continue the pregnancy, management for a high-risk pregnancy, preparation for the child, and plans for delivery at an appropriate medical facility.

4. Folate deficiency is a risk factor for NTD, although the exact mechanism is unknown. The U.S. Preventive Services Task Force (USPSTF) recommends 0.4 to 0.8 mg (400–800 mcg) of folic acid supplement daily at least 1 month before conception and throughout the first trimester for all individuals at average risk for NTD. To be effective, the supplement must be ingested during the first 4 weeks after conception for proper formation of the neural tube. In addition, advise patients to eat a well-balanced diet with green leafy vegetables and fortified grains. Recommend folic acid as a single supplement or prescribe a multivitamin containing 0.4 to 0.8 mg folic acid. Because nearly 50% of pregnancies in the United States are unplanned, clinicians should advise all individuals capable of pregnancy to take folic acid supplements.

5. Individuals at high risk for NTDs because of a previous pregnancy complicated by NTD or a close relative with NTD are advised to take 4 mg of folic acid daily before conception and throughout the first trimester.

6. The primary screening test for NTDs is the measurement of MSAFP, which is elevated in 89% to 100% of pregnancies complicated by NTDs. The screening test should be offered to all pregnant individuals between 15 and 22 weeks gestation (optimally between 16 and 18 weeks). The MSAFP is 85% predictive for NTDs in pregnancies with a single fetus and 80% predictive for twin pregnancies. Although AFP screening is primarily intended for the detection of anencephaly and open spina bifida, the test can also identify abdominal wall defects (e.g., gastroschisis or omphalocele), and aneuploidy. The test does not detect closed spina bifida. MSAFP results are reported as multiples of the median (MoM); a value above 2.0 or 2.5 MoM is an abnormal result (positive screen).

7. Factors that affect the correct interpretation of the MSAFP results include maternal weight, ethnicity, maternal diabetes, tobacco use, and multifetal pregnancy. Because the MSAFP results depend on accurate gestational age, an ultrasound performed before MSAFP screening can verify gestational age and identify multiple gestations, thereby lowering the false positive rate. If the MSAFP test is completed prior to ultrasound and results are abnormal, the provider should first confirm gestational age with ultrasound, and if the ultrasound shows that the gestational age was not accurate, the test results should be recalculated or the test repeated if performed prior to 15 weeks. If the elevation persists, the next step is to obtain a specialized ultrasound to assess whether a NTD or other anomaly is present.

8. Individuals with an elevated (positive) MSAFP should be referred for genetic counseling and consideration of further testing. A specialized ultrasound in the second trimester has been found to increase detection rates of spina bifida to 92% to 95%. If the ultrasound findings are inconclusive, an amniocentesis can be considered to test amniotic fluid for AFP and acetylcholinesterase.

9. Elevated amniotic fluid AFP together with acetylcholinesterase is 96% sensitive for NTD with a false positive rate of 0.14. If an amniocentesis is performed for a fetus with an identified NTD, a karyotype is also advised because of the association of NTD with chromosomal abnormalities.

10. An elevated MSAFP in the second trimester that cannot be explained is associated with an increased risk of fetal death, especially in pregnancies complicated by hypertension. Increased antepartal testing has been recommended for these pregnancies (see Chapter 6).

MSAFP testing is one of the components of the triple, quad, or penta screen offered for aneuploidy testing. If a pregnant individual opts for first-trimester aneuploidy screening only, the MSAFP will still need to be offered in the second trimester to screen for NTD.

Prenatal Genetic Carrier Screening

Two autosomal recessive hemoglobinopathies commonly screened during pregnancy are SCD and the thalassemias. However, there are other autosomal recessive disorders of concern. All pregnant individuals and those planning pregnancy should be given information about genetic carrier screening (ACOG, 2017a, 2017b). If a patient is found to be a carrier for a genetic condition, the partner should be offered testing. If both partners are found to be carriers, genetic counseling should be offered. Online resources for parents concerned about specific genetic conditions are provided in Appendix A.

A. SCD OR SICKLE CELL ANEMIA

1. Definition and background: Hemoglobin consists of four subunits, two alpha chains and two beta chains, plus an attached heme molecule. Normal adult hemoglobin is genotypically designated as Hb A or AA (homozygous Hb A). Sickle cell trait (SCT) occurs when a person has one abnormal allele of the beta-globin chain (heterozygous) and therefore produces both normal and abnormal hemoglobin. However, if a person has two abnormal alleles (homozygous), he or she only produces abnormal hemoglobin, which results in fragile, sickle-shaped cells and a reduced ability to carry oxygen. This condition is known as *sickle cell anemia* (SCA) or SCD. The most severe form of the disorder is Hb SS; however, sickle cell disorders are also found in those who have Hb S and one other abnormality of the beta-globin chain, such as Hb C or beta-thalassemia (discussed in Section IV.B).

2. SCD most commonly affects those of African heritage. Approximately one in 10 African Americans has SCT (ACOG, Committee on Genetics, 2017a). However, SCT is also found in families that come from Southeast Asia, India, the Mediterranean and Caribbean areas, Saudi Arabia, and South and Central America. Carriers of SCT will have a higher amount of S or C hemoglobin but also adequate amounts of normal hemoglobin with genotypic pattern of AS or AC.

3. All pregnant individuals at risk because of known carrier status, ancestry, or family history should be offered screening with hemoglobin electrophoresis in addition to a complete blood count (CBC). Hemoglobin electrophoresis is preferred compared to the sickle cell test, which only tests for abnormal S hemoglobin and will not test for C or for the thalassemias (discussed in Section IV.B).

4. If a pregnant individual is found to have SCT, the father of the baby needs to be tested. If both parents are found to carry SCT or another beta-hemoglobinopathy trait, the family should be referred to a genetic counselor to discuss whether a prenatal diagnosis of SCD would be beneficial.

5. In the United States, testing for SCD is included in the newborn screening panel completed shortly after the baby is born.

B. ALPHA- AND BETA-THALASSEMIAS

1. Definition and background: Thalassemia occurs when there is a defect in either alpha-globin or beta-globin chains. They are classified according to the globin chain affected, most commonly alpha-thalassemia or beta-thalassemia. The resulting disorder can be mild to life threatening, depending on the severity of the defect. Thalassemias are characterized by microcytic anemia.

2. Thalassemias are more common in families that come from Mediterranean countries, Southeast Asia, China, India, Pakistan, the Philippines, Middle Eastern countries, and those of African descent. Individuals of these ancestries may be carriers of a thalassemia trait. Carrier testing begins with a CBC; CBC with microcytosis (low mean corpuscular volume [MCV]) in the absence of iron deficiency may identify a patient who is a carrier for alpha- or beta-thalassemia.

3. Pregnant individuals at risk because of suspected or known mild disease or carrier status, ancestry, or family history should have a CBC and, if abnormal, be offered screening with hemoglobin electrophoresis and serum ferritin. A low MCV (<80 fL) is significant for one of the thalassemia traits. If the hemoglobin electrophoresis is normal, further DNA testing may be needed to detect alpha-globin gene deletions.

4. If a pregnant individual is a carrier for thalassemia, the father of the baby needs to be tested. If the father is also a carrier or is a carrier of SCT, refer to a genetics counselor. Beta-thalassemia and SCT can coexist, resulting in a serious hemoglobinopathy with most of the symptoms and complications of SCD.

5. In the United States, testing for thalassemia is included in the newborn screening panel, completed shortly after the baby is born.

C. CYSTIC FIBROSIS

1. Definition and background: CF is an autosomal, recessive disorder that causes the body to produce abnormally thick, sticky mucus in the cells that line the lungs, pancreas, and other organs, resulting in problems with breathing and digestion. CF is caused by a mutation in the CF transmembrane regulator (CFTR) gene located on chromosome 7 and is one of the more common inherited diseases, affecting about one in 2,500 births (Russo, 2020).

2. Genetic screening for CF should be offered to all pregnant individuals and their partners. CF carrier testing requires a small sample of blood or a swab of cheek cells.

3. CF is most common among the non-Hispanic Caucasian and the Ashkenazi Jewish population. It also occurs in other ethnic populations (see Table 2.1). If there is no family history of CF, sequential testing is usually done for the patient and then for the partner if the patient is a carrier. Concurrent screening of both parents can be done if there is a time constraint.

TABLE 2.1 ETHNICITY, CYSTIC FIBROSIS DETECTION RATES, AND RISK OF BEING A CARRIER

ETHNICITY	CF DETECTION RATE (23-MUTATION PANEL)	CF CARRIER RISK	CF CARRIER RISK AFTER NEGATIVE TEST
Ashkenazi Jewish	94%	1/24	1/384
Non-Hispanic Caucasian	88%	1/25	1/206
Hispanic Caucasian	72%	1/58	1/203
African American	64%	1/61	1/171
Asian American	49%	1/94	1/183

CF, cystic fibrosis

Modified from the American College of Medical Genetics and Genomics (2006). Reprinted with permission.

4. CF carrier testing is used to determine if a person carries one or more mutations of the CF gene. More than 2,100 mutations of the CF gene have been identified (Russo, 2020). A pan-ethnic panel for the most common 23 mutations is recommended for initial screening. A positive carrier test, meaning that the person has a mutation of the CF gene, is more than 99% accurate; however, a negative carrier test is not as accurate. A negative result shows a greatly reduced but not completely "zero" risk of being a CF carrier because some of the rare mutations may not be identified. The sensitivity of CF carrier testing varies by ethnicity (ACOG, Committee on Genetics, 2017a).

5. If there is a family history of CF or if the pregnant individual and/or father is a known carrier, refer the patient for genetic counseling. If indicated, a complete analysis of the CFTR gene by DNA sequencing can be performed. If both parents are carriers, DNA analysis of the embryo or fetus can be accomplished by CVS or amniocentesis. Genetic counseling is recommended to review prenatal testing options.

6. In the United States, testing for CF is included in the newborn screening panel, completed shortly after the baby is born. This testing is only for CF disease and does not provide carrier testing for the infant.

D. TAY–SACHS DISEASE

1. Definition and background: Tay–Sachs disease (TSD) is caused by a defect on chromosome 15 that results in a lack of hexosaminidase A in the body and accumulation of gangliosides in the central nervous system. It is an autosomal, recessive disorder that manifests with severe progressive destruction of nerve cells in the brain and spinal cord and death in early childhood.

2. The rate of TSD carriers is approximately 1 in 30 in individuals with Ashkenazi Jewish heritage (Eastern and Central European) and is also more common in certain French Canadian populations of Quebec, Amish communities in Pennsylvania, and those of Cajun descent. The carrier rate for non-Jewish individuals is approximately 1 in 300. Couples at risk because of their heritage and those with a family history of TSD should be offered screening.

3. Carrier screening can be performed by molecular analysis with a DNA-based test, biochemical analysis for hexosaminidase A, or both. Carrier tests are approximately 98% sensitive in the high-risk populations but are not as sensitive in a low-risk population. Biochemical analysis should be used in low-risk populations because it is more accurate. The results of biochemical carrier screening using serum are not accurate when performed in pregnant individuals or those taking oral contraceptives and may misclassify a patient as a carrier. Therefore, biochemical testing in these individuals must be accomplished with leukocyte testing (ACOG, 2017).

4. If one partner is at high risk because of heritage but the other partner is not, screen the high-risk partner first. If this individual is found to be a carrier for TSD, the other partner should be offered screening. If both parents are carriers or if results are inconclusive, refer them for genetic counseling for additional testing and DNA analysis. Prenatal diagnosis by CVS or amniocentesis may be indicated.

E. CANAVAN DISEASE

1. Definition and background: Canavan disease is an autosomal recessive disorder caused by a defect on chromosome 17 that causes a lack of the enzyme aspartoacylase. The buildup of N-acetylaspartic acid in the brain causes progressive damage to nerve cells and early death.

2. Canavan is relatively rare in the general population; it is most common in individuals of Ashkenazi Jewish heritage (Eastern and Central European).

3. Carrier testing includes a DNA analysis for two mutations. The test is 98% sensitive.

4. If the pregnant individual is a carrier for Canavan disease, the father needs to be tested and considered for a genetic counseling referral. If both parents are carriers, DNA testing can be accomplished by CVS or amniocentesis.

F. ADDITIONAL CARRIER SCREENING FOR INDIVIDUALS OF ASHKENAZI JEWISH ANCESTRY

1. Familial dysautonomia, a disorder of the sensory and autonomic nervous system, causes autonomic dysfunction and significant morbidity. Carrier frequency is 1 in 32 in the target population. Carrier testing involves DNA analysis for one mutation and is 99% sensitive. Assess whether either the pregnant individual or father is of Ashkenazi ancestry and, if so, offer carrier screening and consider genetic counseling, especially if the family history is positive for the disorder.

2. Carrier testing is also available for mucolipidosis IV, Niemann–Pick disease type A, Fanconi anemia group C, Bloom syndrome, Gaucher disease, dihydrolipoamide dehydrogenase deficiency, familial hyperinsulinism, glycogen storage disease type 1a, maple syrup urine disease, nemaline myopathy, and Usher syndromes type IF and III. Testing has a high degree of sensitivity in the Jewish population. Consult with or refer to a genetic counselor if additional testing is requested or if the family history is positive for any genetic disorders more prevalent in individuals of this background.

3. The prevalence of these disorders in the non-Jewish populations is unknown. Therefore, carrier screening of a non-Jewish partner is of limited value. When only one partner is of Ashkenazi Jewish heritage, screen that person first. If found to be a carrier, consult or refer to a genetic counselor for further discussion of screening options and limitations.

G. FRAGILE X

1. Definition and background: Fragile X is a genetic disorder that results from changes in the fragile X mental retardation 1 (FMR1) gene on the X chromosome. A part of the gene code is repeated in this gene. The number of repeats varies in individuals. A small number of repeats causes no issues; an intermediate number of repeats increases the chance of having offspring with the disorder, and a large number of repeats causes the disorder. The syndrome occurs in approximately 1 in 3,600 males and 1 in 4,000 to 6,000 females from all ethnic backgrounds (ACOG, 2017b). It is the most common inherited form of mental disability and autism. Children with the disorder demonstrate developmental delays and speech and language difficulties. This condition affects both girls and boys. However, a fragile X mutation will result in a more severe effect in males, who have only one X chromosome. Physical features may include distinctive facial features such as a long face, large forehead with prominent ears, large body size, enlarged testicles, and flexible joints with poor muscle tone and coordination.

2. Individuals who are known carriers of fragile X and those with a family history of unexplained mental disability, developmental delay, autism, or early menopause before age 40 without a known cause should be offered genetic counseling and testing for fragile X.

3. Testing for fragile X can be accomplished by DNA-based molecular tests that analyze triplet repetitions in the FMR1 gene. However, interpretation of fragile X testing can be complicated; therefore, genetic counseling is recommended prior to testing. Known carriers of fragile X should be offered amniocentesis or CVS for fetal prenatal diagnosis.

H. SPINAL MUSCULAR ATROPHY

1. Definition and background: Spinal muscular atrophies (SMA) are a group of autosomal recessive inherited disorders caused by deletions of, or mutations in, the survival motor neuron 1 (SMN1) gene on chromosome 5. SMA appears with progressive muscular degeneration and weakness in various degrees of severity with the seriousness of symptoms influenced by several genetic factors. Werdnig–Hoffman disease, or SMA type I, is the most severe form of SMA, leading to death in infancy or early childhood. Type II SMA, the most common subtype, is of intermediate severity with onset before 2 years of age. Type III SMA (Kugelberg Welander) typically has onset after 18 months of age with symptoms and prognosis that are quite variable. The spinal muscular atrophies are autosomal recessive inherited disorders and are the second most common after CF. The incidence of SMA is about 1 in 10,000 live births, and the carrier frequency is 1 in 50 (Tsao, 2015). There is no racial or ethnic variation.

2. Offer genetic counseling if either partner has a family history or symptoms of SMA, or requests carrier screening. Carrier testing involves a quantitative polymerase chain reaction assay that measures SMN1. However, patients need to be counseled that the test is not 100% sensitive, and approximately 3% to 4% of carriers will not be detected. Couples who are both known carriers for SMA should be referred for genetic counseling and consideration of CVS or amniocentesis.

3. ACOG (2017b) recommends that screening for SMA should be offered to all patients who are considering pregnancy or are currently pregnant.

Teratogen Recognition

1. A teratogen is an agent that can permanently disturb the development of an embryo or fetus, causing a birth defect in the child, growth retardation, or pregnancy loss. Classes of teratogens include drugs, radiation, maternal infections, maternal metabolic disorders (e.g., maternal PKU, diabetes, folate deficiency), and chemicals or environmental exposures. Effects on the fetus are influenced by the dose, duration, and gestational age at the time of exposure. In some cases, the combination of two exposures may increase teratogenic risk. First-trimester exposures are generally of greatest concern as this is the most rapid period of organogenesis. However, exposure at other times in the pregnancy may also present a serious risk to the fetus, depending on the specific agent.

Because nearly 50% of pregnancies are unplanned, pregnant individuals are often exposed to drugs in the first trimester. In addition, many patients need medication therapy to treat chronic health conditions. Many individuals are reluctant to use any medications or receive vaccines during pregnancy out of fear of possible harm to their unborn child. However, many medical conditions if left untreated, such as asthma, major depression, or seizure disorder, can harm both the patient and the baby. Although most exposures during pregnancy are not teratogenic, patients often perceive that medications and environmental exposures are a major cause of birth defects and greatly overestimate risks; therefore, counseling must be accurate and based on the latest evidence to prevent unnecessary anxiety. Whenever possible, multidisciplinary management involving the patient's prenatal provider, primary and specialty care providers, and pediatric provider is recommended. Alternative treatments that might be relatively safe during pregnancy should be considered. In most cases, counseling about exposures during pregnancy can provide reassurance that the concerning agent is not known to be teratogenic.

A list of known teratogens is presented in Box 2.1. This list is not comprehensive and will continue to expand as knowledge grows. Research is now addressing the effect, if any, of paternal exposure to medications preconceptionally and during a partner's pregnancy. Some exposures are known to affect the quality of the sperm, which results in pregnancy loss or difficulty conceiving. However, based on current

BOX 2.1 POTENTIAL TERATOGENIC EXPOSURES DURING PREGNANCY*

COMMONLY PRESCRIBED MEDICATIONS
Aminoglycoside antibiotics Amiodarone Anticonvulsants Antineoplastic agents Antiretroviral medications: efavirenz Antithyroid agents Atenolol (always) and other beta-blockers used late in pregnancy Benzodiazepines Coumadin anticoagulants Fluconazole (high doses, prolonged exposure) Folic acid antagonists Hormonal medications such as oral contraceptives, androgens, and drugs with anti-androgen activity (such as finasteride), DES, and hormone replacement agents Immunologic drugs, live attenuated vaccines (MMR, varicella, influenza nasal spray), and HPV vaccine Isotretinoin and oral tretinoin Nicotine aids for smoking cessation NSAIDs in the third trimester Select psychiatric medications: imipramine, lithium, valproic acid, paroxetine Statins Tetracycline antibiotics Thalidomide
Recreational Drugs
Alcohol Cocaine or crack Hallucinogens Methamphetamines Opioids Tobacco use or secondhand smoke exposure
Environmental and Occupational Exposures
Heavy metals such as arsenic, cadmium, and mercury Herbicides Hyperthermia (temperature of 101°F or higher) Industrial solvents Ionizing radiation in high doses Lead PCBs

(continued)

BOX 2.1 POTENTIAL TERATOGENIC EXPOSURES DURING PREGNANCY* (*CONTINUED*)

COMMONLY PRESCRIBED MEDICATIONS
Maternal Infections and Health Conditions
Addiction CMV Diabetes mellitus (pregestational) Genitourinary infections HSV I and II HIV Influenza Maternal NTD Parvovirus B-19 PKU Rubella Syphilis Toxoplasmosis Varicella

CMV, cytomegalovirus; DES, diethylstilbestrol; HPV, human papillomavirus; HSV, herpes simplex virus; MMR, measles, mumps, and rubella; NSAIDs, nonsteroidal anti-inflammatory drugs; NTD, neural tube defect; PCBs, polychlorinated biphenyls; PKU, phenylketonuria.

*This list is not all inclusive. Up-to-date online information about other medications is available through MotherToBaby fact sheets, a service of the Organization of Teratology Information Specialists (OTIS), and through resources listed in Appendix A.

evidence, teratogenic agents to which the father is exposed do not seem to directly interfere with normal fetal development with a few exceptions. Paternal alcohol and tobacco use have been associated with heart defects in the newborn, and paternal chemotherapy or radiation therapy exposure may increase the risk of chromosomal abnormalities of the fetus (Bastow, 2016). The major classes of teratogens follow.

A. DRUGS

Prescription and nonprescription drug use is common in pregnancy. Although some medications are known to be harmful when taken during pregnancy, the safety of the majority of medications during pregnancy has not been determined. The U.S. Food and Drug Administration (FDA) regulates all medications to ensure their general safety and effectiveness. The Pregnancy and Lactation (Drugs) Labeling Final Rule went into effect June 30, 2015, eliminating the letter categories—A, B, C, D, and X—and instead require content to assist healthcare providers to assess benefit versus risk in pregnant and lactating individuals. See Chapter 5 for more information.

1. Advise individuals who are pregnant or planning pregnancy to talk with their provider before stopping or starting any type of prescription or over-the-counter medication. Shared decision-making is recommended. Consider whether the medication can be safely continued or a different medication could be substituted and advise the patient of the risks.

2. If a patient has been taking medication while pregnant, determine how much medication was taken, when the medication was taken, other medications taken, and the health condition. Although it is best to avoid or minimize exposure to potentially teratogenic agents during pregnancy, in some health conditions, the benefits of continuing medication outweigh risks to the fetus (i.e., asthma, high blood pressure, seizure disorder, or psychiatric illness).

3. Resources are available to determine effects of medications during pregnancy. These resources are listed in Appendix A and include the Teratology Society (www.teratology.org/OTIS_fact_Sheets.asp), American Academy of Pediatrics (AAP), ACOG, National Birth Defects Prevention Study (NBDPS; www.nbdps.org), March of Dimes, FDA, and the National Institutes of Health (NIH; www.nih.gov).

B. RADIATION, CHEMICALS, AND ENVIRONMENTAL EXPOSURES

1. Ionizing radiation exposure may cause fetal effects, including growth restriction, malformations, impaired brain function, and cancer. As the maternal abdomen protects the fetus, the dose would need to be relatively high to result in adverse effects.
2. Individuals requiring x-rays during pregnancy should use a lead apron to protect against radiation exposure. If exposure occurs, consult with experts in radiation dosimetry to estimate fetal dose and determine risk. In general, radiation exposure through x-ray, CT scans, or nuclear medicine imaging is at a lower dose than exposure associated with fetal harm. Ultrasound and magnetic resonance imaging are the best choices as they are not associated with fetal risk (ACOG, 2016b).
3. Adverse lifestyle exposures (see Chapter 3)
   a. Alcohol is a known teratogen that causes permanent problems manifested as fetal alcohol spectrum disorder (FASD). FASD manifestations typically include mental disability, craniofacial and other birth defects, vision and hearing problems, learning disabilities, intrauterine growth restriction (IUGR), and prematurity. There is no known amount of alcohol that is safe to drink, so pregnant individuals and those planning pregnancy should be advised not to drink any alcohol.
   b. Tobacco use during pregnancy is the single most preventable cause of illness and death among mothers and infants (Centers for Disease Control and Prevention, 2015). Smoking increases the risk of miscarriage, placental abruption and placenta previa, prematurity, IUGR, low birth weight, preterm prelabor rupture of membranes, ectopic pregnancy, decreased maternal thyroid function, stillbirth, certain birth defects such as cleft lip and palate, and sudden infant death syndrome in early life. Secondhand smoke is a health risk for some of these problems.
   c. Substance abuse with any illegal substance, such as cocaine, methamphetamines, marijuana, and heroin, or any other opioids, is not safe during pregnancy and pregnant individuals should be counseled against any usage. If complicated by addiction, refer to a recovery program as soon as possible to minimize exposure to the child.
4. Hyperthermia: A temperature of 101°F (38.3°C) or higher can be of concern, especially if it lasts for a while. Some studies have shown an increased risk for miscarriage, NTDs, heart and abdominal wall defects, or oral cleft when a high fever occurs early in pregnancy, but the results are not conclusive. Hot tubs and saunas should be avoided during pregnancy, and fever should be reduced with acetaminophen. Heat can also have a negative effect on sperm production and is a potential cause of male infertility.
5. Work and environmental exposure to heavy metals, such as lead and mercury, pesticides, polychlorinated biphenyls (PCBs), and organic solvents, are concerning and can be researched using the resources listed in Appendix A. Exposures to these agents may result in miscarriage, NTDs, prematurity, low birth weight, limb defects, brain and neuromuscular defects, and other problems.
6. Maternal conditions: Certain maternal infections and health conditions may increase the risk of birth defects (see Box 2.1).

Genetic Counseling and Indications for Referral

A. DEFINITION AND BACKGROUND

In 2006, the Genetic Counseling Definition Task Force of the NSGC developed the following definition of genetic counseling: "Genetic counseling is the process of helping people to understand and adapt to the medical, psychological, and familial implications of genetic contributions to disease. This process integrates the following three components:

1. Interpretation of family and medical histories to assess the chance of disease occurrence or recurrence

2. Education about inheritance, testing, management, prevention, resources, and research

3. Counseling to promote informed choices and adaptation to the risk or condition (National Society of Genetic Counselors' Task Force, 2006, p. 79)

B. LOCATE A COUNSELOR THROUGH THE NSGC WEBSITE (WWW.NSGC.ORG)

The following are some, but not all, of the standard indications for genetics referral or consultation.

1. Family history of a chromosome abnormality, genetic disorder, or congenital defect

2. Pregnant individuals of age 35 years and older at delivery, which presents an increased risk for Down syndrome and other chromosomal abnormalities

3. Abnormal results from a triple marker or quad screen test

4. Abnormal fetal ultrasound

5. Positive results in both parents as carriers for CF, Tay–Sachs, SCT or other hemoglobinopathies, and all other genetic disorders

6. Familial history of serious X-linked disorders

7. Patient and/or family concern about a familial genetic disease or issue uncovered in initial history

C. DIRECT-TO-CONSUMER GENETIC TESTING

ACOG has published recommendations for clinicians who encounter patients presenting with direct-to-consumer genetic test results. ACOG advises these patients be counseled by a healthcare professional with the appropriate knowledge, training, and expertise in interpreting test results, and confirmatory testing in a clinical laboratory is advised prior to any medical intervention.

D. RESCREENING BEFORE SUBSEQUENT PREGNANCY

In 2015, the American College of Medical Genetics and Genomics, American College of Obstetricians and Gynecologists, NSGC, Perinatal Quality Foundation, and SMFM issued a joint statement that carrier rescreening typically is not recommended unless the patient's medical or family history has changed (Edwards et al., 2015). With screening panels and molecular techniques improving and rapidly evolving, potential differences exist for the results of the conditions screened and the interpretations. Research is ongoing to determine on population levels how expanded carrier testing should be integrated into clinical care for patients with previous targeted or ethnic-based testing. If a patient requests repeat screening, ACOG recommends referral to a provider with genetics expertise to review previous results and determine the benefits and limitations of the request for subsequent rescreening.

Bibliography

Advani, P. (2015). *Beta thalassemia.* http://emedicine.medscape.com/article/206490-overview

American College of Medical Genetics and Genomics. (2006). *American college of medical genetics standards and guidelines for clinical genetics laboratories: Technical standards and guidelines for CFTR mutation testing.* Author. http://www.acmg.net/docs/CFTR_Mutation_Testing_2011.pdf

American College of Obstetricians and Gynecologists. (2003). Neural tube defects (Practice Bulletin No. 44, reaffirmed 2014). *Obstetrics & Gynecology, 102,* 203–213.

American College of Obstetricians and Gynecologists. (2007). Hemoglobinopathies in pregnancy (Practice Bulletin No. 78, reaffirmed 2015). *Obstetrics & Gynecology, 109,* 229–237. https://doi.org/10.1097/00006250-200701000-00055

American College of Obstetricians and Gynecologists. (2008). Use of psychiatric medications during pregnancy and lactation (Practice Bulletin No. 92, reaffirmed 2014). *Obstetrics & Gynecology, 111,* 1001–1020. https://doi.org/10.1097/AOG.0b013e31816fd910

American College of Obstetricians and Gynecologists. (2016a). Prenatal diagnostic testing for genetic disorders (ACOG Practice Bulletin No. 162). *Obstetrics & Gynecology, 127,* e108–e122. https://doi.org/10.1097/AOG.0000000000001405

American College of Obstetricians and Gynecologists. (2016b). Guidelines for diagnostic imaging during pregnancy and lactation (Committee Opinion No. 656). *Obstetrics & Gynecology, 127,* e75–e80. https://doi.org/10.1097/00006250-201602000-00055

American College of Obstetricians and Gynecologists. (2017). Counseling About Genetic Testing and Communication of Genetic Test Results (Committee Opinion No. 693). *Obstetrics & Gynecology, 126,* e96–e101. https://doi.org/10.1097/AOG.0000000000002020

American College of Obstetricians and Gynecologists. (2020). Screening for fetal chromosomal abnormalities (ACOG Practice Bulletin No. 226). *Obstetrics & Gynecology, 136*(4), e48–e69. https://doi.org/10.1097/AOG.0000000000004084

American College of Obstetricians and Gynecologists, Committee on Genetics. (2011). Family history as a risk assessment tool (Committee Opinion No. 478, reaffirmed 2015). *Obstetrics & Gynecology, 117,* 747–750. https://doi.org/10.1097/AOG.0b013e318214780e

American College of Obstetricians and Gynecologists, Committee on Genetics. (2017a). Carrier screening in the age of genomic medicine (Committee Opinion No. 690). *Obstetrics & Gynecology, 129,* e35–e40. https://doi.org/10.1097/AOG.0000000000001951

American College of Obstetricians and Gynecologists, Committee on Genetics. (2017b). Carrier screening for genetic conditions (Committee Opinion No. 691). *Obstetrics & Gynecology, 129,* e41–e55. https://doi.org/10.1097/AOG.0000000000001952

American College of Obstetricians and Gynecologists, Committee on Genetics and Committee on Ethics. (2009). Ethical issues in genetic testing (Committee Opinion No. 410, reaffirmed 2014). *Obstetrics & Gynecology, 111,* 1495–1502. https://doi.org/10.1097/AOG.0b013e31817d252f

American College of Obstetricians and Gynecologists, Committee on Genetics and Society for Maternal–Fetal Medicine. (2015). Cell-free DNA screening for fetal aneuploidy (Committee Opinion No. 640). *Obstetrics & Gynecology, 126,* e31–e37. https://doi.org/10.1097/01.AOG.0000471172.63927.b6

Bastow, B. D. (2016). *Teratology and drug use during pregnancy.* http://emedicine.medscape.com/article/260725-overview

Centers for Disease Control and Prevention. (2014). *Radiation and pregnancy: A fact sheet for clinicians.* http://emergency.cdc.gov/radiation/prenatalphysician.asp

Centers for Disease Control and Prevention. (2015). *Tobacco use and pregnancy.* . https://www.cdc.gov/reproductivehealth/Pregnancy/index.htm

Centers for Disease Control and Prevention. (2016). *Fetal alcohol spectrum disorders (FASDs).* http://www.cdc.gov/ncbddd/fasd/index.html

Dolan, S. M. (2009). Prenatal genetic testing. *Pediatric Annals, 38,* 426–430. https://doi.org/10.3928/00904481-20090723-05

Dolan, S. M., & Moore, C. (2007). Linking family history in obstetric and pediatric care: Assessing risk for genetic disease and birth defects. *Pediatrics, 120*(Suppl. 2), S66–S70. https://doi.org/10.1542/peds.2007-1010E

Edwards, J. G., Feldman, G., Goldberg, J., Gregg, A. R., Norton, M. E., Rose, N. C., Schneider, A., Stoll, K., Wapner, R., & Watson, M. S. (2015). Expanded carrier screening in reproductive medicine—points to consider. *Obstetrics & Gynecology, 125*(3), 653–662. https://doi.org/10.1097/AOG.0000000000000666.

Hochberg, L., & Stone, J. (2016). *Prenatal screening and diagnosis of neural tube defects. UpToDate.* http://www.uptodate.com

Malm, H., Artama, M., Gissler, M., & Ritvanen, A. (2011). Selective serotonin reuptake inhibitors and risk for major congenital anomalies. *Obstetrics & Gynecology, 118,* 111–120. https://doi.org/10.1097/AOG.0b013e318220edcc

National Society of Genetic Counselors' Task Force. (2006). A new definition of genetic counseling: National society of genetic counselors' task force report. *Journal of Genetic Counseling, 15,* 77–83. https://doi.org/10.1007/s10897-005-9014-3

Nava-Ocampo, A. A., & Koren, G. (2007). Human teratogens and evidence-based teratogen risk counseling: The Motherisk approach. *Clinical Obstetrics and Gynecology, 50*(1), 123–131. https://doi.org/10.1097/GRF.0b013e31802f1880

Norrgard, K. (2008). Medical ethics: Genetic testing and spinal muscular atrophy. *Nature Education, 1*(1), 88. http://www.nature.com/scitable/topicpage/medical-ethics-genetic-testing-and-spinal-muscular-666

O'Rahilly, R., & Müller, F. (2001). *Human embryology & teratology* (3rd ed.). Wiley-Liss.

Palomaki, G. L., Messerlian, G., & Halliday, J. (2021). *Prenatal screening for common aneuploidies using cell-free DNA. UpToDate.* http://www.uptodate.com

Russo, M. (2020). *Cystic fibrosis: Carrier screening. UpToDate.* http://www.uptodate.com

Schwarz, E. B., Postlethwaite, D. A., Hung, Y. Y., & Armstrong, M. A. (2007). Documentation of contraception and pregnancy when prescribing potentially teratogenic medications for reproductive-age women. *Annals of Internal Medicine, 147,* 370–376. https://doi.org/10.7326/0003-4819-147-6-200709180-00006

Shur, N., & Abuelo, D. (2009). Genetic syndromes: From clinical suspicion to referral to diagnosis. *Pediatric Annals, 38,* 419–425. https://doi.org/10.3928/00904481-20090723-04

Stevens, B., Krstic, N., Jones, M., Murphy, L., & Hoskovec, J. (2017). Finding middle ground in constructing a clinically useful expanded carrier screening panel. *Obstetrics & Gynecology, 130*(2), 279–284. https://doi.org/10.1097/AOG.0000000000002139

Stewart, D., & Vigod, S. (2016). *Risks of antidepressants during pregnancy: Selective serotonin reuptake inhibitors (SSRIs). UpToDate.* http://www.uptodate.com

Tsao, B. (2015). *Spinal muscular atrophy.* http://emedicine.medscape.com/article/1181436

Uhlmann, W. R., Schuette, J. L., & Yashar, B (Eds.). (2009). *A guide to genetic counseling* (2nd ed.). Wiley-Blackwell.

U.S. Preventive Services Task Force. Agency for Healthcare Research and Quality. (2009). Folic acid for the prevention of neural tube defects: U.S. Preventive services task force recommendation statement. *Annals of Internal Medicine, 150,* 626–631. https://doi.org/10.7326/0003-4819-150-9-200905050-00009

II. Guidelines for Routine Prenatal and Postpartum Care

3. The First Prenatal Visit

MARY LEE BARRON | KELLY D. ROSENBERGER | JANET THORLTON

General Guidelines

The American Academy of Pediatrics (AAP) and the American College of Obstetricians and Gynecologists (ACOG) describe prenatal care as a comprehensive care program involving a coordinated approach to medical care and psychosocial support that optimally begins before conception and extends throughout the antepartum period (AAP & ACOG, 2017). Comprehensive prenatal care is composed of the following elements: (a) preconceptional care, (b) prompt diagnosis of pregnancy, (c) initial prenatal evaluation, and (d) follow-up prenatal visits. Ongoing maternal–fetal assessment, education and support for the pregnant individual, preparation for parenting, and promotion of a positive physical and emotional family experience are all part of quality prenatal care.

A. BACKGROUND

1. National goals from the Centers for Disease Control and Prevention (CDC) for promoting prenatal care are as follows:

- **a.** To increase the percentage of pregnant individuals who receive timely comprehensive screenings for risk factors
- **b.** To increase the percentage of pregnant individuals who receive timely prenatal counseling and education as outlined in the guideline
- **c.** To increase the number of first-trimester patients who have documentation of counseling about appropriate aneuploidy screening
- **d.** To increase the percentage of vaginal birth after cesarean (VBAC)-eligible individuals who receive documented education describing risks and benefits of VBAC
- **e.** To increase the rate of appropriate interventions for identified change in status in individuals with preterm birth risk factors (National Clearinghouse Guidelines, 2012)

B. MEDICAL AND SURGICAL HISTORY, INCLUDING HEALTH MAINTENANCE INFORMATION

1. Endocrine disease: thyroid or diabetes mellitus
2. Hypertension
3. Pulmonary disease, asthma
4. Cardiac disease
5. Anemia, thalassemia, and hemoglobinopathies
6. Kidney or urinary tract disease, repeated urinary tract infection (UTI), and bacteriuria
7. Cancer
8. Seizure disorder
9. Psychiatric or emotional disorder

10. Hepatitis or liver disease
11. HIV or AIDS
12. Autoimmune disease
13. Deep vein thrombosis (DVT), pulmonary embolism (PE), clotting disorder
14. Prior blood transfusions
15. Past surgery

C. OBSTETRIC AND GYNECOLOGIC HISTORY

1. Terminology
   a. Two-digit system
      i. Gravida: number of pregnancies, including current
      ii. Para: number of pregnancies that resulted in the birth of a baby having reached viability (usually past 20 weeks)
   b. Five-digit system
      i. Gravida: number of pregnancies, including current
      ii. Term: number of term (>37 weeks) pregnancies
      iii. Preterm: number of preterm births (past age of viability and <37 weeks)
      iv. Abortion: number of pregnancies ending in spontaneous or elective abortion (less than the age of viability)
      v. Living children: number of children currently alive
2. Menstrual history
3. Family planning history
4. Pap smear history
5. History of sexually transmitted infections (STIs)
6. Previous preterm labor and/or birth
7. Previous pregnancy loss (either spontaneous or elective)
8. Previous ectopic pregnancy
9. Previous cesarean birth
10. Previous low birth weight or macrosomic infant
11. Previous stillborn or neonatal death
12. Previous infant with congenital anomaly, neurological deficit, birth injury
13. Preeclampsia, eclampsia, HELLP (hemolysis, elevated liver enzymes, low platelet count) syndrome
14. Uterine fibroids
15. Rh negative
16. Cervical cerclage or history of incompetent cervix
17. Previous postpartum hemorrhage
18. Gynecologic surgery or breast problems

D. PSYCHOSOCIAL HISTORY

1. Age
2. Marital status
3. Educational level
4. Economic status
5. Religious and cultural beliefs, including whether blood transfusion would be acceptable and whether there are gender restrictions for obstetrics care provider
6. Health maintenance habits
7. Smoking
8. Alcohol consumption
9. Occupation/job

10. Heavy lifting and/or long periods of standing
11. Support systems/household composition
12. Safety issues (e.g., domestic or intimate partner violence [IPV], weapons in the home)
13. Pets
14. Late entry into prenatal care

E. IMMUNIZATIONS/IMMUNE STATUS

1. Rubella
2. Hepatitis A and B
3. Varicella
4. Tetanus or Tdap (tetanus, diphtheria, and pertussis)
5. Polio
6. Influenza
7. Tuberculosis (TB)

F. DRUG HISTORY

1. Over-the-counter (OTC) medications, including nonsteroidal anti-inflammatory drugs, vitamins, and botanical use
2. Current prescription medications
3. Illicit/illegal drug use

G. NUTRITIONAL STATUS

1. Height, weight, body mass index (BMI), and prepregnancy weight
2. Eating habits and usual dietary routine (use 1-to 3-day recall)
3. Eating of nonfood substances
4. Food allergies
5. Caffeine intake
6. Artificial sweetener use
7. Food safety
8. Exercise habits
9. Who does the cooking at home?
10. Risk factors for poor nutrition:
    a. Adolescence
    b. Low income
    c. Cigarette smoking
    d. Frequent dieting
    e. Vegan diet
    f. Pica
    g. High parity
    h. Mental illness, including depression
    i. Use of certain medications such as phenytoin
    j. Intellectual disability
    k. Chronic diseases
    l. Eating disorders
11. Screening for nutritional risk: Based on the 1-to 3-day recall, the nurse practitioner (NP) should assess whether the individual is at high risk nutritionally. If it is determined that the patient is undernourished, underweight, or nutritionally stressed, then active management is indicated (King et al., 2015). If the NP works with a dietician, the patient should be referred. However, many insurers only cover one visit. So, the NP should be prepared to spend time covering nutritional management.
    a. Undernourished: an individual who is deficient in protein intake for pregnancy requirements

b. Underweight: ≥5% below ideal body weight

c. Nutritionally stressed: pernicious vomiting, short interval between pregnancies (<1 year apart), poor obstetrical history, failure to gain 10 lbs. by the 20th week of gestation, serious emotional upset or problems

H. GENETIC HISTORY

(see Chapter 2)

1. Tay–Sachs disease
2. Sickle cell disease (SCD) or trait
3. Phenylketonuria (PKU)
4. Cystic fibrosis
5. Hemophilia, muscular dystrophy, Huntington's chorea
6. Intellectual disability, Down syndrome, fragile X
7. Birth defects, including cardiac and neural tube defects
8. Celiac disease
9. Myotonic dystrophy
10. Ethnic background: Ashkenazi Jewish, African American, Mediterranean, Asian

I. EXPOSURE TO POTENTIAL TERATOGENS

1. Metals (lead or mercury)
2. Organic solvents and their fumes
3. Gases, carbon monoxide
4. Ionizing radiation
5. Pollutants
6. Secondhand smoke
7. Pesticides, herbicides
8. Lead paint
9. Plastics, vinyl monomers
10. Hyperthermia, use of hot tubs
11. Recent travel history for potential teratogenic exposures (may be infectious or others)

J. FAMILY MEDICAL HISTORY

1. Autoimmune disorders such as lupus, rheumatoid arthritis, rashes, and arthralgias
2. Intellectual disability
3. Psychiatric disorders such as schizophrenia, depression, and bipolar disease
4. Diabetes
5. Polycystic ovarian syndrome (PCOS)
6. Hypertension
7. Obstetrical conditions such as preeclampsia
8. Fetal or neonatal death in a family member
9. Substance abuse in family members

Screening Tools

A. SUBSTANCE USE AND ABUSE

1. Because substance abuse or chemical dependency can adversely affect the health of the patient and the fetus, it is essential to include drug use

assessment and education strategies in prenatal and preventative healthcare encounters.

2. The substance-use risk profile pregnancy scale
   a. Have you ever smoked marijuana?
   b. In the month before you knew you were pregnant, how many beers, how much wine, or how much liquor did you drink?
   c. Have you ever felt that you needed to cut down on your drug or alcohol use?

   Scoring: Answering yes to one question = moderate risk; answering yes to two or three questions = high risk of having a positive screen for alcohol or illicit drug use

B. TOBACCO USE

1. Counseling interventions have been shown to increase cessation rates. One evidence-based approach is the "five As." In practices that have used the five As approach, quit rates among pregnant individuals have risen by >30% (Martin et al., 2006) and more recently, over 23%, specifically in individuals enrolled in Women, Infants, and Children (WIC; Olaiya et al., 2015). This approach to smoking cessation is easily integrated into prenatal care.
   a. *Ask:* Ask the patient to choose a statement that best describes smoking status.
   b. *Advise:* Ask permission to share the health message about smoking during pregnancy.
   c. *Assess:* Readiness to change
   d. *Assist:* Briefly explore problem-solving methods and skills for smoking cessation.
   e. *Arrange:* Let the patient know that you will be following up on each visit; assess smoking status at subsequent prenatal visits; affirm efforts to quit (U.S. Preventive Services Task Force [USPSTF], 2021).

C. DEPRESSION

1. There are multiple depression screening tools available, with most taking no more than 10 minutes to complete. Examples of highly sensitive screening tools include the Edinburgh Postnatal Depression Scale, Center for Epidemiologic Studies Depression Scale, Beck Depression Inventory–II, Postpartum Depression Screening Scale, and the Patient Health Questionnaire. However, the two-item screening measure "Over the past 2 weeks have you felt down, depressed, or hopeless?" and "Over the past 2 weeks, have you felt little interest in doing things?" is a sufficient and rapid way to begin identifying individuals at high risk for depression in prenatal care settings. This two-item screening tool, if positive, is then followed by the nine-item tool (PHQ9). "Failure to identify women with symptoms of depression is not a lack of sufficiently sensitive and brief screening measures; rather, it could be a failure to integrate brief depression screening questions such as these into prenatal interviews" (Jesse & Graham, 2005, p. 44).

D. INTIMATE PARTNER VIOLENCE

1. There are a variety of tools available to screen for IPV(see www.nnvawi.org/assessment.htm). There is no evidence that one screening tool is better than another. The first question to ask is whether the patient is safe at home, particularly if injuries are present. The routine history-taking procedure in which a standardized screening protocol is integrated increases

identification, documentation, and referral for IPV. Victims are found among individuals of all ages, socioeconomic classes, and ethnicities. Married individuals living apart from their spouses are more likely to be victims of rape, physical assault, and/or stalking. Separated, divorced, and cohabitating individuals are at a greater risk for IPV. However, there is no single profile of the individual who suffers abuse, and the abuse is likely to continue or escalate during pregnancy (AAP & ACOG, 2017).

2. If abuse is identified or suspected, intervention is essential. At a minimum, referral sources and educational material should be readily available (including phone numbers to a shelter and the police). Documentation (including patient quotes) should include the frequency and severity of present and past abuse, location and extent of injuries, treatments, and interventions. Discuss a plan of escape and document whether shelter assistance was declined or accepted by the patient. Counseling and intervention can reduce IPV and improve pregnancy outcome. See Section VI.M (of this chapter) and Appendix B for screening tools.

Physical Examination

A. AREAS OF ASSESSMENT

1. Vital signs, height and weight, and prepregnancy weight and BMI
2. Skin, hair, and nails
3. Head, neck, and thyroid
4. Eyes, ears, nose, mouth, and throat
5. Chest and lungs
6. Heart
7. Abdomen, including fundal height as appropriate
8. Pelvic examination
   a. External genitalia/perineum
   b. Vagina
   c. Cervix
   d. Uterus
   e. Adnexa
   f. Clinical pelvimetry
   g. Rectal or rectovaginal examination as appropriate
9. Microscopic wet prep of vaginal secretions as appropriate

TABLE 3.1 AREAS OF ASSESSMENT AND COMMENTS

AREA OF ASSESSMENT	PREGNANCY-RELATED FINDING/COMMENTS
Physical characteristics	Physical characteristics such as height, weight, and pelvimetry data can influence pregnancy course and birth, that is, patients of small stature; android-shaped pelvis
Prepregnancy BMI	BMI is the strongest predictor of maternal weight gain occurring outside of the IOM recommendations. Low BMI = highest risk for inadequate weight gain; high BMI = highest risk for excessive weight gain
Cardiovascular changes: blood pressure and pulse	Blood volume increases until about 30–34 weeks and then plateaus; cardiac output increases and peaks at 25–30 weeks gestation at 30%–50% above prepregnant levels Pulse rate increases by up to 10–15 bpm; blood pressure decreases 5–10 mmHg, reaching the lowest point during the second trimester and then gradually increases to near prepregnant levels at term

(continued)

TABLE 3.1 AREAS OF ASSESSMENT AND COMMENTS (*CONTINUED*)

AREA OF ASSESSMENT	PREGNANCY-RELATED FINDING/COMMENTS
	Femoral venous pressure slowly rises with uterine expansion, which leads to a tendency toward venous stasis, dependent edema, and varicose vein formation in the legs, vulva, and rectum. In addition, a reduction of plasma colloid osmotic pressure resulting from reduced albumin promotes lower extremity edema Postural hypotension and supine hypotensive syndrome may occur as a result of uterine pressure on the vena cava. Exaggerated splitting of S1; systolic murmurs are common due to volume expansion
Hair	There is a decrease in the rate of growth and the number of hair follicles in the resting or dormant phase. During the postpartum phase, the number of hair follicles in the resting phase increases sharply so that the patient may notice increased shedding of hair for 1–4 months. Nearly all hair is replaced within 6 months
Skin	Hyperpigmentation of the face (chloasma), areola, and nipples; linea nigra, striae gravidarum, and spider nevi are common; rubor of palms due to estrogen levels; occasionally intrahepatic cholestasis will lead to pruritus, which resolves after delivery
Eyes	Intraocular pressure decreases; corneal sensitivity increases; slight thickening of the cornea that disappears by 6 weeks postpartum; may make it difficult to wear contact lenses comfortably
Nose	Vascular dilation of the nasal mucous membranes due to estrogen may cause stuffiness and nosebleeds
Dentition/gums	Saliva production increases; no demineralization of the teeth; gum tissue becomes hyperemic, spongy, and swollen, which may lead to gingivitis as pregnancy immunosuppression hinders the normal response to bacteria that causes periodontal infections
Thyroid	Slightly enlarged because of glandular hyperplasia
Chest and lungs	Adaptive changes to improve gaseous exchange and promote fetal circulation: respiratory center in the brain is more sensitive to CO_2; dyspnea may occur; lower ribs flare, which increases tidal volume by 30%–40%; slightly increased respiratory rate. Systolic murmurs are common due to volume expansion
Breasts	Increase in size, nodularity, and sensitivity due to estrogen and progesterone; alveolar cells become secretory; bra size increases
Gastrointestinal abdomen	Changes in sense of taste are common. Tone and motility of smooth muscle are lowered (due to progesterone). Gastric secretion of hydrochloric acid and pepsin decreases. Delayed gastric emptying. Nausea, indigestion, reflux, and constipation are common. Gallbladder is hypotonic and distended so that gallstone formation may occur
Musculoskeletal	Joint relaxation due to influence of relaxin; mobility of the sacroiliac, sacrococcygeal, and pubic joints increases; lordosis is common by third trimester
Neuro/reflexes	Fainting or light-headedness common in the first trimester. Carpal tunnel syndrome due to fluid retention; mild frontal headaches are common and may be related to hormonal influences. Deep tendon reflexes become more reactive with preeclampsia

(*continued*)

TABLE 3.1 AREAS OF ASSESSMENT AND COMMENTS (*CONTINUED*)

AREA OF ASSESSMENT	PREGNANCY-RELATED FINDING/COMMENTS
Pelvis	Vagina: pink or dark pink; in multiparas, vaginal folds may become smooth Cervix: softens, more readily bleeds, bluish color (Chadwick's sign); os closed in nulliparas; external os may admit one fingertip in the multipara Uterine size: initial enlargement in the anterior–posterior diameter, softening of the isthmus (Hegar's sign); see Section III.D for further information Adnexae: usually of normal size, nontender (however, a unilateral nontender corpus luteum cyst may be present)
Anus/rectum	Pressure from an enlarging uterus may cause hemorrhoids

BMI, body mass index; bpm, beats per minute; IOM, Institute of Medicine.

10. Back, spine, and extremities
11. Neurological examination, including deep tendon reflexes (Table 3.1)

B. DEVELOPMENTAL DEFINITIONS AND TERMINOLOGY

1. Preembryonic stage: First 14 days of human development. Synchronized development of the endometrium and embryo is necessary for successful implantation.
2. Ovum, zygote (fertilized ovum), morula (when cleavage occurs)
3. Blastocyst: After the cleavage has produced over 100 cells, the embryo is called a *blastula*. The blastula is usually a spherical layer of cells surrounding a fluid-filled or yolk-filled cavity with an inner cell mass that is distinct from the surrounding blastula. The total structure is the blastocyst. The inner cell mass subsequently forms the embryo, and the outer layer of cells, or trophoblast, later forms the placenta.
4. Implantation at 7 to 10 days after fertilization
5. Embryo (8 weeks), fetus (8 weeks until birth)
6. Trimester: First, conception to 13 weeks; second, 14 to 27 weeks; third, 28 weeks to birth (ACOG & AAP, 2017).

C. CONFIRMATION OF PREGNANCY

1. Human chorionic gonadotropin (HCG) testing in urine or blood (Table 3.2)
2. Clinical landmarks: first-trimester bimanual examination of the uterus
3. Presence of the fetal heartbeat

TABLE 3.2 BETA-HCG LEVEL (MIU/L) IN EARLY SINGLETON PREGNANCY AND ULTRASOUND FINDINGS

APPROXIMATE GESTATIONAL AGE (WEEKS FROM LMP)	BETA-HCG LEVEL (MIU/L)	TYPICAL TRANSVAGINAL ULTRASOUND FINDING
5	≥1,000	Gestational sac
6	≥2,500	Yolk sac
7	≥5,000	Fetal pole
8	≥17,000	Fetal heartbeat

HCG, human chorionic gonadotropin; IU, international units; LMP, last menstrual period.

4. Ultrasound confirmation of the presence of the gestational sac/embryo/fetus

D. DATING CRITERIA

Accurate dating of the pregnancy is one of the most important clinical responsibilities.

1. Naegele's rule (dependent on a menstrual cycle of 28 days and an accurate date of the last menstrual period [LMP])
   a. First day of LMP, subtract 3 months, add 7 days
   b. Estimated date of delivery (EDD) wheel is a tool to use representing Naegele's rule
   c. There are many due-date calculation apps available for smartphones or personal digital assistants (PDAs); these are based on a 28-day cycle
   d. If the pregnancy resulted from ART (assisted reproductive technology), the ART-derived gestational age should be used to assign the EDD
2. Ultrasound is highly accurate for dating when performed in the first trimester. Accuracy for dating purposes diminishes with the progress of the pregnancy. Crown–rump length can be used for gestational age from 4 days up to 12 weeks. If ultrasound dating before 14 weeks varies by more than 7 days than dating by LMP, then the EDD should be changed to agree with ultrasound dating. Biparietal diameter (BPD) can be assessed at approximately 14 weeks and is useful until 26 weeks. BPD predicts EDD within 7 to 10 days. After 26 weeks, predicting EDD by BPD is less accurate, usually ±3 weeks.
3. Uterine size
   a. Bimanual examination: This is an essential diagnostic tool to date early pregnancies. Accuracy of this estimate is generally considered to be ±2 weeks because uterine size is affected by fibroids, uterine position (i.e., retroflexed uterus), multiple gestation, and maternal obesity. Using a comparison to various fruit sizes is a rough mental benchmark that is clinically useful, especially for the inexperienced clinician.
      i. 5-week size: small unripe pear
      ii. 6-week size: small orange
      iii. 8-week size: large navel orange
      iv. 12-week size: grapefruit
   b. Fundal height: An indicator of uterine size measuring from the symphysis pubis to the top of the fundus. Correlates with the weeks of gestation after 20 weeks within ±2 cm, that is, 22 weeks = ± 22 cm. May be used up to 36 weeks. If it does not correlate, then an ultrasound exam for fetal growth may be indicated.
4. Serum beta-HCG testing: Serum beta-HCG levels are highly correlated with gestational age during early pregnancy. Beta-HCG can be detected as early as 8 days after the luteinizing hormone (LH) surge, when pregnancy occurs. The beta-HCG concentration in a normal intrauterine pregnancy rises in a curvilinear fashion during the first 6 weeks of pregnancy. Beta-HCG then plateaus at approximately 100,000 IU/L. Doubling time for the hormone is from 48 hours for clinical decision-making purposes. The beta-HCG concentration rises at a much slower rate in most, but not all, ectopic and nonviable intrauterine pregnancies. However, when the beta-HCG level exceeds 3,000 mIU/mL, the absence of a gestational sac strongly suggests that the pregnancy is abnormal.
5. Chadwick's, Goodell's, and Hegar's signs may support a diagnosis of pregnancy but are mainly of historical value and no longer used now that more accurate diagnostic tools are available.

Diagnostic and Laboratory Examination for the First Prenatal Visit

A. SERUM TESTING

1. Complete blood count (CBC): hematocrit (Hct), hemoglobin (Hgb), mean corpuscular volume (MCV), mean corpuscular Hgb concentration (MCHC), platelet count, and white blood cell (WBC)

a. The increased plasma volume, along with the increase in red blood cell (RBC) mass, ultimately expands the maternal blood volume by as much as 35% to 45%, peaking at 32 weeks (Cunningham et al., 2014). Physiologic anemia describes the proportionately greater increase in plasma volume compared with the rise in RBCs. When Hgb levels are <11 g and/or Hct levels are <32%, pathologic anemia is diagnosed. However, Hgb and Hct levels are lower in African American women compared with Caucasian women; therefore, the Institute of Medicine (IOM) recommends lowering the cutoff levels by 0.8 mg/dL for Hgb and 2% for Hct in this population.

b. The nonpregnant woman normally has a platelet count of 150,000 to 400,000/mm^3. Although during normal pregnancy there is a progressive drop in the count, it rarely drops below the range for the nonpregnant woman. The decreased platelet count is due to increased utilization of platelets. A low platelet count is associated with pregnancy-induced hypertension, immunologic thrombocytopenic purpura, disseminated intravascular coagulation, acquired hemolytic anemia, septicemia, and lupus erythematosus (Cunningham et al., 2014).

c. The normal nonpregnant WBC ranges between 5,000 and 10,000 mm^3. During pregnancy, the WBC increases, yielding a range of 5,000 to 12,000 mm^3 (Cunningham et al., 2014).

2. ABO and Rhesus (Rh) typing, antibody screen

a. Hemolytic disease of the fetus and newborn occur when blood incompatibilities between the pregnant individual and fetus exist. The potential for these incompatibilities exists in the following situations in which the maternal and fetal blood types differ.

i. The mother has type O blood; the fetus has type A, B, or AB

ii. The mother is Rh negative; the fetus is Rh positive

iii. The mother is negative for some other RBC antigen, like Kell, for which the fetus is positive

b. Early identification of blood incompatibilities and appropriate medical and nursing management are essential to reducing severity of the disorder. Laboratory assessment at the first prenatal visit includes an antibody screen as well as blood type and Rh. An indirect Coombs test is most often used for the initial antibody screen because this test is sensitive to anti-Rh antibodies. Patients who test positive are then tested for the specific antibody and titer. Management in pregnancy is dependent on the degree to which the specific antibody is known to cause hemolytic disease in the fetus or newborn. Most cases of hemolytic disease are caused by Rh and ABO incompatibilities, with Rh-induced disease causing the most severe cases. The Rh antigens are grouped into three pairs: Dd, Cc, and Ee. The presence of D determines that the person is Rh positive. The absence of D determines that a person is Rh negative. Rh isoimmunization occurs only when Rh-positive erythrocytes enter a Rh-negative person's bloodstream, which then produce anti-D. Anti-D causes hemolytic disease in the Rh-positive fetus. Isoimmunization can result when a patient is transfused with improperly matched blood, or when an individual is exposed to fetal blood through miscarriage or abortion, an ectopic pregnancy, an amniocentesis, antepartal bleeding, or placental separation. In response to exposure to Rh-positive cells, the mother produces antibodies to the Rh antigen that have the potential to cause hemolytic disease in an Rh-positive fetus or newborn in future pregnancies. Specifically, fetal erythrocytes are destroyed by maternal antibodies that cross the placenta and enter fetal blood.

c. Cases that require follow-up include patients who are:

i. Blood type O, positive antibody screen
ii. Rh negative, father is Rh positive
iii. Rh negative, father's type is unknown

d. Cases in which no follow-up is needed include patients who are:

i. Rh positive; blood group A, B, or AB with negative antibody screen
ii. Rh negative; father is Rh negative; both have negative antibody screen
iii. Rh negative, Du positive

e. Fortunately, the process of Rh isoimmunization can usually be prevented with prenatal (at 28 weeks) and postpartum administration of Rho(D) immune globulin such as RhoGAM®. Additional times when RhoGAM may be administered include any possible "leaking" of fetal blood into the maternal system:

i. During or after all pregnancies, including ectopic pregnancies and after early miscarriages
ii. After chorionic villus sampling, amniocentesis, cordocentesis
iii. After external cephalic version
iv. After an injury to the abdomen

f. The Rh blood group system is more complex than what has just been described. There are 35 other antibodies that delineate Rh antigens. Du replacing D is not uncommon and is found more frequently among African Americans. Rarely, a Du-positive mother carrying a D-positive fetus may produce anti-D, which in turn causes hydrops fetalis.

3. Serology: Either rapid plasma reagin (RPR) or venereal disease research laboratory (VDRL) with reflex microhemagglutination assay (MHA-TP) or fluorescent treponemal antibody (FTA-ABS)

a. A serologic test for syphilis should be performed on all pregnant patients at the first prenatal visit. In populations in which the amount of prenatal care delivered is not optimal, RPR card test screening (and treatment, if that test is reactive) should be performed at the time of confirmation of pregnancy. Individuals who are at high risk for syphilis, who live in areas of high syphilis morbidity, or who are previously untested should be screened again early in the third trimester (at approximately 28–32 weeks gestation) and at delivery (Centers for Disease Control and Prevention [CDC], 2021).

b. The VDRL and RPR designed to detect the presence of nonspecific reaginic antibodies elicited by the spirochete are relatively inexpensive, very sensitive, moderately nonspecific, and fast. The false-positive rate for pregnant individuals is 1% to 2% (Williamson & Snyder, 2014). A high titer (>1:16) usually indicates active disease. A low titer (<1:8) indicates a biologic false-positive test in 90% of the cases or occasionally may be due to late or late latent syphilis. A titer is performed before treatment. A fourfold drop in the titer indicates a response to therapy. Treatment of primary syphilis usually causes a progressive decline (i.e., low titers) to a negative VDRL titer within 2 years. In secondary, late, or latent syphilis, low titers persist in approximately 50% of the cases after 2 years despite a fall in the titer. This does not indicate treatment failure or reinfection, and these patients are likely to remain positive even if retreated. Titer response is unpredictable in late or latent syphilis. Rising titer (four times) indicates relapse, reinfection, or treatment failure (Williamson & Snyder, 2014).

c. False positives can occur in individuals with acute and chronic illnesses, such as TB, infectious mononucleosis, rheumatoid arthritis, collagen vascular diseases, chlamydia infection, and hepatitis (Williamson & Snyder, 2014). The presence of anticardiolipin antibodies, which can trigger a reactive VDRL, is particularly significant in pregnancy.

d. The presence of *Treponema pallidum* is confirmed using either the FTA-ABS absorption test MHA-TP or *Treponema pallidum* antibodies to determine whether the individual has developed antibodies to the spirochete. A seropositive result indicates that the individual has been exposed to the spirochete and has developed antibodies. Because this test frequently remains positive after successful treatment, monitoring is accomplished using titers of the VDRL or RPR.

4. Rubella screening

a. The most frequently used test to detect rubella antibodies in serum is the hemagglutination inhibition test. Immunity is confirmed if the rubella antibody titer is 1:8 or more (Williamson & Snyder, 2014). Persons who have an "equivocal" serologic test result should be considered susceptible to rubella.

5. Hepatitis screening

a. Hepatitis B virus (HBV): Pregnant individuals at risk for HBV infection should be vaccinated. To avoid misinterpreting a transient positive HBsAg result during the 21 days after vaccination, HBsAg testing should be performed before vaccine administration. All laboratories that conduct HBsAg tests should use a Food and Drug Administration (FDA)-cleared HBsAg test and perform testing according to the manufacturer's labeling, including testing of initially reactive specimens with a licensed neutralizing confirmatory test. Pregnant patients who are HBsAg positive should be reported to the local or state health department to ensure that they are entered into a case management system and that timely and appropriate prophylaxis is provided for their infants. Information concerning the pregnant patient's HBsAg status should be provided to the hospital in which delivery is planned and to the healthcare provider who will care for the newborn. In addition, household and sexual contacts of individuals who are HBsAg positive should be vaccinated. Patients who are HBsAg positive should be provided with, or referred for, appropriate counseling and medical management. Pregnant individuals who are HBsAg positive should receive information regarding hepatitis B that addresses:

i. Modes of transmission

ii. Perinatal concerns (e.g., breastfeeding is not contraindicated)

iii. Prevention of HBV transmission, including the importance of postexposure prophylaxis for the newborn infant and hepatitis B vaccination for household contacts and sex partners

iv. Evaluation for and treatment of chronic HBV infection

b. Hepatitis C virus (HCV): No treatment is available for pregnant individuals infected with HCV. However, all patients with HCV infection should receive appropriate counseling and supportive care as needed. Because the vertical transmission is so low, routine screening of prenatal individuals is not warranted. No vaccine is available to prevent HCV transmission. HCV antibodies pass transplacentally to the infant, so testing for this antibody in the infant should be delayed until 18 months of age.

6. HIV (see Chapter 20)
   a. The CDC recommends HIV screening for all individuals as a standard part of prenatal care to identify and treat HIV and to prevent transmission of HIV to infants. Patients who test positive for HIV and begin treatment early in their pregnancy reduce the risk of mother-to-child HIV transmission to ≥2%.
   b. Pregnant individuals are likely to get tested if their providers strongly recommend it. In a study of 1,362 pregnant patients, 93% of patients who felt their providers strongly recommended an HIV test decided to get tested.
   c. Screening for HIV early in pregnancy, preferably at the first obstetrical visit, benefits both mothers and babies. Patients with HIV who start treatment early and maintain it throughout their pregnancy protect their own health and rarely pass HIV to their infants. Patients who have not been tested or have an increased risk for HIV should be tested in the third trimester.
   d. It is never too late for pregnant individuals to get tested. Rapid HIV tests allow patients who arrive at delivery rooms with unknown HIV status to receive an HIV test. Preventive medications administered to the mother during labor, and to the infant after birth, can reduce the risk of mother-to-child HIV transmission to about 10%. Some clinicians may also test a pregnant patient late in the third trimester of pregnancy.
7. Blood lead level
   a. In 2019, the USPSTF concluded that the current evidence is insufficient to assess the balance of benefits and harms of screening for elevated blood lead levels in asymptomatic pregnant persons. The prevalence of elevated blood lead levels varies substantially among different communities and populations. Children living with mothers who have elevated levels are at higher risk for elevated lead levels, which lead to neurodevelopmental damage. Children and pregnant individuals share many of the same risk factors for lead exposure. The most predictive factor is living in a home that was built before 1960. Therefore, the NP should decide based on what is known regarding the community lead exposures. The prevalence of levels >15 mcg/dL appears to be quite low in pregnant individuals. There is some evidence that mildly elevated lead levels during pregnancy are associated with small increases in antepartum blood pressure, but only limited evidence indicates that these levels have important adverse effects on reproductive outcomes.
8. Progesterone level may be considered for patients at high risk for preterm delivery and for those with first-trimester spotting or bleeding (see Chapter 15).
9. Thyroid function screening: Maternal and fetal complications are associated with both hypothyroidism and hyperthyroidism. The ACOG, the Endocrine Society, and the American Thyroid Association recommend testing for thyroid dysfunction if the pregnant individual has any of the following:
   a. Symptoms of thyroid disease
   b. Personal or family history of thyroid disease
   c. Characteristics that are associated with developing overt hypothyroidism such as type 1 diabetes, goiter, amiodarone/lithium use, iodine deficiency, history of head, and neck radiation). See Chapter 23 for in-depth information.

10. Type 2 diabetes: Some clinicians universally screen with an HbA1C at the initial prenatal visit and then again at 24 to 28 weeks. Others screen patients at risk with a random glucose (>200 mg/dL is abnormal) and subsequently, an HbA1C to confirm the diagnosis (see Chapter 16).

B. PAP SMEAR

1. Pregnancy is not a reason to do cervical screening. A Pap smear is done according to standardized guidelines at the first prenatal visit. However, if in the past 24 to 48 hours the pregnant individual has douched, had intercourse, or used a vaginal suppository, or there is evidence of vaginal or cervical infection, the Pap smear should be deferred until the next visit.

2. Pregnancy produces changes in the cervix that need to be taken into account when interpreting the results of a Pap smear. During pregnancy, the squamocolumnar junction increases in size. As the pregnancy progresses, squamous epithelium may replace columnar epithelium by a process called *squamous metaplasia*, which may be reflected in the Pap smear result. However, this migration of cells makes the process of colposcopy easier to do in pregnancy than in the nonpregnant state (Cunningham et al., 2014).

3. In pregnancy, the only diagnosis that alters management of an abnormal Pap smear is invasive cancer (ACOG, 2013; American Society for Colposcopy and Cervical Pathology, 2013). Patients with Pap results that are not likely to be associated with cancer (atypical squamous cells) may undergo colposcopy examination either during the pregnancy or at 6 to 12 weeks postpartum. For pregnant individuals with a low-grade squamous intraepithelial lesion, colposcopy is preferred, but deferring to 6 weeks postpartum is acceptable.

C. URINE TESTING

1. Prenatal screening for bacteriuria is essential because of the well-known association between preterm labor and UTI during pregnancy. A complete urinalysis (UA) is generally performed only once during a healthy, low-risk pregnancy at the first or second prenatal visit. Anatomic, physiologic, and hormonal changes predispose a pregnant individual to the development of pyelonephritis, one of the most common medical problems of pregnancy. Pregnant individuals with sickle cell trait or disease, high parity, and diabetes are more likely to develop bacteriuria. However, asymptomatic bacteriuria (ASB) is a major risk factor for the development of pyelonephritis. To screen for symptomatic UTI or ASB, a clean-catch midstream urine is required. The diagnosis of ASB or symptomatic UTI is usually based on a colony count of ≥100,000/mL of a particular organism on a freshly voided clean-catch midstream specimen. The pathogen responsible for 80% to 90% of infection is *Escherichia coli*, followed by *Klebsiella, Proteus*, and the enterococcus. Group B *Streptococcus* and *Staphylococcus saprophyticus* have also been noted as important urinary pathogens (Sweet & Gibbs, 2009).

a. Urine dipstick for nitrites and leukocyte esterase is a less expensive way to screen for UTI after the initial UA and urine culture. The urine dipstick alone is not sensitive enough to be used for a screening test for ASB. Nitrites are by-products of bacterial growth and are frequently present when there is a UTI. However, for best results, the urine must be in the bladder for 4 hours or longer. Gram-negative rods, such as *E. coli*, are more likely to produce a positive test. Leukocyte esterase may not be as useful to the clinician as vaginal contamination readily causes positive leukocyte esterase urine. Those patients at risk for a UTI should have a UA and culture repeated at least once or once in each trimester.

2. In the absence of hypertension, routine urine screening for glucosuria and proteinuria beyond the first prenatal visit has not been found to be useful in identifying patients at risk for gestational diabetes or preeclampsia (Alto, 2005, 2007). A trace amount of protein may be found in a urine specimen during normal pregnancy. In addition, healthy pregnant individuals may manifest glucosuria without abnormal plasma glucose levels.

D. STI SCREENING: CHLAMYDIA AND GONORRHEA

1. Nucleic acid amplification testing (NAAT) is considered the gold standard for the diagnosis of genital *Chlamydia trachomatis* infections. FDA-approved kits are available for endocervical, urine, urethral specimens, and liquid-based Pap test specimens. The NAAT method detects the genetic material of the bacteria, living or dead, and therefore is not used to determine treatment effectiveness. However, the sensitivities reported for NAATs range from approximately 90% to 97%; the specificities are more than 99% (Williamson & Snyder, 2014).
2. Test of cure is not routinely required. However, if the patient had gastrointestinal (GI) side effects as a result of antimicrobial therapy, compliance may have been an issue.

E. TB SKIN TESTING (PROTEIN PURIFIED DERIVATIVE)

1. TB continues to be a public health problem. Untreated TB represents a greater hazard to a pregnant individual and fetus than does its treatment. The tuberculin skin test (TST) is considered both valid and safe to use throughout pregnancy. The TB blood test is safe to use during pregnancy but has not been evaluated for diagnosing *Mycobacterium tuberculosis* infection during pregnancy. Other tests are needed to show whether a person has TB.
2. Testing for TB in Bacille Calmette–Guérin (BCG)-vaccinated persons:
   a. The TST and blood tests to detect TB infection are not contraindicated for persons who have been vaccinated with BCG.
   b. TST: BCG vaccination may cause a false-positive reaction to the TST, which may complicate decisions about prescribing treatment. The presence or size of a TST reaction in persons who have been vaccinated with BCG does not predict whether BCG will provide any protection against TB disease. Furthermore, the size of a TST reaction in a BCG-vaccinated person is not a factor in determining whether the reaction is caused by latent TB infection (LTBI) or the prior BCG vaccination. BCG vaccination should not be given during pregnancy. Even though no harmful effects of BCG vaccination on the fetus have been observed, further studies are needed to prove its safety.
   c. TB blood tests: Blood tests to detect TB infection, unlike the TST, are not affected by prior BCG vaccination and are less likely to give a false-positive result.
3. Persons with no known risk factors for TB may be considered for treatment of LTBI if their reaction to the tuberculin test is at least 15 mm of induration or they have a positive result using a TB blood test. Targeted skin testing programs should only be conducted among high-risk groups. All testing activities should be accompanied by a plan for follow-up care for persons with TB infection or disease.
4. Treatment of pregnant persons should be initiated whenever the probability of TB is moderate to high. Infants born to mothers with untreated TB may be of lower birth weight than those born to mothers without TB, and, in rare circumstances, the infant may be born with TB. Although the drugs used

in the initial treatment regimen for TB cross the placenta, they do not appear to have harmful effects on the fetus.

F. OTHER TESTS

1. Hgb electrophoresis: Sickle cell anemia, thalassemia major, and Hgb C are common autosomal recessive hemoglobinopathies. Like other autosomal recessive disorders, a fetus is at risk for sickle cell anemia and thalassemia major if both parents are carriers of the trait (see Chapter 2). However, a milder form of anemia may exist if the individual has one normal gene and one gene for the trait. There may be a combination of traits as well. An individual has a 25% chance of inheriting sickle–thalassemia or Hgb SCD if one parent carries the sickle cell trait and the other parent carries the trait for either thalassemia or Hgb C. Sickle–thalassemia can be as severe as sickle cell anemia. In Hgb SCD, there is less marked destruction of RBCs and anemia; hence, the disorder is less severe clinically (Williamson & Snyder, 2014). A quick screening test is available to detect sickle cell traits, but it does not differentiate between those who have the disease or the trait. An Hgb electrophoresis provides more detailed information that includes the thalassemias and other hemoglobinopathies. These recessively inherited conditions occur in the United States primarily in families of Asian, Middle Eastern, African, and Mediterranean descent. Pregnant individuals of African descent are routinely screened for these disorders as the prevalence rate for sickle cell trait in these patients is 8% to 12% in the United States.

2. The TORCH acronym is well known in the fields of neonatal/perinatal nursing. Infections acquired in utero or during the birthing process may lead to abnormal growth, developmental anomalies, or multiple clinical and laboratory abnormalities. The O for Other has been expanded to include not only syphilis but also other causes of in utero infection. TORCH: (T) toxoplasmosis, caused by the protozoan parasite *Toxoplasma gondii,* can lead to an increased risk of vision loss, intellectual disability, deafness, seizures, and muscle spasticity; (O) other organisms (parvovirus B19, HIV, Epstein–Barr virus, zika, varicella-zoster virus, syphilis, and enteroviruses), (R) rubella, now rare in the United States due to immunization programs, can lead to an increased risk of deafness, cataracts, cardiac malformations, neurologic disorders, and endocrine sequelae; (C) cytomegalovirus, is common worldwide and is the leading cause of sensorineural hearing loss and other neurodevelopmental disabilities including cerebral palsy, intellectual disability, vision impairment, and seizures; and (H) herpes simplex virus (HSV), with most cases being acquired during the birthing process. HSV infections in newborns may be localized to the skin, eyes, mouth, central nervous system, or disseminated involving multiple organs. Gestational age at the time of any of the TORCH infections greatly influences the effect on the fetus.

3. Vitamin D deficiency: Although recent evidence suggests that vitamin D deficiency is fairly common during pregnancy, there is not enough evidence to support universal screening. An optimal serum level for pregnancy has not been established, but for those individuals thought to be deficient (<32 ng/mL), vitamin D supplementation of 1,000 to 2,000 IU per day is safe (ACOG, 2015).

G. ULTRASOUND EXAMINATION IN THE FIRST TRIMESTER

1. A sonographic examination can be of benefit in many circumstances in the first trimester of pregnancy, including but not limited to the following indications (according to the American Institute of Ultrasound in Medicine):

a. To confirm the presence of an intrauterine pregnancy
b. To evaluate a suspected ectopic pregnancy
c. To define the cause of vaginal bleeding
d. To evaluate pelvic pain
e. To estimate gestational (menstrual) age
f. To diagnose or evaluate multiple gestations
g. To confirm cardiac activity
h. As an adjunct to chorionic villus sampling, embryo transfer, and localization and removal of an intrauterine device
i. To assess for certain fetal anomalies, such as anencephaly, in high-risk patients
j. To evaluate maternal pelvic masses and/or uterine abnormalities
k. To measure nuchal translucency when part of a screening program for fetal aneuploidy
l. To evaluate a suspected hydatidiform mole

2. Limited examination may be performed to evaluate interval growth, estimate amniotic fluid volume, evaluate the cervix, and assess the presence of cardiac activity

3. Components of the basic ultrasound examination include the following:

a. Intrauterine pregnancy
b. The uterus, including the cervix, and adnexa should be evaluated for the presence of a gestational sac. If a gestational sac is seen, its location should be documented. The gestational sac should be evaluated for the presence or absence of a yolk sac or embryo, and the crown–rump length should be recorded, when possible. Embryonic/fetal anatomy is appropriate for the first trimester.
c. Fetal number
d. Cardiac activity
e. The uterus, including the cervix, adnexal structures, and cul-de-sac, should be evaluated
f. Free fluid
g. If possible, the appearance of the nuchal region should be assessed as part of a first-trimester scan when a live fetus is present

4. Order of appearance of structures

a. Gestational sac: 4 to 5 weeks
b. Yolk sac: 5 to 6 weeks
c. Fetal pole: 6 to 7 weeks
d. Cardiac activity: 6 to 7 weeks

Common Discomforts in the First Trimester

A. NAUSEA AND VOMITING

1. Definition: Among the most common complaints, nausea and vomiting occur in 50% to 80% of pregnant individuals. The problem can have a major impact on the quality of life of the pregnant individual, causing missed workdays and affecting job performance. The term "morning sickness," although common, is a misnomer as nausea can occur anytime. The cause is unknown, and there is no evidence to support the notion that psychological factors play a role. Influencing factors include high levels of circulating steroids (estrogen and HCG), slowed peristalsis of the GI tract due to progesterone, pressure from the enlarging uterus, gastric overloading, low blood sugar, and changes in carbohydrate metabolism.

2. History
   a. Sensation of nausea
   b. Loss of appetite
   c. Aversion to certain types of foods
   d. Aversion to the smell or sight of food
   e. Vomiting
   f. Additional information to consider
      i. The patient is between 4 and 16 weeks of pregnancy
      ii. Symptoms occur with fatigue
      iii. Absence of fever, diarrhea, and abdominal pain
3. Physical examination
   a. Unremarkable
      i. Vital signs are within normal limits
      ii. Weight variable depending on the severity of the symptoms
      iii. No evidence of dehydration in mucous membranes, skin turgor, or urine-specific gravity
      iv. Abdominal examination is negative for organomegaly, pain, tenderness, or guarding
      v. Fetal heart tone auscultation is appropriate for gestation
      vi. Fundal height is appropriate for gestation
4. Laboratory examination
   a. Urine negative or positive for ketones; negative or trace proteinuria
   b. CBC, electrolytes may be done for patients who are severely nauseated but will show absence of severe hemoconcentration, normal WBC counts, and absence of acidosis
5. Differential diagnosis
   a. Hyperemesis gravidarum
   b. Multiple gestation
   c. Hydatidiform molar pregnancy
   d. Infectious process (gastric influenza, appendicitis, pancreatitis, intestinal parasites, UTI/pyelonephritis, and hepatitis)
   e. Drug or alcohol effect
   f. Gall bladder disease
   g. Hyperthyroidism
   h. Migraine headache
   i. Food poisoning
   j. Bulimia
   k. Diabetic ketosis
   l. Malaria
6. Treatment
   a. Reassurance that the condition will end
   b. Small frequent meals
   c. Avoid foods with strong odors or tastes (individual preferences/dislikes may change in pregnancy)
   d. Avoid low blood sugar levels; eat high-protein foods frequently; decrease fluid intake with and between meals, or separate fluids and solids (patterned intake)
   e. Avoid high-fat foods
   f. Acupressure wrist bands: Low-tech varieties are available (elastic bands with ball that is placed two fingerbreadths below the bend of the wrist over the tendon on the inner aspect of the forearm, worn bilaterally) as an alternative to the more expensive and higher tech ReliefBand that is worn on one arm and has a transcutaneous electric nerve stimulator unit, which is available at Reliefband.com

g. Ondansetron ODT (Zofran ODT) 4 to 8 mg/d: Data are limited and unclear as to the association with birth defects. There is no clear benefit for using this drug over other agents (Kennedy, 2016). Recent studies analyzed data from more than 88,000 pregnancies in which pregnant individuals took ondansetron during the first trimester to examine the risk of cardiac malformations or oral clefts. The teams report no increased risk of cardiac malformations and a very small increased risk of oral clefts in studies published online in *JAMA* (Huybrechts et al., 2018, 2020).
h. Possibly beneficial: A diet rich in B complex vitamins, vitamin B_6 supplements such as B_6 25 to 50 mg two to three times a day. Unisom (doxylamine) 25 mg at bedtime or twice a day (Briggs et al., 2011).
i. Stop smoking
j. Suck on hard candy (sour or sweet), such as Atomic Fireballs (cinnamon candy)
k. Eat popcorn or melba toast before rising out of bed and then eat a high-protein breakfast
l. Combine sweet and salty foods (potato chips and lemonade)
m. Brush teeth more often; rinse mouth frequently
n. Reduce fat, fried foods, and spices in diet
o. Good posture and nausea-preventing exercise
p. Stop chewing gum
q. Herbal teas: The FDA does not regulate these teas and considers them to be dietary supplements. Safe teas include raspberry leaf tea, ginger, and peppermint. Avoid black or blue cohosh, kava, and St. John's wort as these stimulate uterine activity.
r. Consider that prenatal vitamins may be contributing to the nausea. Have the patient use the "gummy" or "chewable" variety, as these are not upsetting to the stomach for most patients. Doses can be divided.

7. Warning signs/complications
   a. Inability to retain food for 24 hours or more; any weight loss, rule out hyperemesis gravidarum
   b. Ketone bodies in urine suggest severe/prolonged vomiting or prolonged fasting
   c. Dizziness, dry mucous membranes, decreased urination, and other signs of dehydration
   d. Persistent nausea and vomiting after first trimester; rule out hydatidiform mole and/or pregnancy-induced hypertension
   e. If abnormal vital signs, abdominal pain or tenderness, and/or diarrhea are present, rule out infections, pancreatitis, GI conditions such as intestinal obstruction, appendicitis, cholelithiasis, cholecystitis, hepatitis, pyelonephritis, and food poisoning
   f. If there is a lack of heart tones, uterus greater than estimated gestational age, persistent nausea and vomiting, and/or abnormal vaginal bleeding, rule out hydatidiform mole
8. Consultation/referral
   a. If no response to treatment
   b. If complications develop (see previous item Warning Signs)
9. Follow-up
   a. Contact provider if unable to retain fluids for 12 hours or more
   b. Continued weight loss: recheck weight weekly until symptoms subside
   c. Check urine ketones and signs of dehydration until symptoms subside
   d. If symptoms respond to treatment, check at routine intervals, that is, in 4 weeks

B. FAINTING

1. Definition: An abrupt, usually brief loss of consciousness, generally associated with an alteration of normal blood circulation
2. History: The patient complains of slight dizziness, swirling, or a floating sensation and a decrease in the ability to hear or focus attention; accompanied by prolonged standing or being in a warm, crowded room
3. Physical examination: Unremarkable, although supine hypotension can be replicated by placing the patient in a supine position (usually third-trimester phenomenon)
4. Laboratory examination: CBC, random blood sugar only if there is reason to suspect gestational diabetes or a neurologic or cardiovascular problem
5. Differential diagnosis
   a. Heat-causing dilation of blood vessels, which lowers blood pressure
   b. Hyperventilation caused by progesterone acting on the respiratory center of the brain
   c. Hypoglycemia caused by a change in carbohydrate metabolism
   d. Supine hypotension (when supine pressure of gravid uterus on vena cava decreases blood flow to the heart)
   e. Orthostatic hypotension (late pregnancy venous stasis in lower extremities decreases the amount of blood filling the heart when moving from sitting/lying to standing)
6. Treatment: Advise patient regarding the following:
   a. Moderate exercise
   b. Deep breathing
   c. Move slowly and avoid standing still for a prolonged period
   d. Avoid low blood sugar levels by eating five to six small meals per day
   e. Avoid warm crowded areas
   f. If standing, lie down or sit with head in lap
   g. Avoid hot showers or baths
   h. Avoid supine position in the third trimester, use a side-lying position
   i. Wear anti-embolism compression (TED [thrombo-embolic deterrent]) stockings
7. Consultation/referral
   a. Refer or consult with a physician if cardiovascular or neurologic condition suspected

C. FATIGUE

1. Definition: Marked fatigue, out of proportion to the patient's normal pattern
2. Etiology: Thought to be caused by the sleep-inducing effects of progesterone. This is so common that it is one of the presumptive signs of pregnancy
3. History: Reports needing frequent periods of rest, which is different from the usual pattern
   a. Details about the fatigue's duration (recent, prolonged, or chronic)
   b. Onset (sudden or progressive)
   c. Recovery period (short or long)
   d. Type (physical or mental fatigue)
   e. Patient's usual level of physical activity (sedentary or active)
   f. Symptoms began with the pregnancy
4. Physical examination: unremarkable
5. Laboratory examination: usual prenatal panel
6. Differential diagnosis
7. Fatigue is very broad but could include:

a. Iron-deficiency anemia
b. Mononucleosis
c. Depression
d. Chronic fatigue syndrome
e. Sleep disorder
f. Medication use

8. Treatment
a. Reassurance that the condition usually resolves by 16 weeks gestation
b. Plan rest periods, including going to sleep earlier in the evening
c. Partner should be encouraged to assume more responsibilities, so the patient can rest

First-Trimester Education/Anticipatory Guidance

A. NUTRITION, FOOD SAFETY, AND WEIGHT GAIN IN PREGNANCY

1. Periconceptional nutrition is vital to the critical period (first 12 weeks) of organ development. Maintaining optimal nutrition during this period can be a challenge, especially when the patient is nauseated. Simple instructions include advising eating small frequent meals that include all food groups: "Put a lot of color on your plate" and to stay hydrated. Updated and patient-friendly information is available at www.ChooseMyPlate.gov. The current dietary recommendations developed by the IOM (2009a) are as follows:

a. Protein intake is essential, and many women do not take in an adequate amount. The recommended amount is 70 g/d (1.1 g/kg/d) or three to four servings per day. Typical sources include dairy, beans, nuts, legumes, meat, poultry, and fish.

b. Omega-3 fatty acids: Optimal fetal neurodevelopment is dependent on many essential nutrients, including docosahexaenoic acid (DHA) and eicosapentaenoic acid (EPA), which can be obtained only from dietary sources. Essential fatty acids are lipids that cannot be synthesized within the body. The standard Western diet is severely deficient in essential fatty acids because the best sources are cold-water fish, such as salmon, tuna, sardines, anchovies, and herring. Therefore, supplementation with 300 mg of DHA daily is recommended.

i. Omega-3 dietary deficiency is compounded by the fact that pregnant individuals become depleted in omega-3s when the fetus uses omega-3s for its nervous system development. Omega-3s are also used after birth to make breast milk. With each subsequent pregnancy, mothers are further depleted.

ii. Adding omega-3s to the diet of pregnant individuals has a positive effect on the visual and cognitive development of the baby as well as possibly reducing the risk of allergies in infants. Increased intake of EPA and DHA has been shown to reduce the risk of preterm labor and delivery in at-risk populations, may lower the risk of preeclampsia, and may increase birth weight. Omega-3 deficiency may also increase the risk for depression.

iii. Quality fish oil (labeled U.S. Pharmocopeia [USP]) is safe to take during pregnancy. Fresh fish (that is eaten) can often contain environmental toxins like mercury that accumulate during the fish's life span. These toxins can be virtually eliminated during the manufacture and processing of fish oil, with the use of high-quality raw materials and an advanced refining process.

c. Iron: Increase iron intake from 15 to 30 g/d
d. Folic acid: Increased folate consumption from 400 to 800 mcg/d
   i. There are certain special circumstances that may affect these recommendations. For example, if there is a history of a child with a neural tube defect, the folic acid recommendation in a subsequent pregnancy is increased to 4 mg rather than 0.4 to 0.8 mg/d
e. Calcium: The recommended amount of calcium for women aged 19 to 50, pregnant or not, is 1,000 mg/d; for adolescents up to age 18, it is 1,300 mg daily
f. Vitamin D: 600 IU/d
g. Add 340 additional calories per day in the second trimester and 452 calories per day in the third trimester
h. Fiber: 28 g/d
i. Water intake: Water is important not only to prevent dehydration, but recent research suggests the importance of sufficient water consumption (mean consumption is about four and a half 8-oz glasses/day) during early pregnancy to decrease the risk of birth defects, including neural tube defects, cleft lip, gastroschisis, and congenital heart defects (Alman et al., 2017).

2. Caffeine use in pregnancy: Data remains inconsistent, with controversy regarding caffeine safety and consumption during pregnancy (National Academies of Sciences, Engineering, and Medicine, 2020). Caffeine metabolism and pharmacokinetics are influenced by many factors, including genetic variability (Hale, 2019; Langer, 2018; Nehlig & Alexander, 2018). Polymorphisms of the CYP1A2 enzyme determine whether caffeine will be metabolized rapidly or slowly by an individual (Langer, 2018).

Relevant to the NP:

a. Consumption of up to 400 mg caffeine/d in healthy adults and 300 mg caffeine/d in healthy pregnant women is generally recognized as safe (Hale, 2019; Rosenfeld et al., 2014; Wikoff et al., 2017).
b. Pregnant women, preterm, and newborn infants metabolize caffeine more slowly; therefore, reduced maternal caffeine intake to <200 mg is often recommended (LactMed®).
c. Smoking stimulates caffeine clearance and oral contraceptives decrease clearance (Langer, 2018, Nehlig & Alexander, 2018).
d. There is no requirement by the FDA to list the amount of caffeine on product.

Regulation, Labeling, and Safety of Caffeinated Products:

Caffeine is naturally found in coffee, tea, chocolate, and may be an additive to medications, foods, beverages, weight-loss products, and cosmetics (IOM, 2014; National Academies of Sciences, Engineering, and Medicine, 2020). The market of caffeinated products is proliferating, and patterns of consumer use are not well understood (National Academies of Sciences, Engineering, and Medicine, 2020). Estimating caffeine exposure in these products is challenging (Kallmyer, 2019; Leviton, 2018). Federal regulations surrounding product labeling are complex. The USFDA regulates caffeine levels in foods and dietary supplements; however, there is no requirement to list the amount of caffeine on product labels (Foster, 2017; USFDA & Center for Food Safety and Applied Nutrition, 2018). American Beverage Association (ABA) member companies—representing 95% of energy drinks sold in the

United States—comply with the ABA Guidance for Responsible Labeling and Marketing of Energy Drinks and voluntarily include cautionary labels advising against use by children, pregnant/lactating women, and individuals sensitive to caffeine (ABA, 2020; Rosenfeld et al., 2014). Caffeine content varies by product and serving size. The Center for Science in the Public Interest (2021) provides a caffeine chart containing approximate content in foods and beverages:

i. A 20-ounce coffee may contain up to 398 mg
ii. A 16-ounce iced or regular tea may contain up 98 mg
iii. A 16-ounce energy drink may contain up to 300 mg and indeterminate amounts of herbal stimulants
iv. Varied sizes of caffeinated shakes and waters may contain from 30 to100 mg
v. Assorted sizes of chocolate candy/drinks may contain from 2 to 600 mg
vi. OTC weight-loss supplements and medications may contain from 64 to 300 mg

3. Weight gain in pregnancy: Approximately 60% of American pregnant individuals do not gain the appropriate amount of weight during pregnancy, with the majority gaining too much, especially those with a high prepregnancy BMI (Olson, 2008). The U.S. Department of Agriculture created an interactive web-based site, which is now known as "ChooseMyPlate." The website provides food intake and physical activity recommendations for persons age 2 and older, replacing healthy foods for unhealthful, diet tracking, menu planning, nutrition information, and personalized advice. The strategies are easy to understand for the lay public. The information should be used to complement and not substitute for prenatal education (Shieh & Carter, 2011). The NP is encouraged to explore the website for use with preconception, prenatal, and lactating individuals (www.choosemyplate.gov) (Table 3.3).

TABLE 3.3 RECOMMENDATIONS FOR WEIGHT GAIN DURING PREGNANCY

PREPREGNANT STATUS	BMI	WEIGHT GAIN (LB/KG)
Singleton pregnancy		
Underweight	<18.5	28–40 lb (12.7–18.2 kg)
Normal weight	18.5–24.9	25–35 lb (11.4–15.9 kg)
Overweight	25.0–29.9	15–25 lb (7.0–11.5 kg)
Obese	>30	11–20 lb (5.0–9 kg)
Twin pregnancy		
Underweight	<18.5	No recommendation due to insufficient data
Normal weight	18.5–24.9	37–54 lb (16.8–24.5 kg)
Overweight	25.0–29.9	31–50 lb (14.1–22.7 kg)
Obese	>30	11–20 lb (11.4–19.1 kg)

BMI, body mass index.

Source: Adapted from www.iom.edu/Reports/2009b/Weight-Gain-During-Pregnancy-Reexamining the-Guidelines.aspx.

B. VITAMINS, HERBAL SUPPLEMENTS, AND MEDICATION (PRESCRIPTION AND OTC)

1. Prenatal vitamin supplements vary in composition. Generally, the vitamin should contain
   a. 400 mcg of folic acid
   b. 400 IU of vitamin D
   c. 200 to 300 mg of calcium
   d. 70 mg of vitamin C
   e. 3 mg of thiamine
   f. 2 mg of riboflavin
   g. 20 mg of niacin
   h. 6 mcg of vitamin B_{12}
   i. 10 mg of vitamin E
   j. 15 mg of zinc
   k. 17 mg of iron
   l. Fish oil can be added as a separate supplement or is added to some brands for an added cost. Some patients become nauseated from the prenatal vitamin. Using a children's chewable or "gummy" or prenatal "gummy" allows for dividing the dose and is usually well tolerated.
2. Anemia: In addition to taking an iron supplement, patients who are anemic should be counseled to consume iron-rich foods such as (heme source) spinach, beef, beef or chicken liver, clams or mollusks, oysters, cooked turkey, and (nonheme source) breakfast cereals enriched with iron, beans, dried apricots, baked potato, enriched egg noodles, tofu, pumpkin, sesame, or squash seeds (see Chapter 10).
3. Herbal supplements: There is a large variety of herbal supplements being marketed to pregnant individuals. Many (1%–87%) pregnant individuals use complementary and alternative medicine, but this practice is not well studied. Common modalities include massage, vitamin and mineral supplements, herbal medicine, relaxation therapies, and aromatherapy. Therefore, an open discussion should be initiated with the patient concerning alternative therapies. Patients should be advised to consult their NP or nurse midwife before ingesting or using these supplements. The following substances have the potential to harm during pregnancy when used in a concentrated formulation (not as a spice in cooking).
   a. Oral supplements: arbor vitae, beth root, black cohosh, blue cohosh, cascara, chaste tree berry, Chinese angelica (dong quai), cinchona, cotton root bark, feverfew, ginseng, goldenseal, juniper, kava kava, licorice, meadow saffron, pennyroyal, poke root, rue, sage, St. John's wort, senna, slippery root, tansy, white peony, wormwood, yarrow, yellow dock, and vitamin A (large doses can cause birth defects)
   b. Aromatherapy essential oils: calamus, mugwort, pennyroyal, sage, wintergreen, basil, hyssop, myrrh, marjoram, and thyme
   c. Further resource: www.pregnancy.org/article/herbs-avoid-during-pregnancy
4. Food safety: For example, norovirus, which causes acute gastroenteritis; *Salmonella*; listeriosis; *E. coli*; hepatitis A. Pregnant individuals have increased susceptibility to listeriosis. Listeriosis can lead to spontaneous abortion, preterm delivery, stillbirth, or serious infection in infants. The FDA provides advice on food safety (www.fda.gov/food/resourcesforyou/healtheducators/ucm081785.htm).
5. The March of Dimes also provides patient-friendly materials at www.marchofdimes.com/pregnancy/nutrition_foodsafety.html. To reduce the risk of food-borne illness, it is important for the pregnant individual to:

a. Practice good personal hygiene (handwashing and care of kitchen utensils, cookware, and surfaces)
b. Consume meats, fish, poultry, and eggs that are fully cooked
c. Avoid unpasteurized dairy or juice, fruit/vegetable products
d. Wash fresh fruits and vegetables prior to eating
e. Avoid raw sprouts (alfalfa, clover, radish, and mung bean)
f. Avoid listeriosis by refraining from unheated processed/deli meats and hot dogs, soft cheeses like feta or brie, smoked seafood, meat spreads, and pâté
g. Avoid certain types of seafood: king mackerel, swordfish, tilefish, and shark. The FDA recommends that pregnant individuals eat up to 12 oz a week (two average meals) of a variety of fish and shellfish that are lower in mercury, such as canned light tuna, salmon, pollock, and catfish. No more than 6 oz a week should be consumed of canned "solid white" or albacore tuna or if the fish in question is caught privately in local waters and health authorities are unable to provide any relevant safety information.

C. EXERCISE

1. Preexercise medical screening: A clinical evaluation of the pregnant patient should be conducted prior to prescribing an exercise regimen. At least 30 minutes of moderate exercise on most days is a reasonable activity level for most pregnant individuals. The factors to include in screening are as follows:

a. Age
b. General physical condition
c. Exercise history
d. Risk factors for coronary artery disease
e. Musculoskeletal risks
f. Medication use
g. History of pulmonary disease
h. Anticipated type of exercise
i. Handicaps or disability
j. Current or previous obstetrical history

2. Some activities carry more risk in pregnancy than others, for example, contact sports or skiing. Scuba diving is to be avoided completely. Pregnant individuals who pursue activities that increase the risk of falls or contact (soccer, basketball) or joint stress (jogging) should be cautioned. Many pregnant individuals will benefit from a walking regimen, especially those who were not active prior to pregnancy. Activities that promote musculoskeletal fitness include strength training, resistance training, and flexibility exercises. Water exercise appears to have benefits that include the reduction of edema, thermoregulation, and buoyancy, which reduces the risks of joint injuries during pregnancy. Pregnancy should not be thought of as a time to "get in shape." Patients who exercised before pregnancy should be able to continue to do so as long as the pregnancy is healthy and uncomplicated. The CDC recommends that healthy pregnant and postpartum individuals get at least 150 minutes of moderate-intensity aerobic activity per week, such as brisk walking and should be cautioned to remain hydrated.

3. Pregnant individuals with gestational diabetes who exercise may improve their glucose control. Obese pregnant individuals who exercise reduce the risk of developing gestational diabetes. Pregnant patients who exercise are at lower risk for developing preeclampsia.

Absolute Contraindications to Aerobic Exercise During Pregnancy

a. Hemodynamically significant heart disease
b. Restrictive lung disease
c. Incompetent cervix/cerclage
d. Multiple gestation at risk for premature labor
e. Persistent second-or third-trimester bleeding
f. Placenta previa after 26 weeks of gestation
g. Premature labor during the current pregnancy
h. Ruptured membranes
i. Preeclampsia/pregnancy-induced hypertension

Signals to Stop Exercising While Pregnant

i. Vaginal bleeding
ii. Dyspnea prior to exertion
iii. Fatigue
iv. Dizziness
v. Headache
vi. Chest pain
vii. Muscle weakness
viii. Calf pain or swelling (need to rule out thrombophlebitis)
ix. Preterm labor
x. Decreased fetal movement
xi. Amniotic fluid leakage
xii. Pain in back, hips, or pubic bone
xiii. Difficulty walking
xiv. Significant swelling in feet or legs

D. SEXUAL INTERCOURSE

(www.marchofdimes.com/pregnancy/physicalactivity_sex.html)

E. ITEMS TO AVOID

1. Hot tubs and sauna
2. Hair dyes (unless vegetable based)
3. Tobacco
4. Alcohol
5. Illicit drugs
6. Workplace/occupational hazards

F. DISCOMFORTS TO EXPECT

1. Nausea
2. Fatigue
3. Frequent urination
4. Breast tenderness

G. TRAVEL DURING PREGNANCY

1. Air travel: Long-haul air travel is associated with an increased risk of venous thrombosis. Advise the patient to wear correctly fitted compression stockings as this is effective at reducing the risk.

2. Car travel: Pregnant individuals should be informed about the correct use of seat belts (i.e., three-point seatbelts "above and below the bump, not over it").

3. Traveling abroad: If a pregnant individual is planning to travel abroad, she should be informed regarding infectious disease prevalence, such as Covid-19, Zika or Chagas disease, vaccinations, airline policies, and travel insurance.

4. See www.acog.org/womens-health/faqs/travel-during-pregnancy for additional information on travel recommendations during pregnancy.

H. DANGER SIGNS IN PREGNANCY

1. Vaginal bleeding
2. Nausea and excessive vomiting that lasts more than 24 hours
3. Fever (more than 100.4 °F)
4. Dizziness; sudden and extreme and associated with pelvic or uterine pain
5. Preterm labor signs and symptoms (see Chapter 18)
6. Leaking of fluid from the vagina
7. Preeclampsia symptoms:
  a. Rapid weight gain
  b. Headaches
  c. Visual disturbances, vomiting, epigastric pain, irritability, scanty urine output (see Chapter 16)
8. Decreased fetal activity (see Appendix A and Chapter 6)
9. Symptoms of a UTI:
  a. Dysuria
  b. Severe backache
  c. Fever (see Chapter 12)

I. INDICATIONS FOR CONSULTATION/REFERRAL

1. A pregnant individual who by medical/family history is considered high risk
  a. Maternal cardiac disease
  b. Maternal hypertensive disease
  c. Diabetes mellitus and glucose intolerance of pregnancy
  d. Maternal pulmonary disease (asthma not controlled)
  e. Maternal renal disease
  f. Maternal collagen disease
  g. Hemoglobinopathies
  h. Anemia
  i. Psychiatric illness
  j. Rh sensitization or other isoimmunization
  k. Habitual abortion (three or more)
  l. Previous second-or third-trimester pregnancy loss
  m. Known substance abuse
  n. Serious maternal infectious disease (e.g., HIV, hepatitis, TB)
  o. Prior early preterm delivery (before 34 weeks)
  p. Prior infant with a genetic abnormality or major congenital anomaly
2. Abnormal findings on the physical or ultrasonic examination
  a. Multiple gestation
  b. No fetal heart activity
  c. Ectopic pregnancy
  d. Breast mass
  e. Short cervix (<25 mm)
3. Abnormal laboratory findings
  a. Positive HIV test result
  b. Abnormal Pap smear with higher atypical squamous cells of undetermined significance (ASCUS)
  c. Anemia (Hgb <10 mg/dL)
  d. Positive screen for significant antibody

4. The following may be indications for a social service consultation/referral
   a. Financial problems
   b. History of abuse (either by an intimate partner or as a child)
   c. Family/marital issues
   d. History of psychiatric/mental illness
   e. Need for community resources such as food stamps, WIC; placement for adoption

J. **FOLLOW-UP CARE**
1. As indicated by gestation
   a. Every 4 weeks until 28 weeks gestation, every 2 weeks until 36 weeks, every week until delivery

Special Considerations

A. INTIMATE PARTNER VIOLENCE

1. IPV is defined broadly as including emotional degradation, threats, and intimidation, as well as a physical or sexual assault from an intimate partner (Ulrich et al., 2006). IPV often starts, or if already occurring, may increase during pregnancy. The incidence is estimated to occur in 1% to 20% of pregnancies, depending on the way IPV is assessed. There is a threefold higher risk for IPV in unintended pregnancy versus intended pregnancy. Although women of all socioeconomic status (SES) have suffered IPV, women of lower SES have an increased risk in both pregnant and nonpregnant populations. Younger women, unmarried, separated or divorced, and those from minority groups are also at an increased risk for IPV. There is also an increased risk if the couple is cohabitating rather than married. Married women who live apart from their spouses are also more likely to be victims of rape, assault, and/or stalking (Tjaden & Thoennies, 2000).

   Adverse pregnancy outcomes are many and varied. Pregnant individuals who are abused (physical, sexual, or emotional) are more likely to deliver preterm and/or low-birth-weight babies, have a cesarean delivery, be hospitalized for premature labor, pyelonephritis, and trauma as a result of blows to the abdomen or falling. These patients also have a threefold higher risk for becoming a victim of attempted/completed homicide. Total healthcare costs from IPV run into the billions in the United States.

   a. Risk profile: There is no single profile of the individual who suffers abuse (see nicic.gov/intimate-partner-violence-risk-assessment-tools-review). Presenting patterns may include the following:
      i. Unwanted pregnancy
      ii. Late entry into prenatal care, missed appointments
      iii. Substance use or abuse
      iv. Poor weight gain and nutrition
      v. Multiple, repeated somatic complaints (AAP & ACOG, 2013)

2. Screening tools: Given the high rates of IPV in the perinatal period and the associated negative health outcomes, NPs should routinely screen for IPV; without such screening, few IPV cases are likely to be detected, and patients cannot be appropriately referred to resources. Assessing for IPV should be performed in different ways (written and verbally) using culturally appropriate language. Assessment strategies and interventions must be appropriate to age, culture, and ethnicity as well as specific to the stage in an abusive relationship. Abuse in a relationship is not a "discrete" event but rather a process. Some patients may resist the label of "abuse" but will acknowledge that there

are problems in their relationships. This may be culturally mediated as the behavior is viewed as "normal" for the environment in which the patient lives. Families and friends do not intervene even with knowledge of the abusive activity. Coping strategies that the patient uses can be elicited. How the patient interprets the situation may make the individual more vulnerable to depression as well as an escalation of violence and danger.

Six screening instruments designed to detect current or recent IPV demonstrated high diagnostic accuracy (Nelson et al., 2012).

a. Hurt, Insult, Threaten, and Scream (HITS) instrument: Both English and Spanish versions of the four-item HITS instrument have sensitivity and specificity greater than 85%. HITS consists of the following four screening questions:

i. "Over the past 12 months, how often did your partner: physically hurt you; insult you or talk down to you; threaten you with physical harm; and scream or curse at you?" Patients responded to each of these items with a five-point frequency format: never, rarely, sometimes, fairly often, and frequently. Score values can range from a minimum of 4 to a maximum of 20 (Sherin et al., 1998).

b. The Ongoing Violence Assessment Tool

i. At the present time, does your partner threaten you with a weapon?

ii. At the present time, does your partner beat you so badly that you must seek medical help?

iii. At the present time, does your partner act like he or she would like to kill you?

iv. My partner has no respect for my feelings (never, rarely, occasionally, often, always).

c. Ongoing Abuse Screen (OAS) or Abuse Assessment Screen (five items). Both use the same category of items, but the OAS is targeted to ongoing IPV.

i. Are you presently emotionally or physically abused by your partner or someone important to you?

ii. Are you presently being hit, slapped, kicked, or otherwise physically hurt by your partner or someone important to you?

iii. Are you presently being forced to engage in sexual activities?

iv. Are you afraid of your partner or any one of the following (circle if applicable): husband/wife, ex-husband/ex-wife, boyfriend/girlfriend, stranger?

v. (If pregnant) Have you been hit, slapped, kicked, or otherwise physically hurt by your partner or someone important to you during pregnancy (Weiss et al., 2003)?

d. The Humiliation, Afraid, Rape, Kick (HARK) instrument

i. H—Humiliation. Within the past year, have you been humiliated or emotionally abused in other ways by your partner or your ex-partner?

ii. A—Afraid. Within the past year, have you been afraid of your partner or ex-partner?

iii. R—Rape. Within the past year, have you been raped by or forced to have any kind of sexual activity with your partner or ex-partner?

iv. K—Kick. Within the past year, have you been kicked, hit, slapped, or otherwise physically hurt by your partner or ex-partner?

v. One point is given for every yes answer; a score of greater than 1 is positive for IPV (Sohal et al., 2007).

e. The Woman Abuse Screening Tool had sensitivity of 88% and specificity of 89%.

i. In general, how would you describe your relationship?
A lot of tension some tension no tension

ii. Do you and your partner work out arguments with . . .?
Great difficulty some difficulty no difficulty

iii. Do arguments ever result in you feeling put down or bad about yourself?
Often sometimes never

iv. Do arguments ever result in hitting, kicking, or pushing?
Often sometimes never

v. Do you ever feel frightened by what your partner says or does?
Often sometimes never

vi. Has your partner ever abused you physically?
Often sometimes never

vii. Has your partner ever abused you emotionally?
Often sometimes never

viii. Has your partner ever abused you sexually?
Often sometimes never

To score this instrument, the responses are assigned a number. For the first question, "a lot of tension," gets a score of 1 and the other two get a 0. For the second question, "great difficulty" gets a score of 1 and the other two get 0. For the remaining questions, "often" gets a score of 1, "sometimes" gets a score of 2, and "never" gets a score of 3 (Brown et al., 1996).

f. STAT (Slapped, Threatened, and Throw)

Have you ever been in a relationship where your partner has pushed or slapped you?

Have you ever been in a relationship where your partner has threatened you with violence?

Have you ever been in a relationship where your partner has thrown, broken, or punched things?

3. Disclosure: No screening tool should be used in lieu of good clinical judgment. As always, clinical judgment should outweigh test scores if there appears to be a discrepancy between the two. There are several considerations when a disclosure of abuse is made:

a. Respecting client confidentiality is a critical aspect of the nurse–client relationship. It is important for nurses to realize when there are ethical, professional, and legal exceptions to client confidentiality within client relationships. Although state requirements vary, nurses should be guided by the American Nurses Association (ANA) Code of Ethics and the profession's practice standards regarding confidentiality and health information.

b. Knowledge of community services and referral services; provide resources for patient safety

c. Provide emotional support; reassure the patient is not alone

d. Teach about the cycle of abuse

e. If postpartum, arrange for a home care visit if possible. Home visiting interventions addressing IPV in nonperinatal population groups have been effective in minimizing IPV and improving outcomes. This suggests that perinatal home visiting programs adding specific IPV interventions may reduce IPV and improve maternal and infant health.

f. Duggan et al. (2000) developed the Hawaii Healthy Start tool, which has since been validated in a number of studies. The following factors raise the risk for IPV in the perinatal setting:

i. Unmarried
ii. Partner employed
iii. Inadequate income
iv. Unstable housing
v. No phone
vi. Education less than 12 years
vii. Inadequate emergency contacts
viii. History of substance use
ix. Inadequate prenatal care
x. History of abortions
xi. History of psychiatric care
xii. Abortion unsuccessfully sought or attempted
xiii. Adoption sought or attempted
xiv. Marital or family problems
xv. History of depression

g. Hawaii Risk Indicators Screening Tool: Based on the medical record or interview; score true, false, unknown. Based on the medical record or interview, score each factor as true, false, or unknown. A positive screen: True score on item number 1, 9, or 12; two or more true scores; seven or more unknown.

B. IMMUNIZATIONS DURING PREGNANCY

The CDC has an excellent reference on immunizations in pregnancy to keep the NP updated (www.cdc.gov/vaccines/pubs/preg-guide.htm).

Risk to a developing fetus from vaccination of the mother during pregnancy is primarily theoretical. No evidence exists of risk from vaccinating pregnant individuals with inactivated virus or bacterial vaccines or toxoids. Live vaccines pose a theoretical risk to the fetus. Benefits of vaccinating pregnant individuals usually outweigh potential risks when the likelihood of disease exposure is high, when infection would pose a risk to the mother or fetus, and when the vaccine is unlikely to cause harm. Generally, live virus vaccines are contraindicated for pregnant individuals because of the theoretical risk of transmission of the vaccine virus to the fetus. If a live virus vaccine is inadvertently given to a pregnant patient, or if an individual becomes pregnant within 4 weeks after vaccination, the patient should be counseled about the potential effects on the fetus. But vaccination is not ordinarily an indication to terminate the pregnancy. Whether live or inactivated vaccines are used, vaccination of pregnant individuals should be considered on the basis of risks versus benefits, that is, the risk of the vaccination versus the benefits of protection in a particular circumstance.

Screening for rubella and hepatitis B is recommended for all pregnant individuals. Individuals susceptible to rubella should be vaccinated immediately after delivery. A patient known to be HBsAg positive should be followed up carefully to ensure that the infant receives hepatitis B immune globulin and begins the hepatitis B vaccine series less than 12 hours after birth and that the infant completes the recommended hepatitis B vaccine series. No known risk exists for the fetus from passive immunization of pregnant individuals with immune globulin preparations.

1. Recommended during pregnancy
   a. Influenza (regardless of the gestational age) during the flu season (October through March in the United States). Do not administer live attenuated influenza vaccines (LAIV) to pregnant individuals.
   b. Tdap (tetanus, diphtheria, acellular pertussis administered during the late second or third trimester): all pregnant individuals should receive the Tdap (vaccine) regardless of whether or not they've had the Tdap before. If not administered during pregnancy, Tdap should be administered immediately postpartum (AAFP, 2013).
2. Contraindicated/not recommended during pregnancy
   a. Anthrax
   b. BCG
   c. Measles
   d. Mumps
   e. Rubella
   f. Varicella
   g. Yellow fever
   h. Zoster
3. Not routinely recommended (risk vs. benefit)
   a. Human papillomavirus
   b. Polio
   c. Plague
   d. Typhoid
4. Contraindicated but no adverse outcomes if given in pregnancy
   a. Varicella (because the effects on the fetus are unknown, pregnant individuals should not be vaccinated)
5. Indications for vaccine that are not altered by pregnancy
   a. Cholera
   b. Hepatitis A
   c. Hepatitis B
   d. Meningococcus
   e. Pneumococcus
   f. Rabies
   g. Tetanus, diphtheria, pertussis
      i. Routine booster: If a tetanus and diphtheria booster vaccination is indicated during pregnancy for a patient who has previously not received Tdap (i.e., more than 10 years since previous Td), then healthcare providers should administer Tdap during pregnancy, preferably during the third or late second trimester (after 20 weeks gestation).
      ii. Wound management: If a Td booster is indicated for a pregnant individual who previously has not received Tdap, Tdap should be administered.
      iii. Unknown or incomplete tetanus vaccination: To ensure protection against maternal and neonatal tetanus, pregnant individuals who never have been vaccinated against tetanus should receive three vaccinations containing tetanus and reduced diphtheria toxoids. The recommended schedule is 0 weeks, 4 weeks, and 6 to 12 months. Tdap should replace one dose of Td, preferably during the third or late second trimester of pregnancy (after 20 weeks gestation). For pregnant individuals who have previously received a dose of Tdap, Td should be used in these situations.

iv. Providers are encouraged to report the administration of Tdap to pregnant individuals, regardless of trimester, to the appropriate manufacturer's pregnancy registry: for Adacel® to Sanofi Pasteur, telephone 1-800-822-2463 and for Boostrix® to GlaxoSmithKline Biologicals, telephone 1-888-825-5249.

Recommended Reading

1. *What to Expect When You Are Expecting* by Eisenberg, Murkoff, Hathaway (Workman Publishing)
2. *Pregnancy, Childbirth, and the Newborn* by Simkin, Whalley, Deppler (Meadowbook Press)
3. Literature specific to the practice, office, or clinic

Bibliography

Alexander, E. K., Pearce, E. N., Brent, G. A., Brown, R. S., Chen, H., Dosiou, C., Grobman, W. A., Laurberg, P., Lazarus, J. H., Mandel, S. J., Peeters, R. P., & Sullivan, S. (2017). Guidelines of the American thyroid association for the diagnosis and management of thyroid disease during pregnancy and the postpartum. *Thyroid, 27*, 315–389. https://doi.org/10.1089/thy.2016.0457

Alman, B. L., Coffman, E., Siega-Riz, A. M., & Luben, T. J. (2017). Associations between maternal water consumption and birth defects in the national birth defects prevention study (2000–2005). *Birth Defects Research Part A: Clinical and Molecular Teratology, 109*, 193–202. https://doi.org/10.1002/bdra.23569

Alto, W. A. (2005). No need for glycosuria/proteinuria screen in pregnant women. *Journal of Family Practice, 54*, 978–983.

Alto, W. A., & Yetman, C.A. (2007). Routine prenatal urine dipstick testing. *Journal of Reproductive Medicine, 52*(10), 984.

American Academy of Pediatrics and American College of Obstetricians and Gynecologists. (2013). *Guidelines for perinatal care* (8th ed.). Author.

American Academy of Pediatrics and American College of Obstetricians and Gynecologists. (2017). *Guidelines for perinatal care* (8th ed.). Elk Grove Village, IL. https://www.acog.org/clinical-information/physician-faqs/-/media/3a22e153b67446a6b31fb051e469187c.ashx

American Association of Family Physicians. (2013). *ACIP now recommending DTAP for all pregnant women*. https://www.aafp.org/afp/2013/1015/p507.html

American Beverage Association. (2020, March 4). *Guidance for responsible labeling and marketing of energy drinks*. https://www.energydrinkinformation.com/resources/guidelines/

American College of Obstetricians and Gynecologists. (2013). ACOG Practice Bulletin No. 140: Management of abnormal cervical cancer screening test results and cervical cancer precursors. *Obstetrics & Gynecology, 122*(6), 1338–1367. https://doi.org/10.1097/01.AOG.0000438960.31355.9e

American College of Obstetricians and Gynecologists. (2014). Committee Opinion No. 611: Method for estimating due date. *Obstetrics & Gynecology, 124*(4), 863–866. https://doi.org/10.1097/01.AOG.0000454932.15177.be

American College of Obstetricians and Gynecologists. (2015). *Vitamin D: Screening and supplementation during pregnancy* (ACOG Committee Opinion No. 495). Author.

American College of Obstetricians and Gynecologists. (2020). ACOG Practice Bulletin No. 223: Thyroid disease in pregnancy. *Obstetrics & Gynecology, 135*, 3261. https://doi.org/10.1097/AOG.0000000000003894

American College of Obstetricians and Gynecologists Committee on Obstetric Practice. (2015). *Physical activity and exercise during pregnancy and the postpartum period* (ACOG Committee Opinion No. 650). Author.

American Society for Colposcopy and Cervical Pathology. (2019). *Updated consensus guidelines on the management of women with abnormal cervical cancer screening tests and cancer precursors*. https://www.asccp.org/management-guidelines

Bardwell, J., Sherin, K., Sinacore, J., Zitter, R., & Shakil, A. (1999). Screening for domestic violence in family medicine. *Journal of Advocate Health Care, 1*(1), 5–7.

Bishop, J. L., Northstone, K., Green, J. R., & Thompson, E. A. (2011). The use of complementary and alternative medicine in pregnancy: Data from the Avon longitudinal study of parents and children. *Complementary Therapeutic Medicine, 19*, 303–310. https://doi.org/10.1016/j.ctim.2011.08.005

Black, C. M., Marrazzo, J., Johnson, R. E., Hook, E. W., Jones, R. B., Green, T. A., Schachter, J., Stamm, W. E., Bolan, G., St Louis, M. E., & Martin, D. H. (2002). Head-to-head multicenter comparison of DNA probe and nucleic acid amplification tests for chlamydia trachomatis infection in women performed with an improved reference standard. *Journal of Clinical Microbiology, 40*, 3757–3763. https://doi.org/10.1128/JCM.40.10.3757-3763.2002

Bonati, M., Bortulus, R., Marchetti, F., Romero, M., & Tognoni, G. (1990). Drug use in pregnancy: An overview of epidemiological (drug utilization) studies. *European Journal of Clinical Pharmacology, 38*, 325–328. https://doi.org/10.1007/BF00315569

Branson, B. M., Handsfield, H. H., Lampe, M. A., Janssen, R. S., Taylor, A. W., Lyss, S. B., & Clark, J. E. (2006). *Recommendations for HIV testing of adults, adolescents, and pregnant women in health-care setting*. https://www.cdc.gov/mmwr/preview/mmwrhtml/rr5514a1.htm

Briggs, G. G., Freeman, R. K., & Yaffee, F. J. (2011). *Drugs in pregnancy and lactation: Reference guide to fetal and neonatal risk* (8th ed.). Williams & Wilkins.

Brown, J. B., Lent, B., Brett, P., Sas, G., & Pederson, L. (1996). Development of the woman abuse screening tool for use in family practice. *Family Medicine, 28*, 422–428.

Center for Science in the Public Interest. (2021). *Caffeine chart*. https://cspinet.org/eating-healthy/ingredients-of-concern/caffeine-chart

Centers for Disease Control and Prevention. (2014). *Tuberculosis (TB) and pregnancy*. http://www.cdc.gov/tb/publications/factsheets/specpop/pregnancy.htm

Centers for Disease Control and Prevention. (2021). *Sexually transmitted infections treatment guidelines*. Retrieved from https://www.cdc.gov/std/treatment-guidelines/default.htm

Chen, P. H., Rovi, S., Vega, M., Jacobs, A., & Johnson, M. S. (2005). Screening for domestic violence in a predominantly Hispanic clinical setting. *Family Practice, 22*, 617–623. https://doi.org/10.1093/fampra/cmi075

Cunningham, F. G., Leveno, K. J., Bloom, S. L., Spong, C. Y., Dashe, J. S., Hoffman, B. L., Casey, B. M., & Sheffield, J. S. (2014). *William's obstetrics* (24th ed.). McGraw-Hill Medical.

Davidson, M., London, M., & Ladewig, P. (2015). *Maternal newborn nursing & women's health across the lifespan* (10th ed.). Pearson.

De Groot, L., Abalovich, M., Alexander, E. K., Amino, N., Barbour, L., Cobin, R. H., Eastman, C. J., Lazarus, J. H., Luton, D., Mandel, S. J., Mestman, J., Rovet, J., & Sullivan, S. (2012). Management of thyroid disfunction during pregnancy and postpartum: An endocrine society clinical practice guideline. *Journal of Clinical Endocrinology and Metabolism, 97*, 2543–2565. https://doi.org/10.1210/jc.2011-2803

De Vigan, C., De Walle, H. E., Cordier, S., Goujard, J., Knill-Jones, R., Aymé, S., Calzolari, E., & Bianchi, F. (1999). Therapeutic drug use during pregnancy: A comparison in four European countries. *Journal of Clinical Epidemiology, 52*(10), 977–982. https://doi.org/10.1016/S0895-4356(99)00091-8

Duggan, A., Windham, A., McFarlane, E., Fuddy, L., Rohde, C., Buchbinder, S., & Sia, C. (2000). Hawaii's healthy start program of home visiting for at-risk families: Evaluation of family identification, family engagement, and service delivery. *Pediatrics, 105*, 250–259.

Foster, J. (2017). Caffeine intake safety laws. *Caffeine Informer*. https://www.caffeineinformer.com/caffeine-safety-laws

Hale, T. W. (2019). *Hale's medications & mothers' milk ™ 2019: A manual of lactational pharmacology*. Springer Publishing.

Huybrechts, K. F., Hernandez-Diaz, S., & Bateman, B. T. (2020). Ondansetron use in pregnancy and congenital malformations- Reply. *JAMA, 323*, 2097–2098. https://doi.org/10.1001/jama.2020.5067

Huybrechts, K. F., Hernandez-Diaz, S., Straub, L., Gray, K. J., Zhu, Y., Mogun, H., & Bateman, B. T. (2020). Intravenous ondansetron in pregnancy and risk of congenital malformations. *JAMA, 323*, 372–374. https://doi.org/10.1001/jama.2019.18587

Huybrechts, K. F., Hernández-Díaz, S., Straub, L., Gray, K. J., Zhu, Y., Patorno, E., Desai, R. J., Mogun, H., & Bateman, B. T. (2018). Association of maternal first-trimester ondansetron use with cardiac malformations and oral clefts in offspring. *JAMA, 320*, 2429–2437. https://doi.org/10.1001/jama.2018.18307

Institute of Medicine. (2009a). *Nutrition during pregnancy: Part 1: Weight gain, Part 2: Nutrient supplements*. National Academies Press. https://www.ncbi.nlm.nih.gov/books/NBK235228/

Institute of Medicine. (2009b). *Weight gain during pregnancy: Reexamining the guidelines*. National Academies Press. https://www.nap.edu/resource/12584/Report-Brief---Weight-Gain-During-Pregnancy.pdf

Institute of Medicine. (2011). *Clinical preventive services for women: Closing the gaps*. National Academies Press. https://www.nap.edu/openbook.php?record_id=13181

Institute of Medicine. (2014). *Caffeine in food and dietary supplements: Examining safety: Workshop summary*. The National Academies Press. https://www.nap.edu/catalog/18607/caffeine-in-food-and-dietary-supplements-examining-safety-workshop-summary

Jesse, D., & Graham, M. (2005). Are you often sad and depressed? Brief measures to identify women at risk for depression in pregnancy. *American Journal of Maternal Child Nursing, 30*(1), 40–45.

Johnson, K. E. (2020). *Overview of TORCH infections*. http://www.uptodate.com

Johnson, K. E., Posner, S., Biermann, J., Cordero, J. F., Atrash, H. K., Parker, C. S., Boulet, S., Curtis, M. G., CDC/ATSDR Preconception Care Work Group, & Select Panel on Preconception Care. (2006). Recommendations to improve preconception health and health care—United States: A report of the CDC/ATSDR preconception care work group and the select panel on preconception care. *MMWR Recommendations and Reports, 55*(RR–6), 1–23. http://www.cdc.gov/mmwr/preview/mmwrhtml/rr5506a1.htm

Kallmyer, T. (2019, December 10). Caffeine sensitivity. *Caffeine Informer*. https://www.caffeineinformer.com/caffeine-sensitivity

Kennedy, D. (2016). Ondansetron and pregnancy: Understanding the data. *Obstetric Medicine, 9*(1), 28–33. https://doi.org/10.1177/1753495X15621154

King, T. L., Brucker, M. C., Kriebs, J. M., Fahey, J. O., Gegor, C. L., & Varney, H. (2015). *Varney's midwifery* (5th ed.). Jones & Bartlett.

Koletzko, B., Lien, E., Agostoni, C., Bohles, H., Campoy, C., Cetin, I., Decsi, T., Dudenhausen, J. W., Dupont, C., Forsyth, S., Hoesli, I., Holzgreve, W., Lapillonne, A., Putet, G., Secher, N. J., Symonds, M., Szajewska, H., Willatts, P., Uauy, R., & World Association of Perinatal Medicine. (2008). The roles of long-chain polyunsaturated fatty acids in pregnancy, lactation and infancy: Review of current knowledge and consensus recommendations. *Journal of Perinatal Medicine, 36*, 5–14. https://doi.org/10.1515/JPM.2008.001

Koren, G. (2003). Hair treatments: Drugs, pregnancy, and lactation. *Ob/Gyn News, 38*, 8.

LactMed® Drugs and Lactation Database. (2019, June). *Caffeine*. National Library of Medicine. https://www.ncbi.nlm.nih.gov/books/NBK501467/

Langer, J. W. (2018, June). *Expert report: Genetics, metabolism, and individual responses to caffeine*. Institute for Scientific Information on Coffee. www.coffeeandhealth.org

Leviton, A. (2018). Biases inherent in studies of coffee consumption in early pregnancy and the risks of subsequent events. *Nutrients, 10*(9), 1152. https://doi.org/10.3390/nu10091152

Li, D. K., Janevic, T., Odouli, R., & Liu, L. (2003). Hot tub use during pregnancy and the risk of miscarriage. *American Journal of Epidemiology, 158*, 931–937. https://doi.org/10.1093/aje/kwg243

Machtinger, R., Gaskins, A. J., Mansur, A., Adir, M., Racowsky, C., Baccarelli, A. A., Hauser, R., & Chavarro, J. E. (2017). Association between preconception maternal beverage intake and in vitro fertilization outcomes. *Fertility and Sterility, 108*(6), 1026–1033. https://doi.org/10.1016/j.fertnstert.2017.09.007

Margulies, R., & Miller, L. (2001). Fruit size as a model for teaching first trimester uterine sizing in bimanual examination. *Obstetrics & Gynecology, 98*, 341–344. https://doi.org/10.1016/S0029-7844(01)01406-5

Martin, J. A., Hamilton, B. E., Sutton, P. D., Ventura, S. J., Menacker, F., & Kirmeyer, S. (2006). Births: Final data for 2004. *National Vital Statistics Reports, 55*(1), 1–102.

National Academies of Sciences, Engineering, and Medicine. (2020). *Nutrition during pregnancy and lactation: Exploring new evidence: Proceedings of a workshop*. The National Academies Press. https://www.nationalacademies.org/our-work/nutrition-during-pregnancy-and-lactation-exploring-new-evidence-a-workshop

National Clearinghouse Guidelines. (2012). *Routine prenatal care*. https://www.guideline.gov/summaries/summary/38256/routine-prenatalcare?q=prenatal+care

Nehlig, A., & Alexander, S. P. (2018). Variation in caffeine metabolism. *Pharmacological Reviews, 70*(2), 384–411. https://doi.org/10.1124/pr.117.014407

Nelson, H. D., Bougatsos, C., & Blazina, I. (2012). Screening women for intimate partner violence: A systematic review to update the 2004 U.S. preventive services task force recommendation. *Annals of Internal Medicine, 156*(11), 796–808. https://doi.org/10.7326/0003-4819-156-11-201206050-00447

Olaiya, O., Sharma, A. J., Tong, V. T., Dee, D., Quinn, C., Agaku, I. T., Conrey, E. J., Kuiper, N. M., & Satten, G. A. (2015). Impact of the 5As brief counseling on smoking cessation among pregnant clients of special supplementation nutrition program for Women, Infants, and Children (WIC) clinics in Ohio. *Preventive Medicine, 81*, 438–443. https://doi.org/10.1016/j.ypmed.2015.10.011

Olson, C. M. (2008). Achieving a healthy weight-gain during pregnancy. *Annual Review of Nutrition, 28*, 411–423. https://doi.org/10.1146/annurev.nutr.28.061807.155322

Paranjape, A., & Liebschutz, J. (2004). STaT: A three-question screen for intimate partner violence. *Journal of Women's Health, 12*(3), 233–239. https://doi.org/10.1089/154099903321667573

Rosenfeld, L. S., Mihalov, J. J., Carlson, S. J., & Mattia, A. (2014). Regulatory status of caffeine in the United States. *Nutrition Reviews, 72*, 23–33. https://doi.org/10.1111/nure.12136

Sharps, P. W., Campbell, J., Baty, M. L., Walker, K. S., & Bair-Merritt, M. H. (2008). Current evidence on perinatal home visiting and intimate partner violence. *Journal of Obstetric, Gynecologic, and Neonatal Nursing, 37*(4), 480–490. https://doi.org/10.1111/j.1552-6909.2008.00267.x

Sherin, K. M., Sinacore, J. M., Li, X. Q., Zitter, R. E., & Shakil, A. (1998). HITS: A short domestic violence screening tool for use in a family practice setting. *Family Medicine, 30*(7), 508–512.

Shieh, C., & Carter, A. (2011). Online prenatal nutrition education. *Nursing for Women's Health, 15,* 27–35. https://doi.org/10.1111/j.1751-486X.2011.01608.x

Sohal, H., Eldridge, S., & Feder, G. (2007). The sensitivity and specificity of four questions (HARK) to identify intimate partner violence: A diagnostic accuracy study in general practice. *BMC Family Practice, 8,* 49. https://doi.org/10.1186/1471-2296-8-49

Sohoni, A., Bosley, J., & Miss, J. C. (2014). Bedside ultrasonography for obstetric and gynecologic emergencies. *Critical Care Clinics, 30,* 207–226. https://doi.org/10.1016/j.ccc.2013.10.002

Stotland, N. E., Haas, J. S., Brawarsky, P., Jackson, R. A., Fuentes-Afflick, E., & Escobar, G. J. (2005). Body mass index, provider advice, and target gestational weight gain. *Obstetrics & Gynecology, 105,* 633–638. https://doi.org/10.1097/01.AOG.0000152349.84025.35

Sweet, R., & Gibbs, R. (2009). *Infectious diseases of the female genital tract* (5th ed.). Williams and Wilkins.

Thorlton, J., Ahmed, A., & Colby, D. A. (2016). Energy drinks: Implications for the breastfeeding mother. *The American Journal of Maternal Child Nursing, 41*(3), 179–185. https://doi.org/10.1097/NMC.0000000000000228

Tjaden, P., & Thoennies, N. (2000). The role of stalking in domestic violence crime reports generated by the Colorado springs police department. *Violence and Victims, 15*(4), 427–441. https://doi.org/10.1891/0886-6708.15.4.427

Ulrich, Y. C., McKenna, L. S., King, C., Campbell, D. W., Ryan, J., Torres, S., Lea, P. P., Medina, M., Garza, M. A., Johnson-Mallard, V., Landenberger, K., & Campbell, J. C. (2006). Postpartum mothers' disclosure of abuse, role, and conflict. *Health Care for Women International, 27,* 324–343. https://doi.org/10.1080/07399330500511733

U.S. Department of Health and Human Services-Food and Drug Administration & Center for Food Safety and Applied Nutrition. (2018, April). *Highly concentrated caffeine in dietary supplements: Guidance for industry.* https://www.fda.gov/files/food/published/Guidance-for-Industry--Highly-Concentrated-Caffeine-in-Dietary-Supplements-DOWNLOAD.pdf

U.S. Preventive Services Task Force (2019). *Elevated blood lead levels in children and pregnant women: Screening.* https://www.uspreventiveservicestaskforce.org/uspstf/recommendation/elevated-blood-lead-levels-in-childhood-and-pregnancy-screening

U.S. Preventive Services Task Force. (2021). *Tobacco smoking cessation in adults, including pregnant persons: Interventions.* Retrieved from https://www.uspreventiveservicestaskforce.org/uspstf/recommendation/tobacco-use-in-adults-and-pregnant-women-counseling-and-interventions

WebMD. (2016). *Taking medicine in pregnancy.* http://www.webmd.com/baby/guide/taking-medicine-during-pregnancy#1

Weiss, S., Ernst, A., Cham, E., & Nick, T. (2003). Development of a screen for ongoing intimate partner violence. *Violence and Victims, 18*(2), 131–141. https://doi.org/10.1891/vivi.2003.18.2.131

Wikoff, D., Welsh, B. T., Henderson, R., Brorby, G. P., Britt, J., Myers, E., Goldberger, J., Lieberman, H. R., O'Brien, C., Peck, J., Tenenbein, M., Weaver, C., Harvey, S., Urban, J., & Doepker, C. (2017). Systematic review of the potential adverse effects of caffeine consumption in healthy adults, pregnant women, adolescents, and children. *Food and Chemical Toxicology: An International Journal published for the British Industrial Biological Research Association, 109*(Pt 1), 585–648. https://doi.org/10.1016/j.fct.2017.04.002

Williams, L., Zapata, L., D'Angelo, D., Harrison, L., & Morrow, B. (2011). Associations between preconception counseling and maternal behaviors before and during pregnancy. *Maternal Child Health Journal, 16*(9), 1854–1861. https://doi.org/10.1007/s10995-011-0932-4

Williamson, M. A., & Snyder, L. M. (2014). *Wallach's interpretation of diagnostic tests* (10th ed.). Lippincott Williams & Wilkins.

4. Ongoing Prenatal Care

MARY LEE BARRON | KELLY D. ROSENBERGER

A. INTERIM HISTORY

Prenatal visits should be structured to reflect the dynamic nature of risk assessment during pregnancy.

1. Ask about the following at each visit:
   a. Nutrition
   b. Fetal movement (after quickening has occurred, starting 16–18 weeks' gestation)
   c. Contractions or cramping
   d. Vaginal discharge or bleeding
   e. Edema
   f. Headache
   g. Nausea/vomiting/heartburn
   h. Fever or exposure to infectious disease
   i. Social situation or relationships
2. As indicated by lifestyle:
   a. Smoking/tobacco use/vaping
   b. Drug use
   c. Alcohol use
   d. Use of over-the-counter (OTC) or herbal preparations
   e. Use of medication targeted to a specific condition, for example, asthma and diabetes
   f. Pregnancy discomforts
   g. Concerns
3. As indicated by trimester:
   a. Developmental changes
   b. Acceptance of pregnancy
   c. Readiness for baby
   d. Prenatal education classes in breastfeeding and childbirth
   e. Physical changes experiencing during pregnancy

B. PHYSICAL EXAMINATION

1. Maternal weight
2. Blood pressure and pulse
3. Fundal height measurement
4. Urine dipstick for protein, glucose, leukocyte esterase (LE), nitrites (although there is little evidence to support this practice, it has persisted). Dipstick analysis does not reliably detect proteinuria in patients with early preeclampsia. Trace glycosuria is also unreliable.
5. Fetal heart tones:
   a. Doppler presence of fetal heartbeat should be present by 12 weeks
   b. In some women, the fetal heartbeat may be heard at 10 weeks

6. Edema of lower extremities, hands, and face
7. Cervical and pelvic examination as indicated by gestational age and condition; examination at 36, 38 to 39, and 40 weeks until delivery is common practice

C. LABORATORY/DIAGNOSTIC EXAMINATIONS

1. At least 10 weeks: Prenatal cell-free DNA (cfDNA) screening, also known as noninvasive prenatal screening, is a method to screen for certain specific chromosomal abnormalities. Patients must be at least 10 weeks' gestation and have adequate counseling regarding the options, benefits, and limits of first- and second-trimester screening (see Chapter 2 for further information).
2. 18 to 20 weeks: All pregnant individuals should be offered maternal serum screening for neural tube defects and trisomy 18 or 21. Depending on the laboratory, this could be the triple, quad, or penta screen: alpha-fetoprotein (AFP), human chorionic gonadotropin (HCG), unconjugated estriol, and, for the quad screen, inhibin A. The penta screen adds invasive trophoblast antigen (see Chapter 2 for more information).
3. 24 weeks: Gestational diabetes screening (24–28 weeks unless at higher risk as indicated by medical or obstetric history; see Chapter 16)
4. 28 weeks
   a. Complete blood count (CBC) at 28 weeks unless being followed up for anemia
   b. Rh antibody status if Rh negative
   c. Hepatitis B surface antigen for high-risk groups
   d. Gonorrhea/chlamydia for high-risk groups
   e. Rapid plasma reagin (RPR) or Venereal Disease Research Laboratory (VDRL) test depending on regional recommendations
5. 36 weeks
   a. Culture for group B Streptococcus
   b. CBC
   c. VDRL or RPR depending on regional recommendations
   d. HIV if at risk or depending on regional recommendations
6. Miscellaneous
   a. Urinalysis (UA), possibly urine culture

D. ULTRASOUND EXAMINATION (SECOND AND THIRD TRIMESTER)

1. Indications: The American Institute of Ultrasound in Medicine has published guidelines for ultrasound examination during the second and third trimesters, including but not limited to the following circumstances:
   a. Estimation of gestational (menstrual) age
   b. Evaluation of fetal growth and well-being
   c. Vaginal bleeding
   d. Abdominal or pelvic pain
   e. Cervical insufficiency
   f. Determination of fetal presentation
   g. Suspected multiple gestation
   h. Adjunct to amniocentesis or other procedure
   i. Significant discrepancy between uterine size and clinical dates
   j. Pelvic mass
   k. Suspected hydatidiform mole
   l. Adjunct to cervical cerclage placement
   m. Suspected fetal death
   n. Suspected uterine abnormality
   o. Screening or follow-up evaluation for fetal anomalies

p. Suspected amniotic fluid abnormalities
q. Suspected placental abruption
r. Adjunct to external cephalic version
s. Premature rupture of membranes and/or premature labor
t. Follow-up evaluation of placental location for suspected placenta previa
u. History of previous congenital anomaly
v. Evaluation of fetal condition in late registrants for prenatal care
w. To assess for findings that may increase the risk for aneuploidy
x. In certain clinical circumstances, a more detailed examination of fetal anatomy may be indicated, that is, abnormal biochemical markers

2. Measurements: Accuracy for dating is optimal until approximately 20 weeks' gestation

a. Measurement of crown–rump length of fetus between 7 and 12 weeks' gestation for dating information
b. Biparietal diameter (BPD): Measured after 13 weeks, increasing from about 2.4 cm at 13 weeks to 9.5 cm at term; use for dating in later stage of pregnancy is unreliable
c. Head circumference (HC): Measured at the same level as the BPD; not affected by head shape
d. Fetal nuchal translucency: 11 to 14 weeks to evaluate for risk of trisomy 21. Some centers also perform an early screening of the fetal nasal bone and tricuspid regurgitation.
e. Femur length: Reflects longitudinal growth of the fetus. Usefulness is similar to BPD. Increases from 1.5 cm at 14 weeks to 7.8 cm at term. If used for dating, like the BPD, it should be done as early as feasible.
f. Abdominal circumference (AC): Single most important measurement in late pregnancy as this reflects fetal size and weight rather than age. Serial measurements are made to evaluate fetal growth (intrauterine growth restriction [IUGR] or macrosomia). AC measurements are not used for dating.
g. Fetal weight estimation: Combination of BPD, HC, AC, and femur length are compared to published nomograms. Even the best fetal weight estimation can yield errors as high as ±15%.
h. Biophysical profile: Evaluate fetal movements, tone, and breathing (see Chapter 6)
i. Amniotic fluid index: Evaluate amniotic fluid for polyhydramnios and oligohydramnios (see Chapter 6)
j. Scans for fetal growth can be repeated 2 to 4 weeks apart. Closer intervals may result in interpretation difficulty because they could be a variation in measurement technique rather than a true change caused by growth.
k. Scan may be repeated at 32 weeks to evaluate fetal size, assess fetal growth, verify placental position, or to follow up on possible abnormalities found on an earlier scan.

3. Fetal anatomic survey

a. Best performed at 18 to 20 weeks' gestation
b. At times, some structures are hard to visualize because of fetal position, movement, maternal abdominal wall thickness, and so on
c. A follow-up examination to clarify will usually be recommended by the ultrasonographer/medical doctor (MD)

4. Placental evaluation

a. Localization of the placental site to determine placental previa, marginal insertion, and chorionic bleeding

b. Used to determine abnormalities associated with diabetes, Rh isoimmunization, and/or IUGR

E. PREGNANCY MANAGEMENT

1. Fetal growth

a. Fundal height measurement: McDonald's rule measures the size of the uterus to assess fetal growth. It is measured from the top of the fundus to the top of the pubic bone. Technique is important! The nurse practitioner (NP) should consistently use either a paper or plastic tape measure (i.e., do not switch back and forth as the measurements may be slightly different). Next, turn the tape over so that you cannot see the numbers. This will help to prevent you from anticipating what the measurement should be. The strategy is to be consistent and to note trends. Careful monitoring increases detection rates of small or large fetuses while reducing unnecessary referral for further investigation.

b. The measurement should match the gestational age in weeks (from 20 to 36 weeks) within ±2 cm, that is, at 29 weeks' gestation, the measurement should measure 27 to 31 cm. Prior to 20 weeks, the fundus should be palpated and the location noted. At 16 weeks, the fundus should be approximately three fingerbreadths above the symphysis pubis or midway to the umbilicus.

c. If a discrepancy between fundal height and gestational age occurs, carefully review dating parameters. As the pregnancy progresses, fundal height measurement becomes less accurate. The reasons for true discrepancy include the following:

i. Dating error based on last menstrual period (LMP)
ii. Hydatidiform mole
iii. Twins or multiple births
iv. Fetal descent into the pelvis normally seen 2 to 4 weeks before delivery
v. Fetus is healthy but physically small/large
vi. Oligohydramnios or polyhydramnios
vii. Small for gestational age (SGA)/large for gestational age (LGA)
viii. Breech or transverse lie position

d. There are patients for whom fundal heights are not accurate because of the position of the uterus. For example, a uterine fundus clearly positioned laterally to the left or right of center. The patient who is multiparous or grand multiparous who has poor abdominal muscle tone may have such a uterus. This is an indication to follow up the fetal growth with a monthly ultrasound.

e. Fundal height measurements are difficult to determine in obese patients. An ultrasound should be performed at 28 weeks' gestation and again at 32 weeks' gestation.

F. MODIFIABLE RISK FACTORS

1. Stress

a. Stress has been suggested as a potential contributor to preterm birth and physical complications of pregnancy such as prolonged labor.

b. Stressful events (death of a family member, job loss, and difficult relationship with baby's father) may increase the risk of poor pregnancy outcome.

c. Job stress: Fatigue may be an issue. Assess physicality of the job, that is, whether she sits or stands continuously, lifts heavy objects, is exposed to environmental toxins, and/or is under any psychological pressure. Be willing to write a prescription or letter to show the employer regarding weight limits, the need for break time, and so on. See Appendix D for a summary of federal regulations on this topic.

d. Questions regarding potential stressors asked at the first prenatal visit bear repeating with ongoing prenatal care. A patient may be reluctant to share information until a trusting relationship has been formed.

e. Assess how the patient currently appraises the situation.

f. Reassess social support. This is a dynamic process. Because pregnancy affects the entire family, assessment and intervention must be considered from a family-centered perspective.

g. Psychosocial screening allows the NP to identify areas of concern, validate major issues, and make suggestions for possible changes. Consider depression screening for all women along with the 24- to 28-week laboratory tests.

h. Depending on the nature of the identified problem, a referral may be indicated.

i. Nutrition and weight gain: As an ongoing assessment and based on the 1- to 3-day recall, the NP should assess whether the patient is nutritionally at risk.

a. Identify patients with inadequate or excessive weight gain. The optimal weight gain during pregnancy varies depending on the pre-pregnancy weight as well as height, bone structure, age, and activity level. The mean rate of weight gain is as important as the total gained. A 2- to 4-lb gain is recommended during the first trimester. During the second and third trimester, 1 lb/wk is recommended for individuals of average body mass index (BMI; Institute of Medicine [IOM], 2009). For overweight individuals, 0.6 lb/wk, and for obese individuals, 0.5 lb/wk is recommended. No additional calories are recommended during the first trimester, but additional calories are required (350 and 450) during the second and third trimesters, respectively, no matter the age group (IOM, 2009).

b. Factors to consider regarding weight-gain pattern

i. Nausea and vomiting during pregnancy

ii. Patients should not try to lose weight during pregnancy. Obese or overweight patients may misunderstand or think that this is a healthy adaptation.

iii. Patients with disordered eating or who express resistant attitudes toward weight gain should be referred to a dietician and/or mental healthcare provider.

iv. Access to food: Patients with low incomes should be referred to Women, Infants, and Children (WIC). The NP should assess the household's use of the supplies provided by WIC. At times, the patient may not access the proper nutrients because of sharing the food with family.

v. Screen for depression if weight gain is either too low or too high, as this is a behavior associated with depression.

vi. Some patients limit eating to have a smaller baby to achieve an easier birth. This notion should be explored as the smaller baby may have more morbidity during the first year of life.

vii. Medical problems or infection

viii. Assess breastfeeding plans: Breastfeeding plays an important role in weight loss postpartum. Patients who are overweight or obese are less likely to initiate and have a shorter duration of breastfeeding when compared to normal weight or underweight patients.

c. Talking to patients about their weight can be difficult and uncomfortable. Using terminology that is comfortable for patients is also important. Dutton et al. (2010) surveyed certain phrases used by physicians when speaking with obese patients. The most acceptable term was "weight," whereas "excess fat" was the most unpopular. Other acceptable terms were "BMI," "unhealthy weight," and "weight problem." Other unpopular terms were "obesity," "overweight," "large size," "heaviness," and "fatness" (see Chapter 17).

d. Assessing the patient's readiness to change is a useful approach recommended by the American College of Obstetricians and Gynecologists (ACOG). Pregnancy is a "teachable moment," a life transition that can motivate change.

e. How to best help individuals gain the targeted amount is not certain. An effective approach is to concentrate on healthy eating rather than the number of pounds on the scale. Dietary counseling sessions are effective. Evidence also suggests the best way to help patients gain the appropriate amount of weight includes one-on-one interventions, tailored dietary guidance, and physical activity counseling. If desired, the patient can use a self-monitoring tool, including the guides at www.myplate.gov/life-stages/pregnancy-and-breastfeeding.

f. Consider using the IOM chart to document weight gain and help the patient set goals (www.iom.edu/Reports/2009/Weight-Gain-During-Pregnancy-Reexamining-the-Guidelines.aspx) or the March of Dimes Weight Gain Chart (www.marchofdimes.com/pregnancy/yourbody_trackingweight.html).

2. Physical activity

a. Advise pregnant individuals to continue exercising as this is generally safe. Pregnancy requires only modest increases in calories (350–450 a day on average). Patients are often highly motivated to adopt a healthy lifestyle during pregnancy. The "5 As" as presented in Chapter 3, Section II.B, may also be used for nutrition and exercise when there are no contraindications to exercise.

b. Exercise prescription: Clinical evaluation is the first step to make sure the pregnant individual does not have medical or obstetric reasons to avoid exercise. Contraindications (danger signs) include vaginal bleeding, regular painful contractions, amniotic fluid leak, dyspnea before exertion, dizziness, headaches, chest pain, muscle weakness affecting balance, and calf pain or swelling. For most pregnant individuals, an exercise program goal should be moderate intensity exercise for at least 20 to 30 minutes on most or all days of the week. Pregnant individuals should also be advised to remain well hydrated, avoid lying on the back for long periods, and stop exercising if they experience any of the danger signs listed.

c. Safe physical activities during pregnancy: Walking, swimming, stationary cycling, low-impact aerobics, yoga (modified to avoid impacting venous return), and modified Pilates. Patients who were active before pregnancy, in consultation with an obstetric provider, may be able to continue running, jogging, playing racquet sports, and strength training. However, racquet sports that require balance changes and rapid movements that increase the risk of falling should be avoided.

d. Intensity: The "talk test" is an easy way for patients to measure their intensity level: if one is able to carry on a conversation during exercise, then one is exercising at the desired level; if not, reduce the intensity.

e. Warm-up: Because of increased relaxation of ligaments during pregnancy, flexibility exercises should be individualized. A typical exercise prescription should promote musculoskeletal fitness and address type, intensity and progression, quantity and duration, and frequency. A typical session includes the following:

i. Warm-ups and stretching (5–10 minutes)

ii. Exercise program (30–45 minutes)

iii. Cool down (5–10 minutes)

iv. Encourage additional walking

3. Tobacco use and vaping: The following guidelines are based on ACOG recommendations (www.acog.org/clinical/clinical-guidance/committee-opinion/articles/2020/05/tobacco-and-nicotine-cessation-during-pregnancy)

a. The "5 As" as presented in Chapter 3, Section II.B, include "arrange," which indicates that a follow-up with the patient at each visit will be conducted to assess tobacco use and vaping status and affirm efforts to quit.

b. Patients benefit from a brief motivational interviewing counseling session.

c. Offer referral to a "quit line." Quit lines offer information, direct support, and ongoing counseling and have been very successful in helping pregnant smokers quit and remain smoke free. By dialing the national quit line network (1-800-QUIT NOW), a caller is immediately routed to the state's smokers' quit line.

d. For those who continue to smoke: These smokers are often heavily addicted to nicotine and should be encouraged at every follow-up visit to seek help to stop smoking. They may also benefit from screening and intervention for alcohol use and other drug use because continued smoking during pregnancy increases the likelihood of other substance use. Vaping and electronic cigarettes (EC) are not recommended during pregnancy and should not be used to encourage patients to quit smoking traditional cigarettes. ECs contain nicotine (ACOG, 2020b, Kuehn, 2019).

e. Pharmacotherapy

i. Nicotine replacement products or other pharmaceuticals for smoking cessation during pregnancy and lactation have not been sufficiently evaluated to determine their efficacy or safety.

ii. Alternative therapies, including antidepressants (varenicline and bupropion), have only limited data on effectiveness, and evidence has not established their safe use.

4. Illicit drug use

a. Ongoing assessment

i. Drug misuse in pregnancy is a complex health problem associated with a wide variety of maternal and fetal complications; the prevalence is increasing worldwide.

ii. Many pregnant individuals face stigmatization and rejection from family, friends, and health and social services and, thus, are reluctant to divulge information. Once a trusting relationship has been established, the patient may readily share information. This is key to the success of the management plan.

iii. If a positive drug screen is found, the NP must share those findings with the patient using an approach that is empathetic, flexible, and optimistic, but not approving. The topic must be sensitively explored with the patient.

iv. Polydrug use is very common in pregnant addicts. Assess whether drug use is recreational or dependent, as this is a key factor in management.

v. Stress of pregnancy may escalate drug use in some patients.

vi. Assess for psychiatric comorbidity. Dual diagnosis is common.

vii. In intravenous drug users, the NP should assess injection practices, such as sharing of needles and other paraphernalia, to screen for blood-borne diseases such as HIV, hepatitis B virus, and hepatitis C virus.

viii. Illicit drug use should be considered in the context of the patient's lifestyle. Malnutrition is a frequent comorbidity that contributes to adverse outcomes. Stress and poverty that may accompany the lifestyle will also contribute to its ill effects. However, not all pregnant drug users are poor—the problem crosses socioeconomic lines.

ix. Urine drug screen (UDS): With one exception (alcohol), a UDS is the preferred method to screen for an unknown drug. Alcohol is best detected by blood sampling. Detection times in urine vary by the following factors:

a) Chronicity and frequency of use
b) Metabolic rate
c) Body mass
d) Physical activity
e) Age
f) Overall health
g) Drug tolerance
h) Urine pH

b. Management approaches

i. The multifactorial nature of substance use/abuse requires a coordinated and multidisciplinary approach:

a) Consult with collaborating physician
b) Referral to addiction services is often indicated
c) Know community resources: social workers, drug counselors, and methadone programs

ii. Because the problem isn't limited to pregnancy but has effects on maternal and infant health, parenting skills, and need for social support, a family-oriented approach may be more effective.

iii. Anxiety and depression are frequent comorbidities that require treatment.

iv. Psychosocial interventions include counseling, education, relapse prevention, brief interventions, cognitive behavioral therapy, contingency management, and motivational enhancement therapy.

v. Self-help groups may be recommended and include Alcoholics Anonymous and Opiates Anonymous.

vi. Psychosocial interventions alone have not been found effective for opioid dependence; pharmacological treatment in combination with psychosocial interventions is more effective.

vii. Patient education should include effects of the drug on the fetus/neonate/infant (Table 4.1).

G. PREGNANCY DISCOMFORTS

1. Back pain (lower)

a. Definition: Lumbosacral pain caused by effects of relaxin, pregnancy weight gain, changes in the center of gravity leading to muscular imbalances,

TABLE 4.1 TYPICAL DETECTION TIMES IN URINE OF SELECTED DRUGS OF ABUSE

DRUG	DOSE	TIME	COMMENTS
Amphetamine	10–30 mg/PO	7–34 hr	Half-life variable; depends on urinary pH
Barbiturates	PO	48 hr	All except phenobarbital
Phenobarbital	1–2 pills/wk		
Benzodiazepines	PO	5–7 d	All except flunitrazepam; effects variable because of pharmacokinetics
Methamphetamine	100 mg/PO 22 mg "ice" smoked	87 ± 51 hr 60 hr	Maximum detection is 6 days; doses higher in tolerant subjects
Cannabis	1.5%–3.5% smoked	34–87 hr	Maximum detection is 95 days
Cocaine	100 gm intranasal	48–72 hr	Maximum detection is 22 days
Heroin	10–15 IV/smoked	11–54 hr	Maximum detection is 11.3 days
LSD	50–100 mcg PO	24–48 hr	Maximum detection is 4 days
Phencyclidine	PO, smoked, inhaled, injected	1–2 wk	Longer in chronic users
Oxycodone	PO	24–48 hr	

Note: Ice is the slang term for methamphetamine that is smoked.
LSD, lysergic acid diethylamide; PO, orally.
Source: Adapted from Verstraete, A. (2004). Detection times of drugs of abuse in blood, urine, and oral fluid. *Therapeutic Drug Monitoring, 26*(2), 200–205. https://doi.org/10.1097/00007691-200404000-00020; Williamson, M.A., & Snyder, L. M. (2015). *Interpretation of diagnostic tests* (10th ed.). Lippincott Williams & Wilkins.

and muscle fatigue; usually occurs in the third trimester. Caused by the weight of the enlarging uterus combined with poor posture, lack of support from lax abdominal muscles, and/or relaxation of pelvic joints.

b. History

i. Sharp or dull low back pain

ii. Denies colicky pain

iii. Denies vaginal bleeding, discharge, or leaking of fluid

iv. Posterior pelvic pain during pregnancy can be brought on or exacerbated by the following activities:

a) Rolling in bed

b) Climbing stairs

c) Sitting and rising from a seated position (such as getting in and out of cars, bathtubs, and bed)

d) Lifting, twisting, and bending forward

e) Running and walking

c. Physical examination

i. May include muscle tension and pain on tender trigger insertion sites

ii. Absence of costovertebral angle (CVA) tenderness, numbness, redness, and swelling

d. Laboratory/diagnostic examination

i. UA and culture if upper or lower urinary tract infection (UTI) is suspected

e. Differential diagnoses
   i. Lumbar strain
   ii. UTI
   iii. Preterm labor
   iv. Renal calculi
   v. Trauma

f. Treatment
   i. Wear low-heeled shoes with good arch support
   ii. Wear maternity pants with a low supportive waistband or a maternity belt
   iii. Instruct on proper lifting with bending at the knees
   iv. Sleep in a supported position: Lie on the side with a pillow supporting the abdomen and with knees slightly bent; insert a pillow between the knees
   v. Alternately apply heat or ice compresses to the area
   vi. Exercise regularly; suggest yoga or stretching exercises, pelvic tilt, and/or lower back pain–specific exercises as recommended by physical therapist or chiropractor
   vii. Lower back massage/massage therapy
   viii. Analgesics
   ix. Wear a maternity girdle or belt (especially appropriate for an obese or multiparous patient or with extreme lordosis)

g. Warning signs/complications
   i. Preterm labor
   ii. Severe pain

h. Consultation/referral
   i. Physician if suspicious of infectious process, preterm labor, or renal calculi
   ii. Physical therapist
   iii. Chiropractor

i. Follow-up
   i. As scheduled for gestational age
   ii. As needed for worsening symptoms or nonresponse to therapy

2. Back pain (upper)

a. Definition: Cervicothoracic pain due to relaxin, pregnancy weight gain, changes in the center of gravity leading to muscular imbalances, and muscle fatigue. May be due to increased weight and/or enlargement of the breasts and/or venous stasis. May occur at any gestational age.

b. History: Neck and shoulder pain

c. Physical examination
   i. May include muscle tension and painful tendon insertion sites
   ii. Absence of CVA tenderness, numbness, redness, and swelling

d. Laboratory/diagnostic examination

e. Differential diagnoses
   i. Compression of cervical nerves
   ii. Pyelonephritis/renal calculi
   iii. Carpal tunnel syndrome
   iv. Mastitis
   v. Myofascial pain
   vi. Thoracic herniated disc

f. Treatment
   i. Maintain good posture: Sit and stand up straight; when sitting, keep feet slightly elevated; refrain from crossing the legs.

ii. Sleep in a supported position: Lie on the side with a pillow supporting the abdomen and with knees slightly bent; place a pillow between the knees.
iii. Instruct the pregnant individual to wear a well-fitting bra 24 hours a day.
iv. Apply heat or ice compresses alternately to the area.
v. Exercise regularly; use upper back pain-specific exercises as recommended by physical therapist or chiropractor.
vi. Neck and upper shoulder massage/massage therapy
vii. Analgesics
viii. Wear supportive low-heeled footwear.

g. Warning signs/complications
i. Numbness or pain in the fingers and hands
ii. Severe pain

h. Consultation/referral
i. Physician if neuropathic pain, infectious process, and/or renal calculi are suspected
ii. Physical therapist
iii. Chiropractor

i. Follow-up
i. As indicated by gestational age
ii. As needed for worsening symptoms or nonresponse to therapy

3. Bleeding gums and epulis (pregnancy gingivitis)

a. Definition: Bleeding gums with or without tenderness; epulis is a vascular spongy growth between two teeth thought to be caused by a hormonal influence that accelerates epithelial turnover.

b. History: May occur throughout but usually starts mid pregnancy
i. Assess medication use for known agents that increase gum tissue, for example, phenytoin

c. Physical examination
i. Gums are pink and spongy in appearance. Dark red gums may indicate the presence of periodontal disease. No lesions or masses are noted.

d. Laboratory/diagnostic examination: None

e. Differential diagnoses
i. Physiologic growth of gum tissue secondary to pregnancy
ii. Periodontal disease
iii. Pyogenic granuloma

f. Treatment
i. Instruct the patient to continue to gently brush and floss teeth using a fluoridated toothpaste
ii. Avoid foods that irritate gums
iii. See the dentist for any regularly scheduled cleaning and examination
iv. Dental problems should be treated during pregnancy (see Chapter 9)

g. Warning signs/complications
i. Preterm labor is associated with periodontal disease; treatment of periodontal disease during pregnancy does not reduce preterm birth risk
ii. Excessive bleeding of gums
iii. Interference with chewing
iv. Persistent unexplained anemia
v. Vitamin C deficiency

h. Consultation/referral
  i. Dentist
i. Follow up
  i. As scheduled for gestation

4. Constipation
a. Definition: Irregular and infrequent or difficult evacuation of the bowels (<3 times/wk) usually caused by the slowing of gastrointestinal tract mobility under the influence of progesterone and compression of the intestines by the enlarging uterus
b. History
  i. Patient complains of decreased evacuation frequency, sensation of rectal fullness, straining, or hard stool. Iron supplements may compound the problem
  ii. Reports excess gas and bloating
  iii. Laxative abuse/use
c. Physical examination
  i. Abdomen may be distended
  ii. Hypoactive bowel sounds
  iii. Stool palpable in rectum
  iv. Negative for abdominal tenderness
d. Laboratory/diagnostic examination
  i. None
  ii. CBC if infectious process suspected
  iii. Thyroid-stimulating hormone (TSH) if hypothyroidism suspected
  iv. Serum calcium possibly
e. Differential diagnoses
  i. If abdominal pain is present, rule out:
    a) Appendicitis
    b) Intestinal obstruction
    c) Irritable bowel syndrome
    d) Labor
  ii. Neurological disorder
  iii. Metabolic or endocrine disorder
    a) Diabetes
    b) Hypothyroidism
  iv. Intestinal functional disorder
f. Treatment
  i. Dietary measures include increasing fiber intake (20–35 g each day). High-fiber foods include beans, whole grains, bran cereals, fresh fruits, and vegetables
  ii. Drink eight glasses of water daily
  iii. Exercise (advise walking if the patient has not been previously exercising)
  iv. Switch iron supplement to another brand if contributing to the constipation
  v. Bulk-forming laxative such as Metamucil, Fiberall, and Citrucel
  vi. Stool softener such as Colace or Surfak
  vii. Avoid use of mineral oil as a laxative
g. Warning signs/complications
  i. If abdominal pain occurs, contact provider as pathological condition may be developing
  ii. Rule out labor
h. Consultation/referral
  i. Abdominal pain

ii. Lack of responsiveness to treatment

i. Follow-up

i. As scheduled for gestation

ii. With onset of warning signs

5. Heartburn

a. Definition: A burning sensation, usually centered in the middle of the chest near the sternum, caused by the reflux of acidic stomach fluids that enter the lower end of the esophagus. May be caused by relaxation of the cardiac sphincter resulting from anatomical and hormonal changes and/or delayed emptying of stomach contents; the cause is likely multifactorial. High levels of circulating progesterone in the presence of estrogen may affect the general pressure, or pattern of relaxation, of the lower esophageal sphincter, allowing acid reflux. Progesterone, acting on smooth muscle, may also affect gut motility and delay gastric clearance.

b. History: Heartburn is so common among pregnant individuals that it has been regarded as a normal part of a healthy pregnancy, but patients may not regard the problem as minor. Symptoms tend to become both more severe and frequent as pregnancy progresses. Heartburn is more likely to occur in older pregnant individuals (it increases with age in the general population) and in patients experiencing their second or subsequent pregnancies, independent of age.

c. Physical examination: Unremarkable

d. Laboratory/diagnostic examination: None

e. Differential diagnoses

i. Hiatal hernia

ii. Epigastric preceding eclampsia

iii. Cholecystitis

iv. Cholelithiasis

v. Pyloric ulcer disease

f. Treatment

i. Dietary measures

a) Small, frequent meals

b) Avoid spicy or greasy foods and acidic juices

c) Avoid large meals before bedtime

d) Sit up for at least 1 hour after meals

e) Drink minimally while eating

f) Avoid gastric irritants such as caffeine, alcohol, smoking, and gas-producing foods

ii. Medications

a) H_2 antagonist such as famotidine. Note the Food and Drug Administration (FDA) removed ranitidine (Zantac) from the market in April 2020.

b) Tums or other low-sodium antacids in limited amounts; avoid antacids containing aspirin.

c) Advise client to avoid taking antacids with iron preparations, as this may decrease absorption

d) Avoid antacids containing sodium bicarbonate

iii. Miscellaneous

a) Wear loose-fitting clothes to avoid pressure on the lower esophageal sphincter

b) Raise the head of the bed 4 to 6 in.

c) Avoid tobacco and alcohol (encourage if patient has not already ceased)

g. Warning signs/complications
   i. Severe and persistent heartburn
   ii. Severe heartburn accompanied by fever, nausea, vomiting, or referred pain to back or right shoulder
h. Consultation/referral
   i. Persistent symptoms not responsive to dietary measures and H_2 antagonist
   ii. Constitutional symptoms accompany heartburn
   iii. Signs/symptoms of severe preeclampsia, that is, epigastric pain and hypertension, proteinuria
   iv. Symptoms accompanied by night coughing (rule out asthma)
i. Follow-up
   i. As scheduled for gestation
   ii. With onset of warning signs

6. Hemorrhoids
   a. Definition: An itching or painful mass of dilated veins in swollen anal tissue caused by stasis of blood from pressure by the enlarging uterus; dilation of veins caused by progesterone
   b. History
      i. Acutely painful mass at rectum
      ii. Pruritus
      iii. Rectal bleeding
   c. Physical examination: External anal and perineal findings important to note
      i. Fissures
      ii. Fistulas
      iii. Signs of infection or abscess formation
      iv. Hemorrhoidal prolapse appearing as a bluish, tender perianal mass
      v. Skin tags from old thrombosed external hemorrhoids
   d. Laboratory/diagnostic examination: None
   e. Differential diagnoses
      i. Anal fissure
      ii. Pedunculated polyps
      iii. Perianal abscess
      iv. Pruritus ani
      v. Colorectal or anal cancer
   f. Treatment
      i. Advise the patient to
         a) Avoid constipation
         b) Increase fiber and fluids to soften stool
         c) Avoid straining during defecation
         d) May use hemorrhoidal topical ointments
         e) May use witch hazel compresses or sitz baths
   g. Warning signs/complications
      i. Thrombosis of hemorrhoids
      ii. Acute pain may indicate infection
   h. Consultation/referral
      i. Anal polyps
      ii. Thrombosis
      iii. Perianal infection
   i. Follow-up
      i. As scheduled by gestation
      ii. As indicated by condition

7. Insomnia
   a. Definition: Chronic inability to fall asleep or remain asleep for an adequate length of time; may include early-morning wakefulness
   b. History
      i. Sleep–wake patterns
      ii. Sleep partners (intimate partner and children)
      iii. Interruptions
         a) Nocturia
         b) Pain
         c) Leg cramps or restless legs syndrome
         d) Partner's sleep habits
         e) Environmental noise
      iv. Use of caffeine
      v. Substance abuse
      vi. Meal patterns, especially late-night eating
      vii. Co-symptoms such as heartburn or night coughing
      viii. History of depression and/or anxiety
      ix. Work hours
      x. Support system
   c. Physical examination: Unremarkable
   d. Laboratory/diagnostic examination
      i. Sleep studies possible
      ii. Testing as indicated by symptoms
   e. Differential diagnoses
      i. Insomnia or secondary to
         a. Anxiety
         b. Depression
         c. Substance abuse
         d. Other sleep disorder
   f. Treatment
      i. Sleep hygiene measures
         a. Sleep environment adjustments: maximally darkened room or sleep mask, sound dampened/white noise
         b. Constant sleep–wake times
         c. Avoid watching TV in bed
         d. Avoid eating late at night
         e. Avoid caffeine
      ii. Medications at bedtime
         a. Category B: Benadryl 25 to 50 mg
         b. Category C: Ambien 5 to 10 mg or Ambien CR 12.5, or Lunesta 2 mg (*Note:* These medications were on the market before the ABC style of labeling was changed. The FDA is gradually updating medication risks on labeling. See Chapter 5 for more details.)
      iii. Massage of back, neck, and shoulders
      iv. Warm bath before sleep
      v. Warm milk (tryptophan released)
      vi. Herbal teas: Chamomile or lemon balm
      vii. Yoga
      viii. Increase vitamin B intake
   g. Warning signs/complications
      i. Lack of responsiveness to treatment
      ii. Maternal exhaustion
   h. Consultation/referral
      i. OB/GYN physician

ii. Sleep disorder center/services
iii. Mental health services if mood disorder present
iv. Social services

i. Follow-up
i. As scheduled for gestation
ii. As indicated by evaluating medication use

8. Leg cramps

a. Definition: Spasmodic, painful contractions of the leg muscles typically affecting the gastrocnemius at night. The problem may also affect gluteal, leg, or thigh muscles.

b. Etiology: Idiopathic and/or not well understood but probably multifactorial; pressure on the veins and nerves from the gravid uterus may contribute; may be caused by reduced or elevated calcium levels and/or elevated serum phosphorus levels.

c. History
i. Reports cramping occurring at night
ii. Complains of fatigue in the legs
iii. Dietary assessment may demonstrate very high or very low intake of calcium or excessive intake of phosphates

d. Physical examination
i. Lower extremity examination demonstrates absence of local warmth, redness, or positive Homans sign

e. Laboratory/diagnostic examination: None

f. Differential diagnoses
i. Physiologic leg cramps
ii. Thrombophlebitis
iii. Varicose veins

g. Treatment
i. Thiamine (100 mg) plus pyridoxine (40 mg; Sohrabvand et al., 2006)
ii. Trial elimination of intake of phosphates: carbonated drinks, processed foods
iii. Reduce milk and calcium supplements, particularly if over the recommended daily allowance (RDA) of 1,300 mg/d
iv. Dorsiflexion of foot in response to cramping for relief of spasm; avoid pointing of toes
v. Attempt standing and then walking
vi. Massage
vii. Apply heat; keep legs warm by wearing knee socks while sleeping

Note that in a recent Cochrane Database review of the evidence as to whether any interventions (oral magnesium, oral calcium, oral vitamin B, or oral vitamin C) provide an effective treatment for leg cramps (Zhou et al., 2015) no conclusion could be reached. This was in part due to disparity in design limitations, methodology, and reporting of outcomes.

h. Warning signs/complications
i. Sleep disturbances

i. Consultation/referral
i. None unless thrombophlebitis is present

j. Follow-up
i. As indicated by gestational age
ii. As needed if symptoms unresponsive to treatment

9. Leukorrhea
   a. Definition: A thick, whitish discharge from the vagina or cervical canal caused by hormonal changes of pregnancy
   b. History
      i. Reports increased vaginal discharge and a feeling of wetness but denies itching, burning, or odor
   c. Physical examination
      i. Pelvic examination
         a) pH of vaginal secretion is between 3.5 and 4.5
         b) Cervix: Some friability is present in pregnancy; if marked ectropion is present, there may be increased white blood cells (WBCs)
   d. Laboratory/diagnostic examination
      i. Wet mount
         a) Saline: Normal parameters of lactobacilli, lack of WBCs, normal epithelial cells (no clue cells), no trichomonads
         b) KOH (potassium hydroxide) test: Negative yeast, negative amine odor
   e. Differential diagnoses
      i. Vaginitis
         a) Monilial infection
         b) Bacterial vaginosis
      ii. Sexually transmitted infection
         a) *Chlamydia trachomatis*
         b) *Neisseria gonorrhoeae*
      iii. Spontaneous rupture of membranes
   f. Treatment
      i. Self-treatment of physiologic leukorrhea should be avoided
      ii. Reassurance
      iii. Use cotton underwear and change as needed. Unscented panty liners can be used, but the plastic lining of these products interferes with airflow, disrupting evaporation from the vulvar area.
   g. Warning signs/complications
      i. Onset of symptoms, such as itching, burning, and odor, may indicate a vaginal infection
   h. Consultation/referral: None
   i. Follow-up
      i. As indicated for gestation
      ii. Return for reevaluation if symptoms occur
10. Nasal stuffiness and epistaxis (pregnancy rhinitis)
   a. Definition: Complaint of nasal congestion that may appear anytime in gestation and occurring in 18% to 30% of pregnant individuals. It is thought to be caused by increased estrogen levels; however, placental growth hormone, smoking, and sensitization to house dust mites are also associated factors. Pregnancy rhinitis is defined as a nasal congestion that lasts 6 or more weeks without other signs of respiratory tract infection, with no known allergic cause, disappearing completely within 2 weeks of delivery.
   b. History
      i. Symptoms may occur at any time or just at night
      ii. Congestion
      iii. Sneezing
      iv. Nasal itching
      v. Persistent coughing

vi. Local decongestants give temporary relief but use for more than a few days results in expected rebound swelling

vii. May complain of nosebleeds

c. Physical examination

i. May include nasal edema, crusting, and evidence of bleeding

ii. Negative for evidence of upper respiratory infection: Multicolored nasal discharge, fever, or other constitutional symptoms

d. Laboratory/diagnostic examination: None

e. Differential diagnoses

i. Allergic rhinitis

ii. Upper respiratory infection

iii. Substance abuse

f. Treatment

i. Normal saline nasal spray

ii. Evidence does not support the use of nasal steroids

iii. Neti pot or nasal lavage

iv. Steam inhalation every 4 hours while awake

v. Humidifier in the bedroom as needed

vi. For epistaxis, continuously compress the soft outer portion of the nose against the midline septum for 5 to 10 minutes

g. Warning signs/complications

i. Upper respiratory infection

ii. Active sinusitis

iii. Clotting disorder

iv. Hypertensive disorder

h. Consultation/referral

i. MD, for comorbid condition

i. Follow-up

i. As scheduled for gestation

11. Palpitations

a. Definition: The feeling that the heart is skipping a beat, fluttering, or beating too hard or too fast; may occur in the chest, throat, or neck. During pregnancy, this is caused by the effect of progesterone, which increases the heart rate (25%), with stroke volume and accompanying plasma volume expansion peaking at 28 to 32 weeks. Palpitations are quite common, occurring in more than 50% of pregnant individuals.

b. History

i. Evaluate genetic propensity to life-threatening arrhythmias

c. Physical examination

d. Laboratory/diagnostic examination

i. Electrocardiogram

ii. Echocardiogram

iii. Holter monitor

e. Differential diagnoses

i. Nonpathological palpitations

ii. Structural cardiac disorder such as mitral stenosis or other valvular disease

iii. History of congenital heart disease and exacerbation

iv. Panic attack

v. Anxiety

vi. Hypoglycemia

vii. Thyroid disorder

viii. Anemia

ix. Stress

x. Caffeine use
xi. Substance use/abuse
f. Treatment
i. Rest quietly
ii. Slow deep breathing for several minutes
iii. Relaxation techniques
iv. Avoid all caffeine in diet
v. Stress-reduction measures
g. Warning signs/complications
i. Accompanying dizziness or shortness of breath (SOB) may indicate a cardiac cause
h. Consultation/referral
i. If cardiac disorder is suspected, refer to or consult with a perinatologist; refer to a cardiologist
ii. Send to the ED if episode is ongoing or if accompanied by chest pain, SOB, dizziness, or syncope
i. Follow-up
i. As indicated by condition
ii. As scheduled for gestation

12. Pedal edema
a. Definition: Edema as a result of increased blood volume and impaired venous circulation and/or increased pressure from an enlarging uterus on the lower extremities. Poor posture aggravated by prolonged standing or sitting or hot weather may contribute to the problem.
b. History: Complains that the ankles and feet swell, usually in the late afternoon or early evening; usually occurs in the second or third trimester.
c. Physical examination: Lower extremities are edematous, but the edema is nonpitting.
d. Laboratory/diagnostic examination: Urine dipstick for proteinuria
e. Differential diagnoses
i. Physiological-dependent edema
ii. Preeclampsia
f. Treatment
i. Nonconstrictive clothing
ii. Elevate the legs and hips often throughout the day
iii. Avoid crossing the legs
iv. Use a side-lying position
v. Use support hose (may require a prescription)
vi. Exercise moderately
vii. Consume adequate fluids
g. Warning signs/complications
i. Edema becomes pitting
ii. Accompanying facial or hand edema, increased blood pressure, proteinuria, and sudden large weight gain
h. Consultation/referral
i. If preeclampsia is suspected, consult with MD
i. Follow-up
i. As scheduled for gestation
ii. As necessary if edema worsens or accompanying danger signs occur

13. Pelvic pressure
a. Definition: Pressure in the lower abdomen and pelvic area. Occurs in the third trimester, but in primiparas it will increase up to 2 weeks before

delivery when "lightening" occurs (descent of presenting part into the pelvis).

b. History

i. Complains that the baby is "pushing down"
ii. Urinary frequency
iii. May complain of irregular or occasional contractions
iv. May complain of increased discharge
v. Denies leaking of fluid

c. Physical examination

i. Cervical examination indicates engagement of presenting part

d. Laboratory/diagnostic examination

i. Evaluate for rupture of membranes with nitrazine paper and look for ferning on a slide as indicated by history. May also utilize Amnisure or ROM Plus Fetal Membranes Rupture Test as a rapid, qualitative test for the in vitro detection of amniotic fluid in vaginal secretions.

e. Differential diagnoses

i. Preterm labor

f. Treatment: None

g. Warning signs/complications

i. Onset of labor
ii. Preterm labor

h. Consultation/referral

i. If preterm labor was suspected, consult MD

i. Follow-up

i. As scheduled by gestation and condition

14. Ptyalism

a. Definition: Excessive flow of saliva, or sialorrhea; more common in women suffering from hyperemesis gravidarum and acid reflux

b. History

i. Complains of producing more saliva since becoming pregnant
ii. Complains of bad taste and maintains that swallowing the excessive or thickened saliva perpetuates the sense of nausea
iii. Reports spitting into a cup because of the amount of saliva
iv. Reports accompanying heartburn

c. Physical examination: Unremarkable

d. Laboratory/diagnostic examination: None

e. Differential diagnoses

i. Neurological disorder
ii. Infection of the oropharynx, esophagus
iii. Dental disorder/infection
iv. Toxicity; heavy metal poisoning

f. Treatment

i. Advise the patient to:

a) Avoid irritants like tobacco smoke
b) Brush teeth and use mouthwash after every meal
c) Drink eight glasses of water daily
d) Suck on hard candy but avoid sour candies, as these increase saliva

ii. Medications

a) There is no satisfactory medication treatment. Categories of medications that have been tried include scopolamine patches, central nervous system depressants, anticholinergics, antihistamines, and homeopathic therapies.

g. Consultation/referral
  i. Accompanying pathology like hyperemesis
  ii. Treatment with medication
h. Follow-up
  i. As scheduled for gestation
  ii. With onset of warning signs

15. Round ligament pain
  a. Definition: Type of pelvic pain caused by stretching of the round ligaments, which occurs more commonly on the right side of the pelvis and is associated with sudden movement.
  b. History
    i. Ligament spasm triggers; unilateral sharp pain from the side of the pelvic area extending to the groin
  c. Physical examination
    i. Abdominal examination: Palpate area of reported pain and note the following:
      a) Guarding
      b) Rebound tenderness
      c) Referred pain
    ii. Uterine examination
      a) Fundal height
      b) Fetal heart rate
      c) Presence of contractions
      d) Consistency and position of uterus
    iii. Pelvic examination as indicated
      a) Cervical or vaginal discharge
      b) Dilation/effacement
    iv. Evaluate CVA tenderness
  d. Laboratory/diagnostic examination: The following tests might be performed
    i. CBC with differential
    ii. UA
    iii. Ultrasound
  e. Differential diagnoses
    i. Acute abdomen resulting from
      a) Appendicitis
      b) Pyelonephritis
      c) Cholecystitis
      d) Ovarian torsion
    ii. Ovarian cyst
    iii. Ectopic pregnancy (first trimester)
    iv. UTI
    v. Preterm labor
    vi. Placental abruption
    vii. Inguinal hernia
    viii. Cramps caused by slowed digestion in pregnancy occur in the ascending colon and cecum (right lower quadrant pain)
    ix. Renal calculi
  f. Treatment
    i. Rest, lying on the opposite side with a pillow supporting the lower abdomen may relieve the pain
    ii. Maternity abdominal support or girdle
    iii. Heating pad
    iv. Pelvic tilt exercises

v. Prenatal exercise class, swimming, or yoga

vi. Changing mechanics of movement in rising or sitting; moving slowly and avoiding sudden movement may decrease spasms

vii. Acetaminophen may provide some analgesia

viii. Reassure of normalcy

g. Warning signs/complications

i. Fever

ii. Chills

iii. Pain on urination

iv. Difficulty walking

v. Persistence of pain

vi. Onset of contractions

vii. Onset of nausea and vomiting

viii. Vaginal bleeding or discharge

h. Consultation/referral

i. Physical therapy for evaluation

ii. Abnormal test results

iii. For diagnosis of pathological process

i. Follow-up

i. As scheduled for gestation

ii. With onset of warning signs

16. Shortness of breath

a. Definition: Dyspnea can occur any time in the pregnancy but is felt more often in the third trimester. Progesterone affects the respiratory center in the brain, resulting in lower levels of CO_2 and increased O_2. The feeling of hyperventilation is the result.

b. History

i. Complains of SOB, which may or may not be in relation to activity level

ii. Denies chest pain

iii. Denies wheezing

c. Physical examination

i. Cardiac: As expected for gestational age; increased pulse rate and a systolic murmur are present

ii. Respiratory examination is normal for gestational age: Lungs are clear to auscultation with no adventitious sounds; respiratory rate is mildly increased

d. Laboratory/diagnostic examination: None unless pathology suspected

e. Differential diagnoses

i. Asthma

ii. Cardiac disease

iii. Smoking

iv. Anxiety

f. Treatment

i. Reassurance regarding the reason for the SOB

ii. Maintain good posture

iii. Teach the patient to stretch; raise arms over head and take a deep breath

iv. Do not overload the stomach

v. Avoid restrictive clothing

vi. Wear a supportive bra

vii. Do not smoke

viii. Rest and breathe deeply

ix. Sleep with extra pillows

g. Warning signs/complications
 i. Chest pain
 ii. Severe fatigue
 iii. Signs and symptoms of an upper respiratory condition
 iv. Hemoptysis
h. Consultation/referral
 i. If pathological condition is suspected, consult MD
i. Follow-up
 i. As scheduled for gestation

17. Urinary frequency
 a. Definition: Nonpathological frequency of urination caused by pressure on the bladder from the enlarging uterus in the first trimester or in the primigravida after "lightening" occurs.
 b. History: Urinary frequency, but denies burning, pain, fever, low back pain, or suprapubic pain. May complain of nocturia.
 c. Physical examination
  i. Unremarkable
 d. Laboratory/diagnostic examination: Urine dipstick for nitrites and LE; UA and culture possible
 e. Differential diagnoses
  i. UTI
  ii. Vaginitis
  iii. Premature rupture of membranes
  iv. Diabetes mellitus
 f. Treatment
  i. None
  ii. May decrease fluid intake prior to bedtime to decrease nocturia. However, fluid from dependent edema is mobilized during sleep and may contribute to nocturia.
 g. Warning signs/complications
  i. UTI
  ii. Premature rupture of membranes
 h. Consultation/referral
  i. MD for pathological and/or comorbid condition
 i. Follow-up
  i. As scheduled for gestation

18. Varicosities
 a. Definition: A condition, usually within a vein, distinguished by swelling and repetitive turns or twists; generally results from congenital predisposition and exaggerated by prolonged standing, pregnancy, and advancing age.
 b. History: Varicosities become more prominent as the pregnancy progresses. The patient may complain of mild discomfort, cosmetic blemishes, and/or increasingly severe discomfort that requires elevating the lower extremities.
 c. Physical examination
  i. Presence of varicose veins in the lower extremities, perineum, and/or vulva
  ii. Negative Homans sign
 d. Laboratory/diagnostic examination: None
 e. Differential diagnoses
  i. Thrombophlebitis
 f. Treatment
  i. Periodic elevation of feet for 15 to 30 minutes
  ii. Apply pad soaked in witch hazel for vulvar varicosities

iii. Prenatal cradle V2 supporter

iv. Place thick maxi pads (not the thin ones) in the underwear to support the perineum and help with the discomfort and swelling

v. Toeless compression hose

vi. Yoga

vii. Swimming

g. Warning signs/complications

i. Positive Homans sign

ii. Calf swelling

h. Consultation/referral

i. Rupture of veins causing bleeding

ii. Refer to a vascular surgeon for evaluation; treatment planned after completion of pregnancy

i. Follow-up

i. As indicated by gestation

H. SECOND-TRIMESTER EDUCATION

1. Quickening; fetal movement expectations
2. Pregnancy discomforts
3. Immunizations (see Chapter 3 and/or Centers for Disease Control and Prevention Guidelines for vaccinating pregnant women at www.cdc.gov/vaccines/pubs/preg-guide.htm)
4. Pregnancy testing such as screening tests and ultrasound
5. Danger signs (see Chapter 3)
6. Travel in pregnancy

I. THIRD-TRIMESTER EDUCATION

1. Danger signs; symptoms prompting urgent evaluation
2. Pregnancy discomforts
3. Planning for labor and delivery; childbirth classes
4. Breastfeeding (see Chapter 7)
5. Cord blood donation
6. Circumcision
7. Family planning (see Chapter 7)
8. Immunizations: www.cdc.gov/vaccines/pregnancy/hcp-toolkit/guidelines.html
9. Kick counts
10. Pregnancy testing
    a. Indications for ultrasound and antenatal testing
    b. CBC
    c. Glucose challenge test
    d. Antibody screen (indirect Coombs test)
    e. RPR
    f. Group B Streptococcus culture
    g. UA, urine culture possibly
    h. Screening of sexually transmitted diseases if at risk
    i. Cervical examination

Bibliography

Alhussien, A. H., Alhedaithy, R. A., & Alsaleh, S. A. (2018). Safety of intranasal corticosteroid sprays during pregnancy: An updated review. *European Archives of Oto-Rhino-Laryngology: Official Journal of the European Federation of Oto-Rhino-Laryngological Societies (EUFOS): Affiliated With the German Society for Oto-Rhino-Laryngology - Head and Neck Surgery*, 275(2), 325–333. https://doi.org/10.1007/s00405-017-4785-3

American Academy of Periodontology. (2016). *Expectant mothers' periodontal health vital to health of her baby*. https://www.perio.org/consumer/AAP_EFP_Pregnancy
American College of Obstetricians and Gynecologists. (2020a). Physical activity and exercise during pregnancy and the postpartum period: ACOG committee opinion, number 804. *Obstetrics and Gynecology*, *135*(4), e178–e188. https://doi.org/10.1097/AOG.0000000000003772
American College of Obstetricians and Gynecologists. (2020b). Tobacco and nicotine cessation during pregnancy: ACOG committee opinion summary, number 807. *Obstetrics and Gynecology*, *135*(5), 1244–1246. https://doi.org/10.1097/AOG.0000000000003825
American College of Obstetrics and Gynecologists. (2018). Screening for perinatal depression (Committee Opinion 757). *Obstetrics and Gynecology*, *132*, e208.
American Institute of Ultrasound in Medicine. (2017). *Limited obstetric ultrasound*. http://www.aium.org/officialStatements/19
Dutton, G., Tan, F., Perri, M., Stine, C., Dancer-Brown, M., Goble, M., & Van Vessem, N. (2010). What words should we use when discussing excess weight? *Journal of the American Board of Family Medicine*, *23*(5), 606–613. https://doi.org/10.3122/jabfm.2010.05.100024
Gaby, A. (2007). Nutritional interventions for muscle cramps. *Integrative Medicine: A Clinician's Journal*, *6*(6), 20–23.
Hensley, J. (2009). Leg cramps and restless legs syndrome during pregnancy. *Journal of Midwifery & Women's Health*, *54*(3), 211–218. https://doi.org/10.1016/j.jmwh.2009.01.003
Institute of Medicine. (2009). *Weight gain during pregnancy: Reexamining the guidelines*. National Academies Press. https://www.nap.edu/resource/12584/Report-Brief---Weight-Gain-During-Pregnancy.pdf
Kirkham, C., Harris, S., & Grzybowski, J. (2005). Evidence based prenatal care: Part I. General prenatal care and counseling issues. *American Family Physician*, *71*(7), 1307–1316.
Kuehn, B. (2019). Vaping and pregnancy. *JAMA*, *321*(14), 1344. https://doi-org.libproxy.siue.edu/10.1001/jama.2019.3424
León, R., Silva, N., Ovalle, A., Chaparro, A., Ahumada, A., Gajardo, M., Martinez, M., & Gamonal, J. (2007). Detection of Porphyromonas gingivalis in the amniotic fluid in pregnant women with a diagnosis of threatened premature labor. *Journal of Perodontology*, *78*, 1249–1255. https://doi.org/10.1902/jop.2007.060368
Lester, B. M., ElSohly, M., Wright, L. L., Smeriglio, V. L., Verter, J., Bauer, C. R., Shankaran, S., Bada, H. S., Walls, H. H., Huestis, M. A., Finnegan, L. P., & Maza, P. L. (2001). The maternal lifestyle study: Drug use by meconium toxicology and maternal self-report. *Pediatrics*, *107*(2), 309–317. https://doi.org/10.1542/peds.107.2.309
Lockwood, C. J., Berghella, V., & Barss, V. A. (2020). *Prenatal care: Second and third trimesters*. *UpToDate*. http://www.uptodate.com
Magdula, R. M., Groshkova, T., & Mayet, S. (2011). *Illicit drug use in pregnancy: Effects and management: Assessment of the pregnant drug user*. http://www.medscape.org/viewarticle/738688_2
Metz, T. D., & Khanna, A. (2016). Evaluation and management of maternal cardiac arrhythmias. *Obstetrics and Gynecology Clinics of North America*, *43*(4), 729–745. https://doi.org/10.1016/j.ogc.2016.07.014
Morse, K., Williams, A., & Gardosi, J. (2009). Fetal growth screening by fundal height measurement. *Best Practices Research in Clinical Obstetrics & Gynaecology*, *23*(6), 809–818. https://doi.org/10.1016/j.bpobgyn.2009.09.004
Phupong, V., & Hanprasertpong, T. (2015). Interventions for heartburn in pregnancy. *Cochrane Database of Systematic Reviews*, *19*(9), CD011379. https://doi.org/10.1002/14651858.CD011379.pub2
Shah, R., Diaz, S. D., Arria, A., LaGasse, L. L., Derauf, C., Newman, E., Smith, L. M., Huestis, M. A., Haning, W., Strauss, A., Grotta, S. D., Dansereau, L. M., Roberts, M. B., Neal, C., & Lester, B. M. (2012). Prenatal methamphetamine exposure and short-term maternal and infant medical outcomes. *American Journal of Perinatology*, *29*(5), 391–400. https://doi.org/10.1055/s-0032-1304818
Siega-Riz, A., Deierlein, A., & Stuebe, A. (2010). Implementation of the new Institute of Medicine gestational weight gain guidelines. *Journal of Midwifery & Women's Health*, *55*(6), 512–519. https://doi.org/10.1016/j.jmwh.2010.04.001
Sohrabvand, F., Shariat, M., & Haghollahi, F. (2006). Vitamin B supplementation for leg cramps during pregnancy. *International Journal of Gynaecology and Obstetrics*, *95*(1), 48–49. https://doi.org/10.1016/j.ijgo.2006.05.034
Thaxter Nesbeth, K. A., Samuels, L. A., Nicholson Daley, C., Gossell-Williams, M., & Nesbeth, D. A. (2016). Ptyalism in pregnancy - A review of epidemiology and practices. *European Journal of Obstetrics, Gynecology, and Reproductive Biology*, *198*, 47–49. https://doi.org/10.1016/j.ejogrb.2015.12.022
Widen, E., & Siega-Riz, A. (2010). Prenatal nutrition: A practical guide for assessment and counseling. *Journal of Midwifery & Women's Health*, *55*(6), 540–549. https://doi.org/10.1016/j.jmwh.2010.06.017

Wolff, S., Legarth, J., Vangsgaard, K., Toubro, S., & Astrup, A. (2008). A randomized trial of the effects of dietary counseling on gestational weight gain and glucose metabolism in obese pregnant women. *International Journal of Obesity*, *32*(3), 495–501. https://doi.org/10.1038/sj.ijo.0803710

Zhou, K., West, H. M., Zhang, J., Xu, L., & Li, W. (2015). Interventions for leg cramps in pregnancy. *Cochrane Data Base of Systematic Reviews*, *2015*(8), CD010655. https://doi.org/10.1002/14651858.CD010655.pub2

5. Medication Use in Pregnancy

MARY LEE BARRON | KELLY D. ROSENBERGER

Pregnant individuals and the nurse practitioners (NPs) who care for them are often concerned about the effects of medication on the developing embryo and fetus. Medication use has increased during the past 30 years. Birth defects are common; for example, the Centers for Disease Control and Prevention (CDC) estimates that 3% of births in the United States result in major birth defects. Birth defects are the leading cause of infant mortality in developed countries. Consider that 50% of pregnancies are unintended. There are more than 6 million pregnancies in the United States every year, and pregnant individuals take an average of three to five prescription drugs during pregnancy. Individuals with preexisting medical conditions, such as asthma or hypertension, may need to continue to use prescription drugs to treat those conditions during pregnancy and while breastfeeding. Individuals may also need to take medications for new or acute conditions that may occur during pregnancy or breastfeeding. New labeling format and requirements reorganize information and are structured to help inform healthcare professionals' decisions in prescribing medications and assist in counseling patients using prescription drugs.

The most significant adverse effects of medications may occur early in pregnancy before many even realize that they are pregnant. From conception to 2 weeks after fertilization, teratogens increase the risk of early fetal death and miscarriage. The fetus is at risk of developing major morphologic abnormalities during organogenesis (occurring during weeks 3–8). Later in gestation, teratogenic exposures increase the risk for more subtle morphologic abnormalities and can produce biochemical, behavioral, or reproductive abnormalities. What is important to note is that the consequences of later exposures can still be of great clinical significance (e.g., renal impairment from angiotensin-converting enzyme inhibitor use, which can be fatal for the fetus).

A. FOOD AND DRUG ADMINISTRATION RATING SYSTEM

1. The Food and Drug Administration (FDA, 2014) has discontinued the rating system created in 1979 to categorize the potential risk to the fetus for a given drug: A, B, C, D, and X. The categories may have mislead health-care providers (and the patients they counsel) to believe that risk increases from Category A to B to C to D to X. In fact, that is not the case because Categories C, D, and X were based not just on risk but also risk weighed against benefit. That means a drug in Categories C or D posed risks similar to a drug in Category X. The categories did not always distinguish between risks based on human and animal data findings or among differences in frequency, severity, and type of fetal developmental toxicities. This FDA system did not address the risk of not treating the disease versus the risks of the medication. However, the FDA rating system was easy to use as a quick screening tool for the potential risk to the fetus for a given drug.

The general public often assumes that studies are done on the safety of drugs in pregnancy; when in reality, the opposite is often true because research on pregnant individuals is restricted. Most adverse or teratogenic effects are discovered after the drug is marketed and used by a large number of pregnant individuals. Animal studies have limits in revealing teratogenic effects in humans. There is no postmarketing requirement for reporting teratogenic effects. Therefore, to make an adequate decision in prescribing the medication, the NP must be up to date on what is known about medications that the pregnant individual might use. Tools and texts are available, such as the Epocrates app for cell phones and updated websites.

2. New labeling: On June 30, 2015, and after a period for commentary, the FDA implemented the Pregnancy and Lactation Labeling Rule (PLLR), a major revision to prescription drug labeling intended to more completely inform on the use of medicines during pregnancy and breastfeeding. Labeling gives health-care providers better information to assess risks and benefits to improve necessary information in making prescribing decisions and for counseling patients who are pregnant or breastfeeding, and both men and women of childbearing age.

Prescription drugs and biologic products submitted after June 30, 2015, use the new format, whereas labeling for prescription drugs approved on or after June 30, 2001, is phased in gradually to the new system (Table 5.1). There are many older medications that patients are often prescribed in pregnancy that are exempt from updated labeling, including antibiotics, antiepileptics, antihypertensives, and some analgesics. Although A to D and X categories were to be removed by 2018 on all medications that were FDA approved prior to 2001, other information for pregnant and lactating individuals does not need to be removed. Labeling for over-the-counter (OTC) medicines did not change and OTC drug products were not affected by the final rule.

Pregnancy exposure registries collect and maintain data on the effects of approved drugs that are prescribed to and used by pregnant individuals. Information about the existence of any pregnancy registries in drug labeling has been recommended but was not required until now. Information in the pregnancy subsection includes a risk summary, clinical considerations, and data. Information formerly found in the "Labor and Delivery" subsection is now included in the "Pregnancy" subsection. More information on pregnancy registries can be found at: (www.fda.gov/science-research/womens-health-research/pregnancy-registries). The "Nursing Mothers" subsection was renamed the "Lactation" subsection (8.2) and provides information about using the drug while breastfeeding, such as the amount of drug in breast milk and potential effects on the breastfed infant. The "Females and Males of Reproductive Potential" subsection (8.3), new to the labeling, describes when pregnancy testing or contraception is required or recommended before, during, or after use of the drug, and relevant animal or human data suggest drug-associated fertility effects. The subheadings

TABLE 5.1 PRESCRIPTION DRUG LABEL 8.1–8.3 IN SPECIFIC POPULATIONS

PREVIOUS LABELING	NEW LABELING
8.1 Pregnancy	8.1 Pregnancy
8.2 Labor and Delivery	8.1 Pregnancy
8.3 Nursing Mothers	8.2 Lactation
	8.3 Females and Males of Reproductive Potential

BOX 5.1 FEMALES AND MALES OF REPRODUCTIVE POTENTIAL

TRADENAME can cause fetal harm (see Warnings and Precautions [5.x], Use in Specific Populations [8.1]).

Pregnancy Testing
Verify the pregnancy status of females of reproductive potential prior to initiating TRADENAME therapy.

Contraception
Advise females of reproductive potential to use effective contraception during treatment and for at least 2 months after the final dose of TRADENAME.

Infertility
Based on findings in animals, male fertility may be compromised by treatment with TRADENAME (see Nonclinical Toxicology [13.1]).

include "Pregnancy Testing," "Contraception," and "Infertility." Box 5.1 shows a sample statement for a drug that causes harm. Both the pregnancy and lactation subsections have three principal components: a risk summary, clinical considerations, and a data section. These are discussed in more detail.

3. Pregnancy subsection
   a. Pregnancy exposure registry
   b. Risk summary: The fetal risk summary describes the the likelihood that the drug increases the risk of four types of developmental abnormalities: structural anomalies, fetal and infant mortality, impaired physiologic function, and alterations to growth. An example based on human data is "Human data do not indicate that Drug X increases the overall risk of structural anomalies." Many of the risk conclusions in the PLLR are standardized statements.

      The risk conclusion states whether it was based on animal or human data. More than one risk conclusion may be needed to characterize the risk likelihood for different developmental abnormalities, doses, duration of exposure, or gestational ages at exposure.

      If there are only animal data, the fetal risk summary contains *only* the risk conclusion. However, when there are human data, the risk conclusion is followed by approximately one paragraph describing the most important data about the effects of the drug on the fetus. To the extent possible, this narrative includes the specific developmental abnormality (e.g., neural tube defects); the incidence, seriousness, reversibility, and correctability of the abnormality; and the effect on the risk of dose, duration of exposure, and gestational timing of exposure.
   c. Clinical considerations (omitted if category is not applicable)
      i. Disease-associated maternal and embryo or fetal risk
      ii. Dose adjustments during pregnancy and the postpartum period
      iii. Maternal adverse reactions
      iv. Fetal or neonatal adverse reactions
      v. Labor or delivery
4. Lactation subsection
   a. Risk summary: This is required for all drug and biologic product PLLR labeling. A risk statement (drugs with systemic absorption) summarizing information on the presence of drug or active metabolite in human milk. Animal data are not included if human data are available. Specifically,

i. Effects of the drug on milk production

ii. Whether the drug is present in human milk (and, if so, how much)

iii. The effect of the drug on the breastfed child

iv. Risk-versus-benefit statement (unless there is a recommendation against concomitant breastfeeding and drug use)

b. Clinical considerations: Included only when information is available regarding:

i. Ways to minimize exposure to the breastfed child, such as timing or pumping and discarding milk

ii. Potential drug effects in the child and recommendations for monitoring or responding to these effects

iii. Dosing adjustments during lactation

c. Data (omitted if not applicable)

i. Detailed description of data on which risk summary and clinical considerations are based

B. RISK VERSUS BENEFIT AND OTHER THERAPIES

1. The risks that medical conditions can pose to both the mother and fetus must be balanced against the risks that many medications pose to a fetus. Cardiovascular, poorly controlled diabetes, and renal and thyroid diseases all have potentially adverse effects on a fetus. For example, depression during pregnancy can affect an individual's participation in prenatal care. Furthermore, depression is associated with tobacco and alcohol use during pregnancy and may affect fetal growth and infant behavior. There are higher rates of miscarriage, low birth weight, and babies who are small for gestational age when depression is left untreated during pregnancy. The risk of preeclampsia in pregnant individuals suffering from depression is more than double the general population risk. Some patients with severe depression will need to continue antidepressant medications while pregnant. Selective serotonin reuptake inhibitors (SSRIs) are safer than tricyclic antidepressants, but paroxetine should be avoided because it is most strongly associated with fetal cardiac malformations.

Both the American College of Obstetricians and Gynecologists (ACOG) and the American Society of Addition Medication (ASAM) recommend medication rather than medically supervised withdrawal for treatment of opioid use disorder during pregnancy. The benefits of Medically Assisted Treatment (MAT) include a reduction of fatal overdoses and increases in both retention in treatment programs and social functioning. MAT with methadone or buprenorphine provides the advantages of known dose, purity, safe and steady availability, and improved maternal and neonatal outcomes compared with the continued use of illicit opioids. Although neither is superior for treating opioid use disorder during pregnancy and lactation, use of buprenorphine has demonstrated less severe neonatal opioid withdrawal syndrome compared with methadone and thus is considered better by many clinicians. With opioid use increasing globally, screening and treating for substance use disorders offers NPs an opportunity to provide appropriate prenatal care important for improving outcomes. NPs can find more information, training, mentoring, and how to obtain a MAT waiver at https://pcssnow.org/.

2. There are many occasions for which nonpharmacologic or adjunctive therapies could serve as the first line of treatment. For example, consider an individual with seasonal allergies. Although loratadine and cetirizine are now OTC drugs and not subject to the new PRRL, some patients want to avoid any medication they perceive as unnecessary. Animal studies did not

show any risks to unborn babies whose mothers have taken these medications. Therefore, adjunctive guidance may include the following:

a. Avoid triggers: limit your exposure to anything that triggers your allergy symptoms.

b. Try saline nasal spray: OTC saline nasal spray can help ease nasal dryness, bleeding, and congestion. Use the spray as often as needed.

c. Rinse your nasal cavity with a nasal lavage system. Neti pots (just one brand) are available in most pharmacies. Fill the Neti pot with an OTC saline nasal solution once or twice daily and then tilt your head over the sink, place the spout of the Neti pot in your upper nostril, and gently pour in the saline solution. As you pour, the saline solution will flow through your nasal cavity and out of your lower nostril. Repeat on the other side. Be sure to rinse the Neti pot after each use with distilled, sterile, previously boiled and cooled, or filtered water. Leave the rinsed Neti pot open to air dry.

d. Include physical activity in your daily routine: Exercise helps reduce nasal inflammation.

e. Use nasal strips at night: OTC adhesive nasal strips—such as Breathe Right and Breathe Clear—can help keep your nasal passages open while you are sleeping (adapted from www.mayoclinic.com/health/allergy-medications/AN00314).

C. PROACTIVE GUIDANCE

1. Patients have questions about the OTC medications that are safe to use. A short list could be included in patient education materials reminding them that no drug is 100% safe during pregnancy. The NP can develop a short list of safe and unsafe commonly used medications. To create a long list invites the patient to *not* ask. There are also many consumer-based websites with various lists. For example, itching is a condition listed and, on several websites, hydrocortisone cream is listed as a safe medication to take. However, the NP may not want to include that if concerned that the patient with a dermatological condition associated with pregnancy may not ask about medication use. For example, there are patients who may choose to self-treat prior to proper diagnosis. In regard to medication use generally, the NP may want to ask how often a pregnant individual is taking an OTC medication, for example, acetaminophen. There may be an increased risk associated with daily use that is not present with occasional use. The bigger picture is to evaluate why the patient is using a medication frequently or has a chronic need to use it.

2. Common **safe** medications to take during pregnancy:

a. Allergy
- **i.** Diphenhydramine (Benadryl)
- **ii.** Loratadine (Claritin)
- **iii.** Cetirizine (Zyrtec)

b. Cold and flu
- **i.** Guaifenesin
- **ii.** Chlorpheniramine (Chlor-Trimeton, Efidac, Teldrin)
- **iii.** Saline nasal drops
- **iv.** Warm saltwater gargle

c. Constipation, hemorrhoids
- **i.** Colace
- **ii.** Metamucil
- **iii.** Tucks
- **iv.** Anusol cream

d. Heartburn
  i. Famotidine (Pepcid or Pepcid Complete)
  ii. Cimetidine (Tagamet)
  iii. Tums
e. First-aid ointment
  i. Bacitracin
  ii. Neosporin
  iii. Polysporin
  iv. Triple antibiotic cream
f. Antibiotics without known teratogenic effects include the penicillins, cephalosporins, clindamycin, and amoxicillin-clavulanate.
g. Pregnant patients should not be treated with metronidazole during the first trimester. Animal reproduction studies revealed metronidazole as a carcinogen in rodents, and the FDA advises this drug be used in pregnancy *only* if clearly needed. In pregnant patients in whom alternative treatment has been inadequate, the 1-day course should *not* be used because it results in higher serum levels that cross the placental barrier entering into the fetal circulation (FDA, 2010). Sheehy et al. (2015) concluded via a systematic review that treating bacterial vaginosis or trichomoniasis with metronidazole is effective and offers no teratogen risk.

3. Common medication to ***avoid*** during pregnancy:
a. Aspirin (except when provider prescribed, such as the daily 81-mg dose)
b. Ibuprofen (Motrin)
c. Naproxen (Aleve)
d. Excedrin or Excedrin migraine
e. Cold remedies that contain alcohol
f. Pseudoephedrine
g. Phenylephrine
h. Nicotine patches and gum (check first)

4. The Organization of Teratology Information Specialists (OTIS) is a nonprofit organization made up of individual services throughout North America. They provide accurate evidence-based, clinical information to patients and health-care professionals about exposures during pregnancy and lactation. Counselors are available by calling (866) 626-6847 (see mother tobaby.org).

Bibliography

American College of Obstetricians and Gynecologists. (2017). Opioid use and opioid use disorder in pregnancy. (ACOG Committee Opinion 711). *Obstetrics Gynecology, 130*(2), e81. https://doi.org/10.1097/AOG.0000000000002235

Briggs, G. G., Freeman, R. K., & Yaffee, S. J. (2011). *Drugs in pregnancy and lactation: Reference guide to fetal and neonatal risk* (9th ed.). Lippincott Williams & Wilkins.

Centers for Disease Control and Prevention (CDC). (2008). Update on overall prevalence of major birth defects—Atlanta, Georgia, 1978–2005. *Morbidity and Mortality Weekly Report, 57*(1), 1–5.

Chang, G., Lockwood, C. J., Saxon, A. J., & Eckler, K. (2020). Substance use during pregnancy: Overview of selected drugs. *UpToDate*. http://www.uptodate.com.

Christianson, A., Howson, C. P., & Modell, B. (2006). *Global report on birth defects*. March of Dimes.

El Marroun, H., Jaddoe, V. W. V., Hudziak, J. J., Roza, S. J., Steegers, E. A., Hofman, A., Verhulst, F. C., White, T. J. H., Stricker, B. H. C., & Tiemeier, H. (2012). Maternal use of serotonin reuptake inhibitors, fetal growth, and risk of adverse birth outcomes. *Archives of General Psychiatry, 69*(7), 706–714. https://doi.org/10.1001/archgenpsychiatry.2011.2333

Fantasia, H. C., & Harris, A. (2015). Changes to pregnancy and lactation risk labeling for prescription drugs. *Nursing for Women's Health, 19*, 266–270. https://doi.org/10.1111/1751-486X.12209

Food and Drug Administration (FDA). (2010). https://www.accessdata.fda.gov/drugsatfda_docs/label/2010/012623s061lbl.pdf

Food and Drug Administration (FDA). (2014). *Federal Register, Vol. 79, No. 233*. https://www.gpo.gov/fdsys/pkg/FR-2014-12-04/pdf/2014-28241.pdf

Lockwood, C. J., Berghella, V., & Barss, V. A. (2020). Prenatal care: Patient education, health promotion, and safety of commonly used drugs. *UpToDate*. http://www.uptodate.com

Mayo Clinic. (2015). *Pregnancy week by week: Is it safe to take Claritin or other allergy medications during pregnancy?* www.mayoclinic.com/health/allergy-medications/AN00314

Mitchell, A. A., Gilboa, S. M., Werler, M. M., Kelley, K. E., Louik, C., & Hernandez-Diaz, S. (2011). & The National Birth Defects Prevention Study. *American Journal of Obstetrics and Gynecology, 205*, 51.e1–51.e8. https://doi.org/10.1016/j.ajog.2011.02.029

Moore, K. L., & Persaud, T. V. N. (2008). *The developing human: Clinically oriented embryology* (8th ed.). Saunders/Elsevier.

Mothertobaby.org. (n.d). *Depression per the URL*. http://mothertobaby.org/fact-sheets/depression-pregnancy

Pace, L., & Schwarz, E. B. (2012). Balancing act: Safe and evidence-based prescribing for women of reproductive age. *Women's Healh, 8*(4), 415–425. https://doi.org/10.2217/WHE.12.25

Sheehy, O., Santos, F., Ferreira, E., & Berard, A. (2015). The use of metronidazole during pregnancy: a review of the evidence. *Current Drug Safety, 10*(2), 170. https://doi.org/10.2174/157488631002150515124548

Stewart, D. E. (2011). Clinical practice. Depression during pregnancy. *New England Journal of Medicine, 365*(17), 1605–1611. https://doi.org/10.1056/

6 Antenatal Fetal Surveillance

NANCY J. CIBULKA | KELLY D. ROSENBERGER

The goal of antenatal fetal testing is to prevent fetal neurologic damage or death through the early detection of hypoxic or acidotic infants. Identification of pregnancies at risk and implementation of timely and appropriate fetal surveillance can prevent poor pregnancy outcome. However, antenatal fetal surveillance cannot predict acute events such as cord accidents or placental abruption. Although routine testing in high-risk pregnancies is standard care, antenatal testing is also utilized in certain low- and moderate-risk pregnancies to evaluate fetal well-being.

Most antenatal fetal surveillance techniques have been in clinical use since the 1970s and are based on the assessment of fetal heart rate (FHR) patterns. The most commonly utilized are nonstress test (NST), fetal biophysical profile (BPP), ultrasonography, and umbilical artery Doppler assessments. In general, the fetus responds to hypoxemia first with signs of physiologic adaptation, progressing to signs of physiologic decompensation. Thus, the pattern of response for fetal distress in utero tends to be loss of FHR reactivity (nonreactive NST), followed by an abnormal blood flow in the umbilical artery and other fetal vessels, and then abnormalities in biophysical parameters, such as fetal breathing, movements, and tone. Blood flow is redirected to the brain and heart and away from less vital organs, such as fetal kidneys, leading to decreased fetal urine production and decreased amniotic fluid volume (Signore et al., 2020; Spong, 2016). Pregnancies that require monitoring by surveillance tests should be comanaged with a physician. Indications for antenatal fetal surveillance and commonly used techniques are discussed in this chapter. Fetal movement assessments, or kick counts, are advised for all pregnant individuals beginning at 28 weeks; patient instructions are available in Appendix A.

A. INDICATIONS FOR ANTENATAL FETAL SURVEILLANCE

1. Table 6.1 shows maternal conditions and pregnancy-related conditions that increase the risk for stillbirth.
2. Although certain risk factors can be identified, pregnancy-related circumstances vary; antenatal testing may be initiated for additional reasons at the discretion of the provider based on clinical judgment.

B. GENERAL RECOMMENDATIONS

1. Antenatal surveillance should be used only when intervention is undertaken if indicated by test results.
2. Second- and third-trimester ultrasounds are essential to assess fetal growth. If there is a risk of fetal growth restriction, order an ultrasound to assess growth every 3 to 6 weeks, beginning at 24 to 26 weeks (Washington University School of Medicine, Department of Obstetrics and Gynecology, 2015).

TABLE 6.1 INDICATIONS FOR ANTENATAL FETAL SURVEILLANCE

MATERNAL CONDITIONS	PREGNANCY-RELATED CONDITIONS
Antiphospholipid syndrome	Gestational hypertension or preeclampsia
Poorly controlled thyroid disease	Decreased fetal movement
Hemoglobinopathies (e.g., sickle cell or thalassemia disease)	Oligohydramnios
Cyanotic heart disease	Polyhydramnios
Systemic lupus erythematous	Intrauterine growth restriction (EFW <10th percentile)
Chronic renal disease	Gestational age >40 weeks
Diabetes mellitus (gestational or preexisting diabetes requiring treatment)	Isoimmunization
Hypertensive disorders requiring antihypertensive therapy	Previous fetal demise (unexplained or recurrent risk)
Mild hypertension without medication—serial growth scans with additional testing only for intrauterine growth retardation	Multiple gestations
Severe maternal respiratory illness	Fetal gastroschisis
Maternal venous thromboembolism (current or history)	Unexplained elevated maternal serum alpha-fetoprotein test (>2.5 MoM)
Maternal age 35 or older	Trisomy 21

Note: This list is not comprehensive.
EFW, estimated fetal weight; MoM, multiple of the median.
Source: Reprinted with permission from Washington University School of Medicine, Department of Obstetrics and Gynecology (2015). Data from American College of Obstetricians and Gynecologists (2021).

3. Begin testing at 32 to 34 weeks of gestation in most cases. In pregnancies with multiple high-risk conditions, begin testing at 26 to 28 weeks of gestation or at the time of diagnosis of intrauterine growth restriction (IUGR) or preeclampsia (if viability has been reached).

4. Frequency of testing is determined based on the clinical judgment because no large clinical trials have been completed to address this issue. Antenatal testing is typically repeated weekly or twice weekly, depending on the circumstances. If the indication for testing persists, continue antenatal testing until delivery. However, if maternal status deteriorates or reduced fetal activity is noted, then further evaluation is indicated regardless of the time elapsed since last testing (American College of Obstetricians and Gynecologists [ACOG], 2021).

5. Any abnormal test result requires further evaluation with a different test.

6. If persistent abnormal test results and/or oligohydramnios are found, then prompt delivery should be carefully considered.

C. NONSTRESS TEST

1. NSTs are often the starting point for antenatal testing because they are less costly than other assessment tests and easy to accomplish. With the pregnant individual in a resting position, a continuous FHR tracing is obtained. FHR activity is a good indicator of autonomic function.

2. FHR should temporarily accelerate with fetal movement, indicating that the fetus is not neurologically depressed or acidotic. The patient may be asked to note each fetal movement.

3. A reactive or reassuring NST is defined as two or more FHR accelerations, at least 15 beats per minute above the baseline and lasting at least 15 seconds within a 20-minute period. Because fetal sleep cycles can result in a nonreactive test, vibroacoustic stimulation is sometimes used to elicit accelerations (Mehta & Sokol, 2013). If the test is reactive, then the fetus is considered to be healthy.

4. A nonreactive NST is defined as insufficient FHR accelerations longer than 40 minutes. The reasons for a nonreactive NST include fetal sleep cycle or central nervous system depression with acidosis.

5. If the NST is nonreactive, then further testing, such as a BPP, is indicated.

D. CONTRACTION STRESS TEST

1. The contraction stress test (CST) is based on the fetal response to a brief reduction in fetal oxygen during uterine contractions.

2. With the pregnant individual in a resting position, uterine contractions and FHR are assessed with an external fetal monitor.

3. Contractions are induced with intravenous oxytocin or nipple stimulation. At least, three contractions need to last for a minimum of 40 seconds each over a 10-minute period. A reassuring test occurs if the FHR shows no evidence of hypoxemia.

4. This test is rarely used because of the need to stimulate contractions and the wide availability of other tests. However, the CST has a very low false-negative rate; false-positive and false-negative rates are lower than for the NST.

E. AMNIOTIC FLUID INDEX

1. Amniotic fluid volume is assessed by ultrasound and is an indicator of long-term placental function. Reduced fluid (oligohydramnios) is a sign of fetal compromise. Amniotic fluid volume is reported as the single deepest or maximum vertical pocket (MVP) of fluid or as an amniotic fluid index (AFI). The use of the MVP is preferred over the AFI as the MVP more accurately diagnoses oligohydramnios.

2. The AFI represents the sum of measurements of the deepest cord-free fluid pockets in each abdominal quadrant.

3. Oligohydramnios, defined as AFI less than 5 cm or MVP of 2 cm or less, identifies the fetus at risk of hypoxia resulting from umbilical cord compression.

4. Excessive amniotic fluid (polyhydramnios), defined as AFI greater than 23 cm or MVP greater than 8 cm, can indicate poor diabetic control, presence of fetal anomaly, or may be idiopathic.

F. BIOPHYSICAL PROFILE

1. The BPP test includes the NST and four other components that are assessed under ultrasound:

- **a.** Fetal breathing movements (30 seconds or more in 30 minutes)
- **b.** Fetal movements (three or more in 30 minutes)
- **c.** Fetal tone (one extension/flexion of an extremity)
- **d.** Amniotic fluid volume (normal range of MVP is 2–8 cm in singleton gestations)

2. Each component is given a score of 2 if passing criteria are met or a score of 0 for abnormal, absent, or insufficient. A score of 8 or 10 is normal, a score of 6 is equivocal, and 4 or less is abnormal. See Table 6.2 for a suggested management protocol.

3. The modified BPP combines the NST with amniotic fluid assessment. The test is normal if the NST is reactive and the MVP is greater than 2 cm.

TABLE 6.2 MANAGEMENT PROTOCOL FOR BIOPHYSICAL PROFILE SCORES

SCORE	INTERPRETATION	ADVISED MANAGEMENT
8–10	Reassuring, low risk	No further action is required
6	Equivocal	Repeat testing within 6–24 hr; consider delivery in term infant
4	Suspected fetal compromise	Consider delivery for infants >32–34 wk. Close observation is necessary for very immature infants
0–2	Significant fetal compromise likely	Delivery may be necessary in viable infant

Source: Data from American College of Obstetricians and Gynecologists. (2016). Ultrasound in pregnancy (Practice Bulletin No. 175). *Obstetrics & Gynecology, 128*, e241–e256. https://doi.org/10.1097/AOG.0000000000001815; Manning, F. A. (2016). *The fetal biophysical profile. UpToDate.* http://www.uptodate.com; Washington University School of Medicine, Department of Obstetrics and Gynecology. (2015). *OB guide 2014–2015*. Washington University.

G. TRANSABDOMINAL ULTRASOUND FOR GROWTH

1. Ultrasound measurement of the fetal head, abdomen, and limbs to assess growth is indicated if pregnancy is at risk for IUGR or macrosomia.

2. Ultrasound measurement for growth is needed if the routine assessment of fundal height differs by more than 2 cm compared with number of weeks gestation (either lagging or ahead).

3. Centers for Disease Control and Prevention (CDC) recommends serial ultrasounds for growth for pregnant individuals with positive or inconclusive testing for the Zika virus (McCabe, 2016). The recommendation is also relevant for pregnant individuals with positive or inconclusive testing for many of the TORCH organisms (toxoplasmosis, other [syphilis, varicella-zoster, parvovirus B19], rubella, cytomegalovirus [CMV], and herpes infections).

4. In obese pregnant individuals, the fundal height measurement is not reliable; a third-trimester ultrasound for growth is advised for a more accurate fetal assessment.

5. Serial measurements are performed every 3 to 4 weeks in the third trimester.

H. DOPPLER VELOCIMETRY

1. Measurement of the velocity of blood flow through maternal and fetal vessels provides information about uteroplacental blood flow. A normal systolic-to-diastolic ratio measured at the umbilical artery suggests normal flow and is associated with normal fetal growth.

2. Alterations in vascular development of the placenta, such as in preeclampsia, result in detectable changes in resistance patterns.

3. Doppler results are displayed as waveform patterns and vary according to the vessel that is assessed.

4. Umbilical artery Doppler tests are most useful for monitoring fetuses with IUGR (ACOG, 2021). In a fetus with normal growth, umbilical artery Doppler has not been shown to provide useful information.

5. Can be used to identify a possibly compromised fetus so that additional assessment (e.g., BPP or continuous fetal monitoring) can be undertaken or early delivery considered.

6. Absent or reversed end diastolic flow is sometimes noted in cases of severe growth restriction and is associated with fetal hypoxemia and acidosis. Prompt delivery should be considered.

I. FETAL LUNG MATURITY TESTING

While fetal lung maturity (FLM) testing has been historically utilized in the past, both ACOG and Society for Maternal–Fetal Medicine now have updated statements that a mature FLM profile is not an indication for delivery in the absence of other clinical indications. Demonstration of lung maturity with FLM is not sufficient to ensure the maturity of other fetal organ systems. Additionally, fetal maturity can be inferred from one of the following:

1. Fetal heart tones have been documented for at least 30 weeks by Doppler.

2. At least 36 weeks have passed since a serum or urine human chorionic gonadotropin-based pregnancy test was positive.

3. Sonographic assessment of gestational age was performed before 14 weeks of gestation and supports a gestational age of 39 weeks or more.

Other assessments are not always black and white, and information about lung maturity may sometimes be helpful and infrequently necessary. Several tests are available to measure fetal phospholipids (substances necessary for successful lung function) present in the amniotic fluid. Ultrasound is used to assist in performing amniocentesis for fluid samples.

Testing for FLM is no longer commonly performed in most clinical settings for several reasons including: delaying delivery due to lung immaturity would place the mother or fetus at significant risk; or the fetus would benefit from delaying delivery, even if lung maturity is documented, and delaying delivery does not place the mother at significant risk; or a course of antenatal steroids can be given, which will benefit the fetus with immature lungs and has no proven harms (ACOG, 2021).

J. CONCLUSIONS

1. Although fetal surveillance techniques are widely used, evidence regarding outcomes may be limited. The optimal choice of tests, when to start testing, and frequency of testing depends on many factors.

2. Antenatal testing may increase maternal anxiety, thus explanations, reassurance, and support should be offered.

Bibliography

American College of Obstetricians and Gynecologists. (2016). Ultrasound in pregnancy (Practice Bulletin No. 175). *Obstetrics & Gynecology, 128*, e241–e256. https://doi.org/10.1097/AOG.0000000000001815

American College of Obstetricians and Gynecologists' Committee on Practice Bulletins—Obstetrics. (2021). Antepartum fetal surveillance: ACOG Practice Bulletin, Number 229. *Obstetrics and Gynecology, 137* (6): e116–e127. https://doi.org/ 10.1097/AOG.0000000000004410

Manning, F. A. (2016). *The fetal biophysical profile. UpToDate.* http://www.uptodate.com

McCabe, E. (2016). *Zika virus infection: Pregnancy and congenital infection. UpToDate.* http://www.uptodate.com

Mehta, S. H., & Sokol, R. J. (2013). Assessment of at-risk pregnancy. In A. H. DeCherney, L. Nathan, T. M. Goodwin, & N. Laufer (Eds.), *Obstetrics & gynecology* (11th ed., pp. 223–233). McGraw-Hill.

Signore, C., Berghella, V., & Baraa, V. A. (2020). *Overview of antepartum fetal surveillance. UpToDate.* http://www.uptodate.com

Signore, C., & Spong, C. (2016). *Overview of fetal assessment. UpToDate.* http://www.uptodate.com

Washington University School of Medicine, Department of Obstetrics and Gynecology. (2015). *OB guide 2014–2015.* Washington University.

7 Postpartum Care in the Ambulatory Setting

NANCY J. CIBULKA | KELLY D. ROSENBERGER

Definitions

The *postpartum period* is the time beginning immediately after the birth of the child until the anatomic and physiologic changes of pregnancy are reversed and the body returns to its nonpregnant state. *Puerperium* is another term that refers to this time period. Although the postpartum period is traditionally considered to last for 6 weeks, the time needed for recovery from pregnancy and childbirth varies. The postpartum period has been arbitrarily divided into three phases: the immediate puerperium, or first 24 hours after the delivery when acute post-delivery complications may occur; the early puerperium, extending through the first week; and the remote puerperium after the first week through the recovery of the reproductive organs and return of first menses, usually from 6 to 12 weeks. While the postpartum period begins with the delivery of the infant, the end is less distinct since all organ systems may return to baseline at various times. The American College of Obstetricians and Gynecologists (ACOG) now considers the postpartum care time frame as the "fourth trimester" extending up to 12 weeks after delivery (ACOG, 2018).

In the United States and other developed countries, where most births take place in the hospital, a patient may choose to leave the hospital as soon as becoming medically stable. However, in most cases, discharge occurs 48 hours after a normal vaginal delivery (NVD) and 96 hours after a cesarean section. During the time the patient is in the hospital, monitoring for bleeding, pain, urinary and bowel functions, breast problems, signs of infection, and maternal interactions with the newborn occurs. Historically, the first postpartum visit is scheduled from 4 to 6 weeks after childbirth for individuals who have had an uncomplicated vaginal birth. In 2018, ACOG recommended that individuals have an encounter (in person or via phone) with a healthcare provider within the first 3 weeks postpartum to assess for any acute issues and have a comprehensive postpartum visit with a physical exam no later than 12 weeks after delivery. Patients who have had a cesarean section are seen initially at 2 weeks to check the incision for adequate healing and return again at 6 weeks for a full postpartum assessment. Patients should be advised to follow up sooner if they are experiencing a problem.

Nurse practitioners (NPs) are uniquely qualified to address known contributing factors for preventable maternal mortality and to optimize healthcare outcomes. In the United States, pregnancy-related death is defined as one occurring during pregnancy or within 12 months after delivery that is causally related to pregnancy (Petersen et al., 2019). Causality includes deaths related to pregnancy complications, events initiated by pregnancy or aggravation of an unrelated condition due to the physiologic effects of pregnancy. Data from the Centers for Disease Control and Prevention's (CDC) national Pregnancy Mortality Surveillance System (PMSS) report indicated cardiovascular conditions led to >33% of maternal mortality rates with other leading causes including hemorrhage and infection. Federal bills have been introduced to extend Medicaid coverage eligibility to include 1 year of postpartum care. This coverage is important since the PMSS data revealed 51.7% of pregnancy-related deaths occurred in the postpartum period, with 18.6% during days 1 to 6, 21.4% during days 7 to 42, and 11.7% during days 43 to 365 postpartum (Petersen et al., 2019). This section focuses on the postpartum care of a patient in an ambulatory setting. Routine postpartum care along with patient education, breastfeeding support, and health promotion are addressed in this chapter, and postpartum complications are addressed in Chapter 8.

A. COMPREHENSIVE POSTPARTUM ASSESSMENT—HISTORY AND REVIEW OF SYSTEMS

1. Review the prenatal record for identified problems during pregnancy and for prenatal laboratory results, including maternal blood type and Rh, Pap smear, cervical cultures, rubella titer, hepatitis and syphilis antibody tests, complete blood count (CBC) trends, and gestational diabetes screening.

2. Review the intrapartum record for the following:

a. Type of delivery: vaginal birth, cesarean section, and vacuum or forceps assist

b. Analgesia and anesthesia during labor and delivery

c. Presence and extent of an episiotomy or laceration

d. Any maternal and/or infant complications or extended stay

e. Infant gestational age, blood gases, Apgar score, birth weight and length, and any complications

f. Estimated blood loss and postpartum hemoglobin/hematocrit

g. Medications given in hospital and at discharge

h. Discharge orders

3. Review maternal interval history since hospital discharge

a. Note any complications, calls to provider, ED visits, and/or resolved illness episodes

b. Determine any acute illness, fever, or abdominal pain that might indicate postpartum infection

4. Assess for pelvic pain or discomfort: If present, determine location, duration, intensity, and other characteristics. Use a pain scale. Elicit comfort measures and analgesics used. Pelvic pain may indicate a complication such as subinvolution or endometritis (see Chapter 8).

5. Assess for breast pain and, if present, investigate further. Breast pain may indicate engorgement, sore nipples, plugged duct(s), or mastitis (see Section IV.D of this chapter and Chapter 8).

6. Assess for bleeding problems: Lochia, vaginal discharge comprising blood, tissue, and mucus, follows a distinct pattern as the uterus shrinks in size, and returns to its nonpregnant condition (involution). The expected pattern for lochia flow is continual decrease in amount and change in character as follows:

a. Lochia rubra consists mainly of bright red blood and cellular debris, lasting 1 to 3 days

b. Lochia serosa becomes increasingly more watery and appears pale in color, pinkish or brown; consisting of old blood, serum, leukocytes, and cellular debris and is present from day 4 up to 3 weeks

c. Lochia alba appears whitish or yellowish and mucoid; consists of leukocytes, mucus, serum, and cellular debris and usually begins around day 10 and may last up to 4 or 5 weeks

d. Foul-smelling lochia may indicate an infection, whereas blood color beyond 2 weeks may indicate subinvolution and endometritis (see Chapter 8)

7. Infant feeding and temperament: Determine whether the patient is breastfeeding or bottle-feeding. If breastfeeding, assess the maternal perception of effort and success. If bottle-feeding, assess comfort and satisfaction with method as well as absence of breast engorgement. Inquire about sleep and activity patterns, crying and consolability patterns, as well as stooling and voiding patterns.

8. Assess for breast problems: If breastfeeding, assess for pain or aching in breasts, nipple cracks or soreness, or any symptoms of mastitis or nipple problems (see Section IV.D).

9. Assess for elimination problems: Voiding and defecation patterns, any discomfort with bowel movements, constipation, signs of urinary tract infection (UTI), and bowel or bladder incontinence. Ask if the patient is using any medications or treatments to assist bowel or bladder function.

10. Assess for healing of episiotomy or laceration: Ask about any perineal discomfort and use of sitz baths or medications.

11. Assess for return of menstruation: Lactating and nonlactating individuals differ significantly in the time before first ovulation occurs and menstruation resumes. Breastfeeding suppresses ovulation because of the persistent elevation of serum prolactin levels that accompany milk production. Ovulation may occur as early as 25 days after delivery with the return of menses in 6 to 12 weeks in nonlactating women (Jackson & Glasier, 2011). In lactating individuals, return of menstruation is affected by the frequency and duration of breastfeeding as well as the amount of supplementary feeding, with most ovulating by 6 months. Because ovulation can occur before the first menses, contraceptive options should be discussed early in the postpartum period. The first menstrual flow is usually heavier than normal but thereafter returns to the prepregnancy pattern.

12. Assess for resumption of sexual relations: Many, but not all, patients wait until after their postpartum visit to resume sexual intercourse with their partner. It is safe to resume intercourse when perineum discomfort has resolved and lochia flow has lightened, indicating that the placental attachment site is adequately healed. If sexually active, ask about any associated discomfort, libido, use of safer sex protections, and contraception.

13. Nutritional assessment: Ask about eating pattern and appetite. If lactating, determine adequacy of key nutrients and enrollment in the Women, Infants, and Children (WIC) supplemental food program, if eligible. A 24-hour dietary recall may be useful. Assess maternal perception of weight and plans for maintenance or weight loss.

14. Assess alcohol, tobacco, and illicit drug use, if indicated

15. Assess the patient's general overall adjustment to childbirth and new role as mother. Inquire about the following areas:

a. Response to birth experience

b. Family and partner support/assistance

c. Family functioning: fatherhood, sibling adjustment, and housing and finances

d. Stress level and coping mechanisms

e. Rest and sleep patterns

f. Activity, exercise, and taking time for one's self

g. Adjustment to motherhood and role adaptation

h. Healthcare system coordination with pediatrician, primary care provider, WIC, and other community resources as indicated

i. Plans to return to work and childcare arrangements

16. Assess for postpartum blues, postpartum depression, and any other psychologic disturbances (see Chapter 8 for more in-depth information and links to depression screening tools): There are multiple screening tools available for use, and most can be completed in less than 10 minutes. The ACOG (2015) and the Association of Women's' Health, Obstetric and Neonatal Nurses (AWHONN, 2015a) encourage screening for postpartum depression.

17. Assess for the history of adverse childhood experiences (ACEs): Traumatic childhood and adolescent life experiences have lasting consequences for adult health, emotional well-being, parenting behavior, and family stability. They are relatively common (Campbell et al., 2016; Felitti et al., 1998). The groundbreaking ACEs study, published more than 20 years ago, included 10 items that assessed emotional, physical, and sexual abuse, neglect, and family dysfunction that occurred before age 18. The questionnaire was designed for use with adult members of the Kaiser Health Plan in San Diego, California, who were mostly White, middle-class, and employed. The tool has since been revised by various researchers and clinicians to include child adversities that may occur when growing up in disadvantaged families and/or unsafe communities (Rariden et al., 2020). To date, there is no final updated version of the ACEs tool, and ACE screenings have not been widely incorporated into practice; however, recent studies have shown that screening can be successfully completed in a variety of settings, including primary care, pediatric care, prenatal care, and during home visits. Trauma-sensitive education of clinicians and support staff, appropriate follow-up care, and resources for positive ACEs identified are essential. Refer to resources within the individual's own community. Resources from the CDC are available www.cdc.gov/violenceprevention/aces/index.html?CDC_AA_refVal=https%3A%2F%2Fwww.cdc.gov%2Fviolenceprevention%2Facestudy%2Findex.html)

18. Review of systems: The provider should complete a review of systems with focus on those that are most relevant: general well-being, breasts, respiratory, cardiovascular, peripheral vascular, gastrointestinal, urinary, genital, and psychiatric. Include others as indicated by presenting complaints.

Physical Examination at the 4- to 6-Week Postpartum Visit

A. GENERAL ASSESSMENT

1. Record the patient's weight, blood pressure, and pulse. Record temperature if needed. Vital signs should be within the normal limits. Observe mood and affect. If the infant is with the mother, observe mother–child interaction.

2. Auscultate heart and lungs.

B. BREAST EXAMINATION

1. Examine nipples for cracks and breasts for redness, firm or hard masses, tenderness, and engorgement (see Section IV.D). In lactating women, breasts may feel full, depending on the time elapsed since the infant's last feeding. In nonlactating individuals, breasts should feel soft without tenderness, masses, or nipple discharge. If nipple discharge persists, instruct the patient to wear a supportive bra and avoid any breast stimulation; recheck in 1 month. Instruct all patients in self-examination of breasts.

C. THYROID EXAMINATION

1. Check size, consistency, and presence of nodules or tenderness to palpation. Postpartum thyroid dysfunction occurs in 2% to 5% of women, typically as thyroiditis or hypothyroidism (Bonnerman, 2013, see Chapter 23).

D. ABDOMEN EXAMINATION

1. Tearing or overstretching of the abdominal muscles during pregnancy can result in hernias and diastasis of the rectus muscles, a separation between the right and left side of the rectus abdominis muscle.
   a. After auscultating bowel sounds, palpate to assess for diastasis recti by having the supine patient lift the head.
   b. Gently check at midline for tenderness and for separation between the muscle bands using your fingers.
   c. Measure separation in fingerbreadths.
   d. Observe and palpate for umbilical hernia.
2. Involution of the abdominal musculature may require 6 to 7 weeks; vigorous exercise is not advised until after healing. Diastasis rectus usually, but not always, resolves without treatment. Refer to physical therapy for persistent diastasis recti. Refer to a surgeon for hernia repair.
3. If delivery was by cesarean section, examine the incision for redness, drainage, or separation. The incision should be intact, nontender, and healing. Patients may report areas of neurogenic pain or numbness for several months after surgery because of neurologic disruption from surgery.

E. PERINEUM AND PELVIC ORGANS EXAMINATION

1. Perform a complete speculum and bimanual examination
   a. Perineum and external genitalia
      i. Examine the episiotomy or laceration for signs of inadequate healing such as erythema, swelling, discharge, and wound separation.
      ii. If lochia is present, note the color and odor.
   b. Vagina and pelvic floor muscles
      i. The vagina may never return completely to its prepregnant state but should return to its approximate antenatal condition by the third postpartum week.
      ii. Estrogenic changes, such as the return of rugae, thickening of the mucosa, and cervical mucous production, will be delayed in lactating women.
      iii. The muscles of the pelvic floor will gradually regain tone (see Section III.D.7).
      iv. Check for lax tone, rectocele, cystocele, and other signs of loss of integrity of the pelvic floor structures.
   c. Cervix
      i. Check for any signs of lacerations of vaginal walls or cervix. If delivery was by vaginal birth, the cervix will now appear as a transverse slit or "fishmouth."
      ii. Check for abnormal discharge, cervical motion tenderness, and other key signs of infection.
   d. Uterus
      i. Involution of the uterus proceeds quickly after delivery with a decrease in weight from 1,000 g to 100 to 200 g at about 3 weeks postpartum (Hobel & Zakowski, 2016).
      ii. After the 10th day, the uterus can no longer be palpated abdominally.
      iii. Upon examination, note the size, shape, consistency, position, tenderness, and mobility.
      iv. Bimanual examination of the uterus should reveal nearly complete involution by 4 to 6 weeks postpartum.
   e. Adnexa: During the bimanual examination, palpate for size, shape, tenderness, and any abnormalities.

f. Rectum
i. Check for normal sphincter tone and for intactness of the rectovaginal septum.
ii. Note any masses, fistulas, and hemorrhoids.
iii. Hemorrhoids often occur during pregnancy as a result of constipation and venous congestion from the enlarging uterus.
iv. If unable to resolve with conservative management, refer for evaluation for surgical treatment.

F. EXTREMITIES

Individuals are at increased risk for deep vein thrombosis (DVT) during the puerperium. Assess for varicosities, swelling, redness, warmth, pain, and/or tenderness in one or both legs.

G. LABORATORY EXAMINATION

1. Hemoglobin/hematocrit or CBC; obtain if there is a history of anemia or hemorrhage, signs of infection, or positive screen for postpartum depression
2. Pap smear, if screening is indicated by current guidelines
3. Chlamydia and gonorrhea test, if indicated by history
4. Urine dipstick, clean voided specimen if suspicion for UTI
5. Thyroid-stimulating hormone (TSH), if signs of thyroid dysfunction and/or a positive screen for postpartum depression

H. DIFFERENTIAL DIAGNOSES

1. Normal postpartum examination (at appropriate number of weeks) versus alteration in postpartum recovery caused by identified problems
2. Effective and adequate lactation versus nonlactating or suppression of lactation accomplished; if problems are identified, describe
3. Incision(s) well healed (episiotomy, laceration, and cesarean section) versus evidence of inadequate healing and/or infection
4. Evidence of adequate mother–child bonding versus mother–child relationship dysfunction
5. Evidence of family adjustment versus identified family maladaptation
6. Adequate knowledge of contraception method selected versus knowledge deficit or absence of effective contraceptive method
7. Adequate and up-to-date health-promotion behaviors versus the need for intervention (e.g., health screenings, adult vaccinations, nutritional counseling, exercise plan, weight loss program, and stress reduction)
8. Emotional well-being and stable mood in transition to motherhood versus evidence of postpartum blues, postpartum depression, postpartum psychosis, or anxiety disorders

Management

A. SURGICAL SITE

1. Incision closure options include sutures (dissolvable or not), staples, Steri-Strips, and surgical glue.
2. If the patient is discharged from the hospital with surgical staples or nondissolvable sutures in place, removal should take place within 7 to 10 days postpartum.
3. Apply Steri-Strips and instruct in wound care.
4. All patients with a surgical incision should be seen at 2 weeks postpartum to assess healing.

B. MEDICATIONS TO CONSIDER FOR THE POSTPARTUM INDIVIDUAL

1. Iron supplementation, if needed; recheck CBC in 1 to 3 months

2. Calcium and vitamin D supplementation, if dietary sources are inadequate

a. The National Academy of Sciences recommends that individuals who are pregnant or breastfeeding consume 1,000 mg of calcium/day, whereas pregnant teens need 1,300 mg of calcium/day.

b. Vitamin D of 600 IU daily is recommended for all women as published in the Institute of Medicine consensus report (www.iom.edu/Reports/2010/Dietary-Reference-Intakes-for-Calcium-and-Vitamin-D.aspx).

3. Vaccines as needed based on the review of immunization status

a. Immunization status can be updated during pregnancy as long as the vaccines do not contain live organisms.

b. Because of a theoretical risk to the fetus, vaccines containing live and attenuated material are postponed until after pregnancy.

c. Unless contraindicated for other reasons, patients can safely receive the following vaccinations during the postpartum period, even if they are breastfeeding

i. Immune globulin

ii. Tetanus, diphtheria, pertussis (Tdap), or tetanus-diphtheria (Td)

iii. Hepatitis B

iv. Inactivated influenza; measles, mumps, and rubella (MMR); meningococcal meningitis; inactivated polio; and varicella (www.cdc.gov/breastfeeding/recommendations/vaccinations.htm)

d. By obtaining the following recommended vaccines, patients will not only protect themselves from potentially serious communicable disease but also protect their infant from exposure:

i. Tdap: Because pertussis remains poorly controlled in the United States and can be a life-threatening illness for infants in their first year of life, the Advisory Committee on Immunization Practices (ACIP) recommends a single dose of Tdap vaccine for adults aged 19 years and older who previously have not received one.

ii. Influenza: Postpartum individuals who have not been vaccinated for the current season should be vaccinated for influenza and can safely receive the inactivated vaccine or, if recommended by the CDC, live attenuated influenza vaccine (LAIV). However, LAIV (administered by nasal spray) is not approved for use during pregnancy or lactation.

iii. MMR and varicella: These live attenuated viruses should be given in the early postpartum period to protect individuals from a potentially serious contagious illness and to prevent fetal exposure to these viruses in a future pregnancy from a harmful exposure.

iv. COVID-19 vaccination (see Chapter 24 for detailed information)

4. Medications specific to identified complications or health problems (see Chapter 8)

C. FAMILY PLANNING/CONTRACEPTION

1. Provide individuals with a safe and effective contraceptive method, if desired. Clinicians should educate patients that a short interval between childbirth and the conception of the next pregnancy has been associated with adverse health outcomes for mother and infant (Zhu, 2005). The greatest risk for adverse pregnancy outcomes has been observed at intervals less than 6 months. The optimal interpregnancy interval for preventing adverse perinatal outcomes is 18 to 23 months. Refer to the latest CDC *U.S. Medical Eligibility Criteria for Contraceptive Use* or update to identify safe contraceptive methods (www.cdc.gov/reproductivehealth/UnintendedPregnancy/USMEC.htm). This document provides recommendations using Categories 1 (safe, no restrictions) to 4 (unacceptable health risk) to indicate whether or not a method is safe for individuals with specific medical conditions. For Categories 1 and 2, benefits generally outweigh the harms.

2. The CDC recommends that postpartum patients should not use combined hormonal contraceptives during the first 21 days after delivery (Category 4) because of a high risk for venous thromboembolism (VTE) during this time. View the CDC recommendation (www.cdc.gov/mmwr/preview/mmwrhtml/mm6026a3.htm). Combined hormonal contraceptives are rated as Category 2 after 21 days postpartum in nonlactating individuals and Category 1 after 42 days (in patients who are not at risk for DVT). In breastfeeding individuals, these choices are rated as Category 2 following 30 days postpartum or thereafter. Clinical studies report conflicting evidence on whether combined oral contraceptives decrease milk supply, resulting in increased supplemental feeding and decreased duration of breastfeeding.

3. Progestin-only hormonal contraceptive methods, including the progestin-only pill, depot medroxyprogesterone acetate (DMPA) injections, and implants (Nexplanon®) are safe for both breastfeeding and nonlactating individuals less than 21 days postpartum (Categories 1 and 2, respectively).

4. Intrauterine devices (IUDs) such as the levonorgestrel-releasing IUD and the copper, hormone-free IUD can be inserted postpartum (Categories 1 and 2) if no evidence of uterine infection exists. Expulsion rates are higher when insertion takes place within 28 days of delivery and uterine perforation rates are higher in breastfeeding individuals before 6 weeks postpartum.

5. Barrier methods, such as condoms and spermicides, can be used any time in the postpartum period (Category 1) once intercourse resumes. The diaphragm and cervical cap can be started at 6 weeks postpartum (Category 1) after fitting for the appropriate size.

6. Fertility awareness-based methods (FABM) of family planning can be used without concern for adverse health effects. The CDC recommends that after 4 weeks postpartum, the symptom-based method is acceptable for individuals who are not breastfeeding; use with caution after 6 weeks postpartum in breastfeeding individuals. Because breastfeeding affects natural indicators of ovulation, additional counseling may be needed to ensure correct use of this method. Previously, the CDC reported a 24% failure rate for FABM. In 2019, the CDC changed this rate to 2% to 23% due to the improved effectiveness of newer proven methods such as the Sympto-Thermal Method and the Ovulation Method. In a 2018 analysis of FABM, the Marquette Method of Natural Family Planning resulted in a low failure rate of 2% to 6.8% with proper use, demonstrating similar effectiveness compared to other birth control methods such as the pill, patch, ring, or injectable (Peragallo et al., 2018). The updated CDC Contraceptive Effectiveness Chart places some of the FABM between the Tier 1 category (<1%, for IUDs and implants) and the Tier 2 category (4%–7%, for pills, patches, rings, and injectables). Note, not all FABM are created equal.

7. Lactational amenorrhea method (LAM) can be a reliable form of contraception for up to 6 months after childbirth, provided the patient's menses have not returned and breastfeeding exclusively with frequent feedings, little to no pacifier use, and no bottle-feeding (Kennedy & Visness, 1992; Panzetta, 2011). If supplementing with formula, pumping breast milk, and/or using pacifiers, then the risk of method failure increases.

8. Permanent sterilization procedures may be an option for couples who are certain they have completed childbearing.
9. A complete discussion of family planning methods is beyond the scope of this book. Please see the resources in Appendix A for more information.

D. GENERAL MEASURES AND PATIENT EDUCATION

1. General postpartum education: AWHONN provides a document "Self-Care Postpartum Discharge Instructions," which is available for free (www.baby.com/jjpi/pregnancy/Self-Care-Postpartum-Discharge-Instructions.pdf)
2. Education about postpartum complications: All patients should be educated about symptoms of common postpartum complications, such as:
   a. UTI
   b. Late postpartum hemorrhage
   c. Infection
   d. Cardiovascular problems
   e. Postpartum depression or psychologic disorders (see Chapter 8)
   f. Prompt recognition and treatment is needed to prevent more serious and long-lasting problems
3. Lactation
   a. The American Academy of Pediatrics (AAP) and ACOG recommend exclusive breastfeeding for 6 months, followed by continued breastfeeding as complementary foods are introduced with continuation of breastfeeding, if possible, for 1 year or longer.
   b. Discuss breastfeeding with nursing mothers and address any concerns.
   c. Provide education for any knowledge gaps and support for any problems that arise (AWHONN, 2015b).
   d. Recommend that a supportive nursing bra be worn daily.
   e. To reduce the risk of nipple confusion, avoid pacifiers, bottles, and supplements of infant formula in the first few weeks unless there is a compelling reason to use them
   f. Refer to a lactation consultant, if needed, to address serious difficulties (see Section IV).
   g. Recommendations for the maternal diet are discussed under nutritional needs (see Section III.D.5).
4. Support for mother–infant dyad
   a. Encourage fathers, partners, and family members to be supportive and helpful.
   b. New mothers need adequate rest and nutrition, time for themselves, and emotional support.
   c. Assistance may be needed with childcare, help around the house, meal preparation, and transportation.
   d. When the mother is supported, she is better able to meet the physical and emotional needs of the infant.
5. Nutritional needs
   a. Use the latest U.S. Department of Agriculture (USDA) MyPlate to help counsel individuals about healthy diet and eating patterns (www.choosemyplate.gov).
   b. Complete up-to-date guidelines are published in the latest Dietary Guidelines for Americans (www.dietaryguidelines.gov/).
   c. Advise individuals to focus on fruits, vegetables, whole grains, lean sources of protein, sufficient fiber, and adequate fluids.

d. Limit beverages with high sugar content, such as soda and fruit drinks.

e. A moderately active, nonlactating postpartum patient can be advised to consume 1,800 to 2,000 kcal/d

f. Diet should be similar in composition to that recommended during pregnancy; breastfeeding individuals should add an additional 500 kcal/d to their diets. Women need 1,000 mg calcium/d (adolescents need 1,300 mg/d) and 600 IU/d vitamin D consumed in foods or by supplement.

g. Individuals who are not anemic after delivery and who breastfeed exclusively may not have a menstrual period for the first 4 to 6 months; thus, iron supplement is usually not needed during this time.

h. Caffeinated drinks are acceptable and should be ingested after breastfeeding rather than before to minimize passage to breast milk and limited to two cups a day.

i. Advise caution regarding alcohol consumption; no more than one drink per day is advised, if ingested at least 4 hours before the next breastfeeding session.

j. The USDA recommends that individuals who are pregnant or breastfeeding consume 8 to 12 oz of seafood weekly from choices that are relatively low in methyl mercury, such as cod, haddock, pollock, shrimp, tilapia, and chunk light tuna. Evidence indicates that intake of omega-3 fatty acids, especially docosahexaenoic acid (DHA), is associated with improved infant health outcomes, such as visual and cognitive development. Avoid tilefish, shark, swordfish, and king mackerel. Seafood contamination with polychlorinated biphenyls (PCBs) is also concerning. Limit consumption of fish that have been found to have high levels of PCBs to no more than 6 to 12 oz per month (as advised during pregnancy), such as farm-raised salmon, herring, albacore tuna, and sardines.

6. Weight loss

a. The infant, placenta, and the amniotic fluid account for approximately 12 lb of weight loss immediately after delivery.

b. Additional weight loss should occur during the postpartum period from loss of excess fluids.

c. A maximum of 4.5 lb/month is the recommended weight loss after the first month of pregnancy.

d. Weight loss should be gradual and occurs as a result of a healthy diet and exercise.

e. The minimum caloric intake should be 1,800 kcal/d, possibly higher if breastfeeding.

f. Individuals who do not consume enough calories are at risk for fatigue and depression.

g. Moderate weight reduction while breastfeeding is safe for mother and infant.

7. Exercise

a. Advise Kegel exercises to improve support and tone of the pelvic floor muscles. Kegel exercises can reduce the occurrence of stress incontinence. Instruct patients to contract their pelvic floor muscles, hold for 10 seconds and then relax; start with 10 contractions four times daily and increase to six times each day. Detailed instructions are available (www.webmd.com/women/guide/kegels-should-i-do-them#1).

b. Because physiologic changes of pregnancy may persist 4 to 6 weeks postpartum, exercise routines should be resumed gradually, as tolerated, and when determined to be medically safe. For many patients, exercises to restore abdominal muscle tone can start within the first week after vaginal delivery. Resuming exercise after a cesarean section is dependent on the rate of recovery and any abdominal soreness.

c. After healing is complete, healthy individuals, even when lactating, should have 30 minutes or more of moderate exercise on all or most days of the week for a minimum of 150 minutes/week. Shorter periods of vigorous exercise are also acceptable. Moderate-intensity exercise may include a wide range of recreational activities, such as running, brisk walking, bike riding, swimming, and others. Providers can offer information on postpartum exercise programs in their local communities, such as at the Young Women's Christian Association (YWCA), health clubs, or neighborhood centers. Downloadable videos are also available from YouTube, public libraries, or commercial businesses.

8. Sleep and rest

a. In the initial weeks after delivery, patients should be advised to get plenty of rest to support their physical recovery.

b. The focus should be on the care of self and infant only, and outside assistance with household duties and/or care of other children is recommended.

c. Counsel patients to try to rest or nap when the baby is sleeping and to limit visitors.

9. General activities

a. Normal activities can be gradually resumed over 6 weeks.

b. Driving is restricted for 1 to 2 weeks or until after the 2-week visit following a cesarean section.

c. In the early postpartum period, the focus should be on recovery, lactation, and the developing mother–child relationship.

d. In most cases, return to work will be 6 to 8 weeks after delivery.

e. Assessment of postpartum recovery is necessary before clearance to return to work is given. Depending on the nature of the work, the individual recovery process, and other circumstances, some individuals may be ready to return to work earlier.

10. Bowels and hemorrhoids

a. Hormones, decreased activity, perineal pain, and other factors may lead to constipation in the early weeks after delivery.

b. An over-the-counter laxative and/or stool softener can be recommended along with increasing fluids and fiber in the diet.

c. Hemorrhoids can be treated with cool compresses, hemorrhoidal pads saturated with witch hazel, and over-the-counter topical creams, ointments, or suppositories containing hydrocortisone.

d. If symptoms are severe or do not improve after 2 weeks of care, refer to a specialist for possible surgical or injection therapy.

11. Sexual relations

a. Intercourse may be resumed when bright red vaginal discharge has resolved, the vaginal area is nontender, the episiotomy or laceration has healed, and the individual feels ready.

b. Discuss the "readiness" factors and provide anticipatory guidance regarding possible differences in sensation, lubrication, and arousal.

c. Gentleness and additional lubrication with commercially available vaginal lubricants may be necessary, especially if breastfeeding.

d. Advise patients that they can conceive even before menstruation has resumed and assist with contraceptive options; discuss safer sex measures.

12. Parenting and infant care
    a. Observe parent–child interaction.
    b. Confirm that the infant has been seen for at least one well-child visit.
    c. Determine that a car seat and appropriate infant bed are in use, that bedding is safe, and that parents and all caretakers are aware of the importance of placing infants on their back for sleep.
    d. Share parenting resources within the community, such as new parent support groups, parenting classes, breastfeeding support groups, and others.
13. Health maintenance and health promotion
    a. Provide anticipatory guidance for continuing recovery, chronic illness prevention, and ongoing risk of postpartum depression.
    b. Encourage the importance of yearly gynecologic care and health screenings at appropriate intervals as indicated by guidelines.
    c. Resources for good nutrition and a healthy lifestyle
       www.niams.nih.gov/health_info/bone/bone_health/nutrition
       www.cdc.gov/physicalactivity/everyone/guidelines/adults.html

Breastfeeding

A. BENEFITS

1. Healthcare providers play a critical role as advocates of breastfeeding in their communities and must be knowledgeable about benefits, essential techniques, and managing common problems to provide support. The WHO/UNICEF (United Nations Children's Education Fund) 1998 publication, "Ten Steps to Successful Breastfeeding" (www.who.int/maternal_child_adolescent/documents/9241591544/en) provides a historical guide for developing strategies to support breastfeeding. Breastfeeding individuals are advised to eat a healthy diet and refrain from tobacco use. Additional up-to-date breastfeeding information can be found at: www.who.int/health-topics/breastfeeding#tab=tab_1.
2. Human milk is the ideal nutritional food for all preterm and term infants during the first year of life, as it contains macro- and micro-nutrients that are essential to support the growth and development of the infant. The CDC promotes and supports breastfeeding (www.cdc.gov/breastfeeding/index.htm).
3. Advantages of breastfeeding for the infant include antibodies that protect against infection and documented lower risk of respiratory tract infections, otitis media, gastrointestinal tract disorders, allergic disease, obesity, diabetes, sudden infant death syndrome, childhood leukemia, and reduced rates of child abuse/neglect. Significant positive effects on long-term neurodevelopment have been observed in preterm infants (AAP, 2012).
4. Maternal advantages of breastfeeding include more rapid involution of the uterus with decreased postpartum blood loss, reduced postpartum depression, decrease in the incidence of breast and ovarian cancer, beneficial effects on weight, decrease in type 2 diabetes, convenience and economy, and fewer missed days at work because of a sick infant.
5. Breastfeeding provides the infant with immune factors and adequate amounts of all nutrients, with the possible exception of vitamin D. The AAP and CDC recommend a supplement of 400 IU/d of vitamin D for all breastfed infants (2008 recommendation, reaffirmed 2020) (www.cdc.gov/breastfeeding/breastfeeding-special-circumstances/diet-and-micronutrients/vitamin-d.html#).

B. CONTRAINDICATIONS TO BREASTFEEDING

1. Maternal conditions
   a. HIV-positive status (in developed countries), human T-lymphotropic virus (HTLV-1), untreated brucellosis, active tuberculosis, active herpes simplex lesions on the breasts (expressed milk is acceptable), varicella or influenza near the time of delivery (expressed milk is acceptable), and active maternal alcohol and substance abuse
   b. This risk of transmission of hepatitis C virus through breastfeeding is not known but is considered minimal.
   c. Hepatitis B infection is not a contraindication to breastfeeding once the infant has received immune globulin (HBIG) and a vaccine.
   d. Patients who have had breast enlargement or reduction surgery will need evaluation with close follow-up for the infant.
2. Infant conditions: Infants with certain metabolic disorders, such as galactosemia and phenylketonuria, should not be breastfed.
3. Maternal medications: All medications appear in small amounts in breast milk; however, only a limited number are contraindicated: cancer drugs, radioactive agents, amphetamines, ergotamines, and statins.
   a. If maternal medications are necessary, minimize infant exposure by having the mother take the medication just after a feeding or before a lengthy sleep period.
   b. Although data are lacking for many psychotropic agents, the following are thought to be acceptable choices: amitriptyline, clomipramine, paroxetine, and sertraline (AAP, 2012).
4. The most up-to-date and comprehensive resource for medications while breastfeeding is LactMed, an Internet source published by the National Library of Medicine, National Institutes of Health (https://www.ncbi.nlm.nih.gov/books/NBK501922/). Helpful reference books are listed in the chapter bibliography (Briggs & Freeman, 2015; Hale & Rowe, 2014; see Appendix A for additional patient and provider resources).

C. BREASTFEEDING TECHNIQUES FOR SUCCESS

1. Positioning
   a. Side-lying, cradle or cross-cradle hold, "football" hold, or semi-reclined "laid-back" are often used (AWHONN, 2015c).
   b. Lift and support breast tissue using the C-hold to direct areola into the infant's mouth.
2. Latch-on
   a. Proper latch-on is very important to successful breastfeeding and for prevention of sore nipples.
   b. Instruct mother to stimulate the rooting reflex by stroking infant's lower lip with the nipple, and when mouth opens widely, center nipple deeply into infant's mouth so that the gums compress the areola, thus positioned to empty the milk ducts.
   c. The tongue should be below the nipple, lips flared outward, and chin touching mother's breast.
   d. Swallowing sounds may be heard.
3. Breastfeeding times and intervals vary, but, in general, breastfeeding should occur often, and breasts should be emptied to maintain or increase milk supply. Feedings may be 15 to 20 minutes or longer per breast. Feeding on demand is recommended.
4. Alternate the starting breasts and their positions for best results and to stimulate the milk supply.

5. Remove infant from breast by breaking suction with finger inserted at the corner of mouth, between gums.

6. Mothers may use a breast pump to express milk for infants who need to be fed through a feeding tube or when there is a need to feed by bottle.

7. Breastfed infants need an assessment at 3 to 5 days of age. The following signs provide evidence of adequate breast milk intake:

- **a.** Six to eight wet diapers in 24 hours
- **b.** Several stools per 24 hours in the first month
- **c.** Breasts feel softer after feeding
- **d.** Infant is content between feedings and is gaining weight appropriately

8. A list of patient/provider resources is available in Appendix A.

D. COMMON BREASTFEEDING PROBLEMS

1. Engorgement

a. *Engorgement* refers to uncomfortable overfilling of the breasts with interstitial edema or excess milk either early or late postpartum. Breasts are swollen, firm or hard, warm to touch, and can be painful.

b. Early engorgement typically occurs with the onset of milk production about 2 to 5 days after delivery. Late engorgement can result from missed feeding or the inability to empty the breasts completely. Problem usually resolves spontaneously within 24 to 48 hours.

c. Engorgement is managed by feeding the infant frequently, whenever they show signs of hunger. A small amount of milk can be expressed to soften the nipples to assure good latch-on. Massage breasts and empty with each feeding. A warm compress or warm shower may help with milk release.

d. Cool compresses or ice packs between feedings may relieve discomfort.

e. Ejection of milk between feedings, such as during a warm shower, may promote milk let-down.

f. Mild analgesics, such as acetaminophen or ibuprofen, are considered safe.

g. Avoid the following, which may worsen the problem or have been found to be ineffective:

- **i.** Use of breast pumps for more than 10 minutes; heat application
- **ii.** Cabbage leaves or extracts
- **iii.** Ultrasound treatments; oxytocin (Spencer, 2015)

h. Advise a well-fitting, supportive bra that is not too tight.

2. Sore nipples

a. This is a common complaint that frequently occurs by postpartum day 2 or 3 and resolves by days 7 to 10. Assess for nipple injury and differentiate from nipple sensitivity, which peaks on the fourth postpartum day and then resolves.

b. Nipple trauma often results from incorrect breastfeeding technique with poor position or latch-on. Nipple abrasion, bruising, cracks, and blisters may result.

c. Assess breastfeeding technique and assist to correct problems that can result in nipple trauma. Try changing positions. Try nursing on the least sore side first.

d. Express a few drops of milk and rub on nipples after feeding to benefit from natural healing properties. Air dry nipples after feeding and change nursing pads often to avoid trapping moisture. Wash breasts only with clean water; avoid soap. Cool or warm compresses and acetaminophen or ibuprofen may also help.

e. If nipple is cracked or abraded, apply an antibiotic ointment (like all-purpose nipple ointment [APNO]) or a hydrogel dressing to facilitate healing.
f. If nipples are too uncomfortable to breastfeed, mother may use an electric pump temporarily and should consult with a lactation specialist.
g. Individuals with injured nipples are at risk of skin or breast infection. Although evidence is not conclusive, purified lanolin or APNO may help. To order APNO, prescribe the following: mupirocin ointment 2% 15 g, betamethasone ointment 0.1% 15 g, and miconazole powder to a concentration of 2% miconazole. Dispense 30 g. Apply sparingly after each feeding. Do not wash or wipe off.
h. Use breast shield to protect nipples between feedings.

3. Plugged milk ducts
   a. Plugged ducts are localized areas where milk has collected and are felt as tender, pea-sized lumps under the skin.
   b. Result from poor latch-on, positioning, and failure to empty the breast completely.
   c. Manage by changing the infant's feeding position, frequent feedings, or use of breast pump. Massage the area and apply heat.
   d. Plugged ducts increase the risk of mastitis. If the problem does not resolve in 72 hours, further evaluation is needed.
4. Inadequate milk supply
   a. May occur because of insufficient milk production or failure to completely empty the breasts, resulting in decreased milk production.
   b. Contributing factors are maternal fatigue, lack of sufficient nutrients, and less fluid intake by the patient.
      i. Infrequent feeding
      ii. Feedings are too short (may be due to sore nipples preventing let-down of the hindmilk, which has higher fat content)
      iii. Poor latch-on—assess infant for ankyloglossia ("tongue-tie")
      iv. Maternal–infant separation
      v. Use of supplemental feedings
   c. Assess for adequate self-care and observe breastfeeding technique. If objective assessment confirms insufficient milk, then counsel the patient about adequate rest, fluid, and nutrient intake for self; increasing frequency and duration of breastfeeding (if needed); and thorough emptying of both breasts. These actions will stimulate breasts to increase milk production.
   d. Avoid use of infant formula or cereal, which may reduce breast milk intake.
   e. Galactagogues, medications thought to assist in increasing milk production, are not recommended because of lack of evidence to support their effectiveness and because of potential safety issues (Spencer, 2015). Metoclopramide 20 mg orally every 8 hours for 2 weeks has been prescribed "off label" to enhance milk production. Domperidone has also been prescribed, though it is not approved in the United States. The AAP has expressed concern about use of these drugs during lactation because of potentially serious effects on the nervous system. The drug manufacturer also advises caution. Avoid use of herbal remedies, as effectiveness and safety during lactation have not been established. Fenugreek is the most widely used herbal agent, and evidence supporting its effect is lacking; reported side effects include diarrhea, flatulence, and others.

E. INDICATIONS FOR CONSULTATION/REFERRAL

1. Excessive and/or abnormal bleeding
2. Uterine subinvolution
3. Signs of pelvic infection, endometritis, or infection of a surgical site
4. Wound separation or delayed healing
5. Signs of DVT or pulmonary embolism
6. Hypertension of stage 2 or higher and signs of late preeclampsia
7. Severe headache with or without visual or neurologic changes
8. Breast mass or abscess
9. Severe postpartum depression or other psychologic disorder
10. Postpartum thyroiditis
11. Abnormal cardiac function
12. Mother–infant bonding dysfunction, neglect, or abuse
13. Any indications for social services or child protective services
14. Maternal substance abuse
15. Nutritional consultation as indicated
16. Lactation consultation for preterm infant and as needed for term infant
17. Follow-up of abnormal Pap smear identified during or prior to pregnancy
18. Identification of health problem requiring further management

F. FOLLOW-UP

1. Follow up on any laboratory work completed at visit
2. Schedule another visit at 1 to 3 months to follow-up on any hormonal contraceptive methods, implants, or IUD initiated at postpartum visit
3. Nursing mothers may need a family planning visit after weaning infant
4. Suggest next visit for recommended vaccinations, health screenings, gynecologic care, and primary care as indicated by patient's age and health risks

Bibliography

American Academy of Pediatrics. (2012). Breastfeeding and the use of human milk. *Pediatrics, 129,* e827–e841. http://doi.org/10.1542/peds.2011-3552

American College of Obstetricians and Gynecologists. (2013). Breastfeeding in underserved women: Increasing initiation and continuation of breastfeeding (ACOG Committee Opinion 570, reaffirmed 2016. *Obstetrics & Gynecology, 122,* 423–428. https://doi.org/10.1097/01.AOG.0000433008.93971.6a

American College of Obstetricians and Gynecologists. (2015a). Physical activity and exercise during pregnancy and the postpartum period (ACOG Committee Opinion #650. *Obstetrics & Gynecology, 1269,* 135–142.

American College of Obstetricians and Gynecologists. (2015b). Screening for depression during and after pregnancy (ACOG Committee Opinion 630, reaffirmed 2016. *Obstetrics & Gynecology, 125,* 1268–1271. https://doi.org/10.1097/01.AOG.0000465192.34779.dc

American College of Obstetricians and Gynecologists. (2016). Optimizing support for breastfeeding as part of obstetric practice (ACOG Committee Opinion #658. *Obstetrics & Gynecology, 1279,* e86–e92. https://doi.org/10.1097/AOG.0000000000001318

American College of Obstetricians and Gynecologists. (2018). Optimizing postpartum care (ACOG Committee Opinion #736. *Obstetrics & Gynecology, 131,* e140–e150. https://doi.org/10.1097/AOG.0000000000002633

Association of Reproductive Health Professionals. (n.d). *Counseling postpartum patients about diet and exercise.* http://www.arhp.org/publications-and-resources/clinical-fact-sheets/postpartum-counseling

Association of Women's Health, Obstetric and Neonatal Nurses. (2015a). Mood and anxiety disorders in pregnant and postpartum women. *Journal of Obstetric, Gynecologic, & Neonatal Nurses, 44,* 687–689. https://doi.org/10.1111/1552-6909.12734

Association of Women's Health, Obstetric and Neonatal Nurses. (2015b). Breastfeeding position statement. *Journal of Obstetric, Gynecologic, & Neonatal Nurses, 44,* 145–150. https://doi.org/10.1111/1552-6909.12530

Association of Women's Health, Obstetric and Neonatal Nurses. (2015c). Top 5 breastfeeding positions. *Healthy Mom & Baby*. http://www.health4mom.org/top-5-breastfeeding-positions

Beck, C. T. (2006). Postpartum depression: It isn't just the blues. *American Journal of Nursing, 106*, 40–50. https://doi.org/10.1097/00000446-200605000-00020

Berens, P., Lockwood, C.J., & Barss, V. A. (2020). Overview of the postpartum period: Normal physiology and routine maternal care. *UpToDate*. http://www.uptodate.com

Bonnerman, C. G. (2013). Thyroid and other endocrine disorders during pregnancy. In A. H. DeCherney, L. Nathan, T. M. Goodwin, & N. Laufer (Eds.), *Current diagnosis & treatment: Obstetrics & gynecology* (11th ed., pp. 519–532). McGraw-Hill.

Briggs, E. G., & Freeman, R. K. (2015). *Drugs in pregnancy and lactation: A reference guide to fetal and neonatal risks* (10th ed.). Wolters Kluwer.

Campbell, J. A., Walker, R. J., & Egede, L. E. (2016). Associations between adverse childhood experiences, high-risk behaviors, and morbidity in adulthood. *American Journal of Preventive Medicine, 50*(3), 344–352. https://doi.org/10.1016/j.amepre.2015.07.022

Centers for Disease Control and Prevention. (2015a). *Breastfeeding: Vaccinations*. http://www.cdc.gov/breastfeeding/recommendations/vaccinations.htm

Centers for Disease Control and Prevention. (2015b). *Healthy pregnant or postpartum women*. http://www.cdc.gov/physicalactivity/everyone/guidelines/pregnancy.html

Centers for Disease Control and Prevention. (2015c). *Breastfeeding*. http://www.cdc.gov/breastfeeding/index.htm

Centers for Disease Control and Prevention. (2016). *Update to CDC's U.S. Medical Eligibility Criteria for Contraceptive use, Revised recommendations for the use of contraceptive methods during the postpartum period*. http://www.cdc.gov/reproductivehealth/UnintendedPregnancy/USMEC.htm

Division of Reproductive Health, National Center for Chronic Disease Prevention and Health Promotion. (2010). U.S. medical eligibility criteria for contraceptive use, 2010: Adapted from the World Health Organization medical eligibility criteria for contraceptive use. *Morbidity and Mortality Weekly Report, 59*(RR-4), 1–86.

Earls, M. F. (2010). & Committee on Psychosocial Aspects of Child and Family Health. *Pediatrics, 126*, 1032–1039. https://doi.org/10.1542/peds.2010-2348

Fehring, R. J., Schneider, M., & Bouchard, T. (2017). Effectiveness of an online natural family planning program for breastfeeding women. *Journal of Obstetric, Gynecologic, and Neonatal Nursing, 46*(4), e129–e137. https://doi.org/10.1016/j.jogn.2017.03.010

Felitti, V. J., Anda, R. F., Nordenberg, D., Williamson, D. F., Spita, A. M., Edwards, V., Koss, M. P., & Marks, J. S. (1998). The relationship of adult health status to childhood abuse and household dysfunction. *American Journal of Preventive Medicine, 14*, 245–258. https://doi.org/10.1016/S0749-3797(98)00017-8

Gjerdingen, D., Crow, S., McGovern, P., Miner, M., & Center, B. (2009). Postpartum depression screening at well-child visits: Validity of a 2-question screen and the PHQ-9. *Annals of Family Medicine, 7*, 63–70. https://doi.org/10.1370/afm.933

Hale, T. W., & Rowe, H. E. (2014). *Medications and mothers' milk: A manual of lactational pharmacology* (16th ed.). Hale Publishing.

Hatcher, R. A., Trussell, J., Nelson, A. L., Cates, W., Kowal, D., & Policar, M. S. (2011). *Contraceptive technology* (20th ed.). Contraceptive Technology.

Hawkins, J. W., Roberto-Nichols, D. M., & Stanley-Haney, J. L. (2016). *Guidelines for nurse practitioners in gynecologic settings* (11th ed.). Springer Publishing Company.

Hobel, C. J., & Zakowski, M. (2016). Normal labor, delivery, and postpartum care. In N. F. Hacker, J. C. Gambone, & C. J. Hobel (Eds.), *Essentials of obstetrics and gynecology* (6th ed., pp. 96–124). Elsevier.

Jackson, E., & Glasier, A. (2011). Return of ovulation and menses in postpartum nonlactating women: a systematic review. *Obstetrics and Gynecology, 117*, 657. https://doi.org/10.1097/AOG.0b013e31820ce18c

Joy, S. (2014). *Postpartum depression reviewed*. http://reference.medscape.com/article/271662

Kennedy, K. I., & Visness, C. M. (1992). Contraceptive efficacy of lactational amenorrhea. *Lancet, 339*, 227. https://doi.org/10.1016/0140-6736(92)90018-X

Kent, J. C., Prime, D. K., & Garbin, C. P. (2012). Principles for maintaining or increasing breast milk production. *Journal of Obstetric, Gynecologic & Neonatal Nursing, 41*, 114–121. https://doi.org/10.1111/j.1552-6909.2011.01313.x

Kim, J. H., & Froh, E. B. (2012). What nurses need to know regarding nutritional and immunobiological properties of human milk. *Journal of Obstetric, Gynecologic, and Neonatal Nursing, 41*, 122–137. https://doi.org/10.1111/j.1552-6909.2011.01314.x

McCoy, S. J. (2011). *Postpartum depression: An essential overview for the practitioner*. http://www.medscape.com/viewarticle/736748

National Academy of Sciences, Institute of Medicine. (2011). *Dietary reference intakes for calcium and vitamin D*. National Academies Press.

Panzetta, S. (2011). Lactational amenorrhea method contraception: Improving knowledge. *Community Practitioner*, *84*(10), 35–37.

Peragallo, U. R., Polis, C. B., Jensen, E. T., Greene, M. E., Kennedy, E., & Stanford, J. B. (2018). Effectiveness of fertility awareness-based methods for pregnancy prevention: A systematic review. *Obstetrics and Gynecology*, *132*, 591–604. https://doi.org/10.1097/AOG.0000000000002784

Pessel, C., & Tsai, M. C. (2013). The normal puerperium. In A. H. DeCherney, L. Nathan, T. M. Goodwin, & N. Laufer (Eds.), *Current diagnosis & treatment obstetrics & gynecology* (11th ed., pp. 190–219). McGraw-Hill.

Petersen, E. E., Davis, N. I., Goodman, D., Cox, S., Mayes, N., Johnston, E., Syverson, C., Seed, K., Shapiro-Mendoza, C. K., Callaghan, W. M., & Barfield, W. (2019). Vital signs: Pregnancy-related deaths, United States, 2011-2015 and strategies for prevention, 13 States 2013-2017. *MMWR*, *68*(18), 423–429. https://doi.org/10.15585/mmwr.mm6818e1

Rariden, C., SmithBattle, L., Yoo, J. H., Cibulka, N., & Loman, D. (2020). Screening for adverse childhood experiences: Literature review and practice implications. *The Journal for Nurse Practitioners*, *17*, 98–104. https://doi.org/10.1016/j.nurpra.2020.08.002 Advance online publication

Schanler, R. J., & Potak, D. C. (2016). Breastfeeding: Parental education and support. *UpToDate*. http://www.uptodate.com

Sparrow Consulting. (n.d). *The Adverse childhood experiences study: A springboard to hope*. http://www.acestudy.org

Spencer, J. (2015). Common problems of breastfeeding and weaning. *UpToDate*. http://www.uptodate.com

U.S. Departments of Agriculture. (2016). *ChooseMyPlate.gov*. http://www.choosemyplate.gov/moms-pregnancy-breastfeeding

U.S. Departments of Agriculture and Health and Human Services. (2016). *Dietary guidelines for Americans, 2015–2020*. http://www.cnpp.usda.gov/dietary-guidelines

U.S. National Library of Medicine. (2013). *LactMED: A new NLM database on drugs and lactation*. https://www.ncbi.nlm.nih.gov/books/NBK501922/

Vieira, F., Bachion, M. M., Delalibera, D., Mota, C. F., & Munari, D. B. (2013). A systematic review of the interventions for nipple trauma in breastfeeding mothers. *Journal of Nursing Scholarship*, *44*(2), 116–125. https://doi.org/10.1111/jnu.12010

Wagner, C. L., & Greer, F. R. (2008). Prevention of rickets and vitamin D deficiency in infants, children, and adolescents. *Pediatrics*, *122*, 1142–1152. https://doi.org/10.1542/peds.2008-1862

Wiener, S. (2006). Diagnosis and management of Candida of the nipple and breast. *Journal of Midwifery and Women's Health*, *51*, 125–128. https://doi.org/10.1016/j.jmwh.2005.11.001

World Health Organization. (1998). *Evidence for the ten steps to successful breastfeeding*. *Author*. http://www.who.int/maternal_child_adolescent/documents/9241591544/en

World Health Organization. (2020). *Breastfeeding overview*. https://www.who.int/health-topics/breastfeeding#tab=tab_1

Zhu, B. P. (2005). Effect of interpregnancy interval on birth outcomes: Findings from three recent U.S. studies. *International Journal of Gynecology & Obstetrics*, *89*(Suppl. 1), S25–S33. https://doi.org/10.1016/j.ijgo.2004.08.002

8. Postpartum Complications

NANCY J. CIBULKA | KELLY D. ROSENBERGER

Nurse practitioners (NPs) providing antepartum and postpartum care are well suited to enhance healthcare outcomes to reduce maternal morbidity and mortality risks. Data from the Centers for Disease Control and Prevention's (CDC) national Pregnancy Mortality Surveillance System (PMSS) report indicated 51.7% of pregnancy-related deaths occurred in the postpartum period, with 18.6% during days 1 to 6 postpartum due to hemorrhage, hypertensive disorders, or infection; 21.4% during days 7 to 42 postpartum due to infection, other cardiovascular conditions, or cerebrovascular accident; and 11.7% during days 43 to 365 postpartum due to cardiomyopathy, other noncardiovascular health conditions or other cardiovascular conditions, respectively (Petersen et al., 2019).

This chapter discusses common postpartum complications with emphasis on problems that may occur after discharge from the hospital following childbirth. Assessment and management of the following complications in the ambulatory care setting are covered: late postpartum hemorrhage (PPH), late-onset endometritis, surgical site infections, postpartum thromboembolism, breast infections, and postpartum depression (PPD).

Postpartum Hemorrhage

A. DEFINITION AND BACKGROUND

1. It is defined as blood loss >500 mL at the time of a vaginal delivery and >1,000 mL following cesarean delivery.
2. Early PPH refers to blood loss that occurs in the immediate postpartum period or within 24 hours of delivery, is managed in the hospital, and accounts for the majority of cases (>99%).
3. Late PPH occurs between 24 hours and 6 weeks after delivery and may be managed in the hospital or in an ED or outpatient setting.
4. PPH is one of the top three causes of maternal mortality (along with embolism and hypertension), accounting for 8% of maternal mortality in developed countries (American College of Obstetricians and Gynecologists [ACOG], 2006). Incidence of late PPH is less than 1%.

B. CAUSES OF PPH

1. Uterine atony
2. Retained placenta
3. Coagulation defects
4. Uterine inversion
5. Subinvolution of placental site
6. Retained products of conception
7. Infection
8. Genital tract trauma or lacerations related to childbirth

9. Placenta previa, abruptio placentae, or placenta accreta
10. Major causes of late PPH are retained placental fragments, subinvolution, and intrauterine infection

C. RISK FACTORS

1. Overdistended uterus (multiple gestations, polyhydramnios, and macrosomia)
2. Prolonged labor
3. Labor induction or augmentation
4. Rapid labor
5. Operative delivery or other uterine surgeries
6. Preeclampsia and magnesium sulfate use
7. Prolonged rupture of membranes increasing risk of infection
8. History of PPH
9. Grandmultiparity (five or more)
10. Chorioamnionitis
11. Asian or Hispanic ethnicity
12. Obesity

D. HISTORY

1. Determine what risk factors are present by reviewing prenatal and intrapartum history.
2. Presenting complaint may include
   a. Lochia rubra that persists beyond 3 days postpartum
   b. Complaint of heavy bleeding, saturating one perineal pad in 30 minutes
   c. Passing large blood clots
   d. Malodorous lochia
   e. Feeling lightheaded, dizzy, weak; syncope
   f. Abdominal or pelvic pain
   g. Fever and chills

E. PHYSICAL EXAMINATION

1. Check vital signs for tachycardia, hypotension, and elevated temperature.
2. General appearance: Observe for pallor, restlessness, tachypnea, diaphoresis, restlessness, and confusion.
3. Inspect vaginal pad for color, odor, and amount of lochia.
4. Palpate for consistency of uterus; massage if boggy and express clots if able.
5. Palpate abdomen for discomfort.
6. Using a speculum, inspect for any perineal, vaginal, or cervical lacerations.

F. LABORATORY AND DIAGNOSTIC STUDIES

1. Complete blood count (CBC) with differential—keep in mind that hemoglobin and hematocrit measurements immediately after acute blood loss are inaccurate. Plasma volume will equilibrate in approximately 2 hours, providing more accurate results.
2. Type and cross-match blood if necessary.
3. Coagulation studies: Prothrombin time (PT), partial thromboplastin time (PTT)
4. Quantitative human chorionic gonadotropin—useful for evaluating for choriocarcinoma, retained products of conception, or a new pregnancy

5. Electrolytes, blood urea nitrogen (BUN) and creatinine, liver function tests (LFTs)
6. Blood cultures if the patient is septic or immunocompromised
7. Transvaginal ultrasound may help to identify retained placental products and is the recommended first-line imaging study.
8. CT or MRI when needed to establish the cause of bleeding

G. DIFFERENTIAL DIAGNOSES

1. Late PPH resulting from subinvolution
2. Late PPH caused by retained placental fragments, with or without intrauterine infection
3. Normal postpartum bleeding

H. MANAGEMENT

1. Massage uterus if boggy and express clots if possible, start an intravenous (IV) if indicated, pack any visible lacerations, give oxytocin by intramuscular (IM) or IV route. Obtain consultation with a physician immediately.
2. Continue to monitor the mother. If signs of hypovolemic shock, provide fluid resuscitation with crystalloids and send to ED by ambulance.
3. Methylergonovine maleate 0.2 mg IM/IV every 2 to 4 hours as needed, no more than five doses; then 0.2 mg orally every 6 hours for 2 to 7 days. Do not give if the patient is hypertensive.
4. Broad-spectrum antibiotics if any signs of infection (see Section II).

I. COMPLICATIONS

1. PPH is a leading cause of maternal morbidity and mortality.
2. Major organ damage caused by massive blood loss
3. Hypopituitarism following severe PPH (Sheehan syndrome)
4. In milder cases, anemia and loss of iron stores

J. CONSULTATION/REFERRAL

1. Massive, acute PPH with hypovolemic shock is a life-threatening emergency and should be managed in the ED.
2. Immediately notify the physician of PPH.
3. Surgical procedures may be necessary to control bleeding, for example, dilatation and curettage (D&C).

K. FOLLOW-UP

1. Reevaluate the patient in 1 week.
2. Repeat hemoglobin/hematocrit and reticulocyte count.
3. The patient will most likely need iron-replacement therapy. Continue iron supplementation and follow up in 4 to 6 weeks for a recheck.

Postpartum Endometritis

A. DEFINITION AND BACKGROUND

1. Infection of the endometrium (lining of the uterus). Infection may also involve the myometrium and extend into the fallopian tubes and pelvic peritoneum. Infections can progress rapidly to severe sepsis, especially in patients with group A *Streptococcal* infections.
2. Occurs in 1% to 3% of vaginal births, up to 10 times more common following cesarean section.

3. Characterized by at least two of the following: fever, lower abdominal (uterine) pain, or tenderness—either unilateral or bilateral, and malodorous lochia.

4. Early onset occurs within 48 hours of delivery and typically follows cesarean section; late onset occurs from 48 hours up to 6 weeks postpartum and is associated with vaginal delivery.

5. Historically known as *puerperal fever*. Postpartum febrile morbidity is defined as an oral temperature of greater than or equal to 38.0°C (100.4°F) occurring on any 2 of the first 10 days postpartum, after the first 24 hours (Adair, 1935).

B. ETIOLOGY

1. Polymicrobial, ascending infection is caused by aerobic and anaerobic vaginal organisms, contamination by bacteria in the gastrointestinal (GI) tract, and/or environmental contaminants.

2. Common causative organisms include group A, B, and D *Streptococcus; Staphylococcus aureus,* and *Staphylococcus epidermidis; Escherichia coli, Enterococcus, Bacteroides* spp., *Peptococcus,* and *Clostridium* spp.

3. Sexually transmitted infections, such as *Chlamydia trachomatis* and *Neisseria gonorrhoeae,* are less common causes of postpartum endometritis.

4. Lochia is an excellent culture medium for bacteria.

C. RISK FACTORS

1. Route of delivery is the most important risk factor; the risk of infection is much increased after a cesarean birth

2. Prolonged rupture of membranes (longer than 24 hours)

3. Prolonged labor (longer than 24 hours)

4. Forceps or vacuum-assisted delivery

5. Vaginitis (bacterial vaginosis or trichomoniasis) or cervicitis prior to delivery

6. Maternal anemia or diabetes

7. Frequent cervical examinations during labor

8. Use of internal fetal-monitoring devices

9. Obesity

10. Low socioeconomic status

11. Colonization with group B *Streptococcus* (GBS)

12. Cervical or vaginal lacerations

13. Retained products or placental fragments and/or manual removal of placenta

D. PREVENTION

1. Careful handwashing and strict aseptic technique

2. Screening and treating any preexisting genital tract infections

3. Minimizing number of cervical examinations in labor

4. Antibiotic prophylaxis during cesarean section

5. Encouraging good nutrition, rest, and adequate vitamin intake

E. HISTORY

1. Determine whether delivery was vaginal or cesarean.

2. Determine whether any risk factors are present.

3. Presenting symptoms may include the following:

- **a.** Abdominal and/or pelvic pain (uterine tenderness)
- **b.** Fever and chills
- **c.** Headache, muscle aches, chills, malaise, and anorexia

d. Malodorous lochia
e. Lochia may be heavy or scant, bloody, purulent

4. Assess other body systems to localize source of infection and exclude other fever-producing diagnoses such as pneumonia, urinary tract infection, or mastitis.

5. Assess the level of pain and relief measures used.

F. PHYSICAL EXAMINATION

1. Check vital signs for temperature elevation, tachycardia, and hypotension.

2. Check general appearance. Observe for chills, diaphoresis, pallor, restlessness, confusion, and generalized rash.

3. Assess heart, lungs, breasts, and costovertebral angle tenderness for coexisting or alternative diagnoses.

4. Inspect incision(s) for separation, purulent discharge, erythema, induration, and tenderness.

5. Palpate for abdominal tenderness, rebound, and rigidity.

6. Perform speculum and bimanual examinations to check for discharge, cervical motion tenderness, adnexal masses, and/or tenderness.

7. Examine lochia for color, odor, and abnormal characteristics.

G. LABORATORY AND DIAGNOSTIC STUDIES

1. CBC with differential

2. Urinalysis and urine cultures

3. Blood cultures, if the patient is septic, immunocompromised, or fails to respond to empiric antibiotic therapy within 24 to 48 hours

4. Cervical or uterine cultures and testing for sexually transmitted infections (DNA probe for *Chlamydia trachomatis* and *Neisseria gonorrhoeae*), if indicated

5. Wet prep and Gram's stain, if indicated; wound cultures, if appropriate

6. Endometrial cultures are *not useful* because of the difficulty of obtaining a pure specimen through the cervix (Chen, 2016).

7. Consider pelvic ultrasound to assess for retained products of conception, pelvic abscess, or infected hematoma.

8. If there is no improvement in 48 hours, consider CT scan or MRI to assess for septic pelvic thrombosis or nonpregnancy sources of infection (e.g., appendicitis or GI conditions).

H. DIFFERENTIAL DIAGNOSES

1. Endometritis

2. Surgical site infection or infected hematoma

3. Tubo-ovarian abscess

4. Urinary tract infection or pyelonephritis

5. Mastitis or breast abscess

6. Septic pelvic thrombophlebitis

7. Deep vein thrombosis (DVT) or pulmonary embolism (PE)

8. Pneumonia

9. Disorders unrelated to pregnancy such as appendicitis, colitis, or viral syndrome

I. MANAGEMENT

1. Moderate to severe infection (temperature >100.4°F) usually occurs within 48 hours postpartum. Treatment involves inpatient care with broad-spectrum parenteral antibiotics, antipyretics, and supportive care.

a. Inpatient antibiotic therapies commonly include gentamicin and clindamycin and have been found to be more effective than other combinations of antibiotics unless resistance to clindamycin is a concern or if the patient is colonized with GBS. If so, ampicillin-sulbactam is a good choice.

b. Rapid improvement (within 48 hours) is anticipated.

2. Late endometritis is identified following hospital discharge, typically between 1 and 6 weeks postpartum, and presents with milder symptoms. Parenteral treatment is usually not necessary; oral therapy is appropriate only for mild endometritis after vaginal birth and may be initiated with one of the following choices:

a. Amoxicillin/clavulanic acid 875/125 mg orally every 12 hours for 10 to 14 days; covers facultative and anaerobic bacteria

b. Amoxicillin 500 mg plus metronidazole 500 mg orally every 8 hours for 10 to 14 days (caution if breastfeeding)

c. Doxycycline 100 mg orally every 12 hours for 14 days—not recommended if breastfeeding

3. General treatment and care include proper hygiene, a healthy diet, adequate rest, fluids, and analgesics/antipyretics for pain and fever.

4. If indications of retained placental fragments (e.g., boggy uterus and heavy bleeding), give methylergonovine maleate 0.2 mg orally every 6 hours for 2 to 7 days.

5. Improvement should be noted within 48 to 72 hours of outpatient treatment.

J. COMPLICATIONS

1. May result in maternal mortality resulting from septic shock or necrotizing fasciitis
2. Sequelae such as pelvic abscess, peritonitis, or salpingitis
3. Septic pelvic thrombophlebitis
4. Scarring and infertility
5. Toxic shock syndrome (rare)

K. CONSULTATION/REFERRAL

1. Notify physician of diagnosis in the ambulatory postpartum patient; patient may require hospitalization.
2. Admit or refer to ED if signs of systemic toxicity or septic shock.
3. Consult with a physician if worsening symptoms within 24 hours or if no improvement in 48 hours of treatment. The patient may need to be admitted to the hospital.

L. FOLLOW-UP

1. Contact patient in 24 to 48 hours for update on status.
2. Advise patient to call if symptoms worsen or are not improving in 24 to 48 hours.
3. Reevaluate the patient in 1 to 2 weeks.
4. Based on home situation, initiate public health or social services referral if needed.

Surgical Site Infections of Abdomen and Perineum

A. DEFINITION AND BACKGROUND

1. Surgical site infections may occur at the cesarean section incision site or at the site of episiotomy or perineal laceration repair. More extensive incisions increase risk for infection and wound breakdown.

2. Most infections occur after hospital discharge and within the first 3 weeks postoperatively; most are treated on an outpatient basis.

3. Occasionally, a seroma (sterile accumulation of fluid) may form below the skin surface. No evidence of fever, erythema, or pus will be present.

B. ETIOLOGY AND RISK FACTORS

1. Endogenous patient flora from skin and GI and genitourinary (GU) tracts

2. Exogenous contamination from the environment and/or break in asepsis

3. Infection with mixed aerobic and anaerobic organisms is common. Usual causative organisms are gram-negative bacilli, *Enterococci*, GBS, anaerobes, and *Staphylococcus aureus.*

4. Obesity is a risk factor for wound infection.

C. PREVENTION

1. Careful handwashing and strict aseptic technique

2. Leave hair intact for delivery. If removal is necessary, remove by clipping or use a depilatory agent; do not shave.

3. Maintain intact vaginal and perineal tissues whenever possible.

4. If an episiotomy is needed, median episiotomy is associated with higher rates of infection and injury to the anal sphincter.

5. Careful attention to perineal hygiene following delivery

6. Encourage good nutrition, rest, and adequate vitamin intake.

D. HISTORY

1. Determine whether the delivery was vaginal or cesarean.

2. Determine whether any risk factors are present.

3. Presenting symptoms may include the following:

- **a.** Pain or discomfort at abdominal incision or perineal site
- **b.** Fever and chills
- **c.** Headache and muscle aches
- **d.** Incontinence of flatus or stool

4. Assess the level of pain and relief measures used.

E. PHYSICAL EXAMINATION

1. Check vital signs noting temperature elevation and tachycardia.

2. Check the general appearance. Observe for chills, diaphoresis, pallor, and pain.

3. Examine heart, lungs, abdomen, and perineum for coexisting or alternative diagnoses.

4. Inspect incision for erythema, induration, presence of serous and/or purulent exudate, edema, and tissue separation with gaping edges.

5. Gently probe cesarean section incision using a sterile Q-tip to determine the depth of separation and to evaluate for fascial integrity or wound dehiscence.

6. For perineal wound, perform a gentle rectovaginal examination to assess for rectal injury, presence of hematoma, and integrity of the anal sphincter.

7. If no improvement in 48 to 72 hours following treatment, consider ultrasound or CT scan to assess for hematoma or abscess formation.

F. LABORATORY AND DIAGNOSTIC STUDIES

1. CBC with differential

2. Wound culture may be indicated.

3. Consider ultrasound or CT scan to assess for hematoma or abscess.

G. DIFFERENTIAL DIAGNOSES

1. Wound infection
2. Seroma
3. Necrotizing fasciitis

H. MANAGEMENT

1. If localized infection and no systemic signs, open and clean the wound, irrigate with normal saline to promote granulation tissue.
2. For cesarean section wounds, do the following:
   a. Debride any devitalized tissue using wet-to-dry gauze dressings two to three times daily.
   b. Once granulation tissue is present, wound fillers, hydrogels, and other absorptive dressings may be used.
3. For a breakdown of a first- or second-degree perineal repair, treat with expectant management, frequent warm sitz baths, and good perineal hygiene.
4. Antibiotics may be needed depending on the extent of wound and culture results. Prescribe cephalosporin, fluoroquinolones, or beta-lactamase inhibitors.
5. Antipyretics and analgesics as needed

I. COMPLICATIONS

1. Necrotizing fasciitis or severe infection
2. Abscess
3. Bleeding with hematoma formation
4. Rectovaginal fistula
5. Prolonged recovery

J. CONSULTATION/REFERRAL

1. Consult with collaborating physician when wound separation occurs.
2. Consult/refer for the following:
   a. Systemic symptoms and purulent drainage
   b. Multiple comorbidities or diabetes
   c. Abscess or hematoma formation
   d. No improvement in signs of infection after 48 hours of antibiotics
   e. Need for surgical debridement
3. Refer if perineal wound closure is needed for perineal integrity.

K. FOLLOW-UP

1. Contact patient in 24 to 48 hours for an update on the status.
2. Advise patient to call if symptoms worsen or are not improving in 24 to 48 hours.
3. Reevaluate the patient in 1 week.
4. Based on home situation, initiate public health or social services referral if needed.

Postpartum Thromboembolism

A. DEFINITION AND BACKGROUND

1. Venous thrombosis is characterized by the formation of a blood clot in a deep vein, usually in the calf or thigh. The clot may break free and travel to the lungs or heart, causing serious damage and possible death. Thromboembolism is one of the leading causes of maternal mortality.

2. Increased risk for thromboembolism during pregnancy and postpartum is the result of circulatory stasis, endothelial damage that may occur at delivery, and hypercoagulability that occurs during the third trimester.

3. Women are at risk for DVT and PE during the postpartum period, especially in the first weeks following delivery; the risk then drops steadily through week 12.

4. Greater than 80% occur in the left lower extremity because of compression of the left iliac vein (Arnett et al., 2013).

B. RISK FACTORS

1. Physiology of pregnancy increases the risk for thromboembolism
2. Multiparity
3. Obesity
4. Cesarean section
5. Maternal age >35 years
6. Tobacco use
7. Prolonged bed rest during pregnancy or postpartum (bedrest is almost never recommended)
8. Any pregnancy-related or severe postpartum complications or trauma
9. Previous episode of thromboembolism
10. Presence of genetic factors for thrombophilia

C. HISTORY

1. Complaints of leg pain or tenderness, redness, and swelling in one or both legs
2. Rapid onset is typical.
3. Complaints of leg fatigue, dull ache, tingling, or pain in leg while standing and/or walking
4. PE: complaints of coughing up blood, chest pain, and shortness of breath

D. PHYSICAL EXAMINATION

1. DVT
- **a.** Vital signs may be normal.
- **b.** Tenderness and swelling in one or both legs
- **c.** Difference in calf circumference of 2 cm or more is highly suggestive of DVT in lower extremity
- **d.** Redness in the affected leg
- **e.** May have a palpable cord
- **f.** Homans sign may be present but is not diagnostic.

2. PE
- **a.** Dyspnea, cough, hemoptysis, pallor; appears anxious
- **b.** Tachypnea, tachycardia, and hypotension
- **c.** Decreased oxygen saturation with oximetry
- **d.** Auscultation of lungs may reveal crackles, rales, and pleural friction rub
- **e.** Abnormal cardiac examination with heave, rub, and/or S3

E. LABORATORY AND DIAGNOSTIC STUDIES

1. DVT: compression ultrasonography with Doppler flow studies (serum D-dimer levels normally increase during the course of pregnancy and slowly decline postpartum; thus, elevated levels are not useful in the diagnosis of DVT during pregnancy or postpartum.)

2. PE: EKG, ventilation-perfusion scintigraphy (V/Q scan), and arterial blood gas

3. CT angiography or MRI may be useful, if initial results are negative or equivocal.

F. DIFFERENTIAL DIAGNOSES

1. DVT
2. Superficial vein thrombosis
3. Septic thrombophlebitis
4. Varicosities
5. Pulmonary emboli
6. Pneumonia
7. Myocardial infarction

G. MANAGEMENT

1. Patient complaints suggestive of DVT or PE must be evaluated promptly; send the patient to the ED.

2. Prompt and prolonged medical management with anticoagulants is required for treatment and will be initiated in inpatient setting.

3. Patient education about the condition, risks, and importance of compliance with management plan

H. CONSULTATION/REFERRAL

1. Refer the patient for immediate emergency care in the ED or order diagnostics with physician collaboration.

2. Referral to vascular medicine may be indicated.

I. FOLLOW-UP

1. Assess for recurrence of thromboembolism at future visits.

2. Future use of estrogen-containing contraceptives and medications is contraindicated.

Lactational Mastitis and Breast Abscess

A. DEFINITION AND BACKGROUND

1. Lactational mastitis is an infection of the breast, a complication of breastfeeding. Clinical presentation includes a hard, red, tender swollen area, usually unilateral, sometimes with fever and flulike symptoms.

2. Occurs in 2% to 10% of lactating women (Dixon et al., 2020).

3. Mastitis may predispose to breast abscess, presenting with symptoms of mastitis and a fluctuant, tender, and palpable mass.

B. ETIOLOGY

1. Most cases are caused by *S. aureus.*

2. Methicillin-resistant *S. aureus* (MRSA) is a common pathogen in patients with lactational mastitis and breast abscess (Dixon et al., 2020).

3. Less common infectious agents include *Streptococcus pyogenes, Bacteroides, Corynebacterium*, and *E. coli.*

C. PREDISPOSING FACTORS

1. Infection typically occurs as a result of trauma to the nipple and introduction of bacteria from the infant to the mother's breasts.

2. Prolonged engorgement

3. Poor latch-on with resulting poor milk removal from breast

4. Maternal stress, fatigue, and/or inadequate nutrition and fluid intake

D. HISTORY

1. Presenting complaints may include:

a. Hard, red, tender, warm, swollen area of breast

b. Myalgia, malaise, chills, headache, and anorexia

c. Fever > 38.5°C

2. Determine onset and duration of the symptoms, pain level, and relief measures tried.

3. Assess frequency and duration of breastfeeding or pumping.

4. Ask whether the woman has cracked or sore nipples.

5. Assess the infant's response to feeding.

6. Determine whether there are any other associated or unrelated symptoms to rule out other causes.

E. PHYSICAL EXAMINATION

1. Check vital signs; temperature may range from 100.0°F to 102.0°F.

2. Inspect breasts for erythema and palpate for hard, tender, warm, swollen quadrant, or lobule.

3. If fluctuant, palpable, tender mass is present with higher fever (102.0°F–104.0°F) and more severe systemic symptoms, suspect a breast abscess.

4. Assess lymph nodes in axillary and upper thorax areas.

5. If possible, observe infant latch-on, suck, and swallow for problems.

6. Examine heart, lungs, abdomen, and perineum for coexisting or alternative diagnoses.

F. LABORATORY AND DIAGNOSTIC STUDIES

1. Laboratories are generally not needed for the diagnosis of mastitis.

2. Culture of breast milk should be obtained if the infection is severe, is hospital acquired, or does not respond to treatment.

3. Ultrasound of the breast should be ordered if breast abscess is suspected or symptoms do not improve within 48 to 72 hours of treatment.

G. DIFFERENTIAL DIAGNOSES

1. Lactational mastitis with or without breast abscess

2. Breast engorgement

3. Plugged milk duct(s)

4. Galactocele (milk retention cysts)

5. Inflammatory breast cancer

H. MANAGEMENT

1. Continue breastfeeding or pumping—it is essential to keep breasts emptied.

2. Improve breastfeeding technique and correct any problems with latch-on.

3. Antibiotic therapy must include coverage against *S. aureus* and should continue for 10 to 14 days to reduce the risk of relapse. The following choices are appropriate for use while breastfeeding:

a. Dicloxacillin 500 mg orally four times daily

b. Cephalexin 500 mg orally four times daily

c. Clindamycin (effective against MRSA) 450 mg orally three times daily (caution for risk of *Clostridioides difficile* colitis)

d. Amoxicillin/clavulanate, 875/125 mg orally twice daily

e. Erythromycin 500 mg twice daily (preferred with beta-lactam hypersensitivity)

4. Symptomatic relief with antipyretics and analgesics such as ibuprofen or acetaminophen

5. General treatment and care should include rest, a healthy diet, increased fluids (minimum of 10 glasses a day of noncaffeinated choices), and analgesic/antipyretics.

6. Cold compresses or ice packs may reduce pain and swelling.

7. Educate/advise family of need for additional support and assistance for at least 48 hours.

I. COMPLICATIONS

1. Breast abscess: Palpable mass, reddened area, may be very firm or fluctuant, possible purulent material from nipple

2. Recurrent mastitis

3. Mastitis that recurs in the same location or does not respond to treatment needs to be evaluated for inflammatory breast carcinoma.

J. CONSULTATION/REFERRAL

1. Refer for ultrasound of the breast if no improvement within 48 to 72 hours of treatment.

2. Refer to a breast surgeon or for surgical consult if breast abscess is suspected or diagnosed.

3. Refer to lactation consultant for assistance with breastfeeding techniques, as needed.

4. Refer if condition is persistent or recurrent.

5. Inform pediatric provider of situation.

K. FOLLOW-UP

1. Contact patient in 24 to 48 hours for an update on the status.

2. Advise patient to call if symptoms worsen or are not improving in 24 to 48 hours.

3. Reevaluate the patient in 1 to 2 weeks.

4. Initiate public health or social service referral if needed for self-care assistance.

Candida Infection of the Breasts

A. DEFINITION AND BACKGROUND

1. Candidiasis of the nipple and/or breast results in significant discomfort during and after breastfeeding

2. Pain with breastfeeding is one of the most common reasons that patients stop nursing and therefore needs to be addressed promptly.

3. Diagnosis is most often based on subjective signs and symptoms.

B. PREDISPOSING FACTORS

1. Vaginal yeast infection at the time of delivery

2. Antibiotic therapy during labor or postpartum

3. Use of bottles and pacifiers

C. HISTORY

1. Take a full history of labor, delivery, and breastfeeding, including any antibiotic use.

2. Presenting complaints may include the following:

a. Burning sensation in nipples before and after breastfeeding
b. Sore nipples, red, inflamed, and tender to touch
c. Stabbing pain in breast associated with breastfeeding

3. Determine the onset and duration of the symptoms, pain level, and relief measures tried.
4. Assess frequency and duration of breastfeeding or pumping and infant's use of pacifiers and bottles.
5. Ask whether the patient has cracked nipples or any lesions (e.g., vesicles and pustules).
6. Ask whether the infant has white, thick coating on the tongue and inner surfaces of cheeks and/or diaper rash.
7. Assess for symptoms of vaginal candidiasis (e.g., itching and burning).
8. Determine whether there are any other associated or unrelated symptoms to rule out other causes.

D. PHYSICAL EXAMINATION

1. Check vital signs—no abnormalities are expected in this condition.
2. Inspect nipples and areola for erythema, shiny and/or flaky skin.
3. Palpate for tenderness and masses.
4. If possible, check infant for thrush (white spots or patches on gums, tongue, or inner cheeks) or characteristic diaper rash.
5. Assess for other causes of sore nipples and breast pain such as cracks in nipples (see Chapter 7 Section IV.D.2) and mastitis (see Section V of this chapter).

E. LABORATORY AND DIAGNOSTIC STUDIES

1. Generally not needed
2. Culture of nipple area and/or breast milk can be obtained but requires the use of specific culture media.

F. DIFFERENTIAL DIAGNOSES

1. *Candida* of the nipple with or without *Candida* of the milk ducts
2. Eczema of the nipple/areola—vesicles and crusting are typical
3. Raynaud's syndrome of the nipples
4. Bacterial infection of the nipples
5. Plugged ducts
6. Lactational mastitis

G. MANAGEMENT

1. For localized *Candida* of the nipples, prescribe one of the following topical medications, applied sparingly after feedings:
   a. Miconazole (Monistat-Derm) 2% cream or
   b. Clotrimazole (Lotrimin) 1% cream or
   c. Nystatin (Mycostatin) 100,000 units/g cream or ointment (more resistance to *Candida* species than listed in points a. or b.)
2. If cracks are present, a topical antibiotic may be included to protect against coexisting *S. aureus* (e.g., mupirocin or triple antibiotic ointment).
3. All-purpose nipple ointment (APNO) contains mupirocin 2% ointment, betamethasone 0.1% ointment, and miconazole powder (see Chapter 7, Section IV.D.2)
4. Continue treatment for at least 10 days, even if symptoms resolve.
5. Infants must be treated simultaneously (usually with oral nystatin suspension, 100,000 units/mL, 0.5 mL to each side of mouth four times daily).

6. One percent gentian violet is effective and inexpensive but is messy. Apply to infant's mouth before a feeding and to nipple/areola after a feeding if not purple. Repeat once daily for 3 to 4 days.

7. Persistent *Candida* of the nipples or presumptive ductal infections should be treated with fluconazole 200 mg orally once daily for 14 days. The medication is considered safe for a nursing infant.

H. PATIENT EDUCATION

1. Continue breastfeeding during treatment.

2. Wash hands well before feedings.

3. Dry breasts thoroughly after each feeding and change disposable breast pads often.

4. Wash all bras and clothing; clean all pumps, nipple shields, or shells.

5. Pacifiers, bottles, and teething rings must be thoroughly cleaned on a daily basis or discarded.

I. CONSULTATION/REFERRAL

1. Refer infant to the primary care provider for treatment.

2. Refer to a lactation consultant for assistance with breastfeeding techniques, as needed.

3. Refer or consult if the condition is persistent or recurrent.

J. FOLLOW-UP

1. Advise patient to call if symptoms worsen or are not improving in 48 to 72 hours.

2. Reevaluate the patient in 2 weeks.

Postpartum Depression

A. DEFINITION AND BACKGROUND

1. PPD is a major depressive mood disorder characterized by moderate to severe depression. Despite the importance of treatment, PPD is often undiagnosed and undertreated.

2. Although the incidence is difficult to determine, it is thought that depression affects one in eight women in the 12 months following delivery of a baby. It is one of the most common complications of childbirth, usually presenting between 2 weeks and 3 months after childbirth and may occur up to 1 year following birth.

3. The Association of Women's Health, Obstetric and Neonatal Nurses (AWHONN), the ACOG, and the American Academy of Pediatrics (AAP) recommend routine screening for PPD. Read the AWHONN position statement (awhonn.org/news-advocacy-and-publications/awhonn-position-statements/) and AAP's clinical report (https://pediatrics.aappublications.org/content/143/1/e20183260). Visit ACOG's Depression Resource Center (www.acog.org/Womens-Health/Depression-and-Postpartum-Depression).

4. Failure to treat PPD can lead to delays in social and cognitive development in the infant that persist into childhood, childhood behavioral problems, and adverse health effects for the mother (Joy, 2014).

5. Suspected causes of PPD include hormonal, psychosocial, and biologic factors, such as changing plasma levels of estrogen and progesterone, thyroid dysfunction, sleep disturbances, and psychosocial risk factors.

B. RISK FACTORS

1. History of depression before or during pregnancy
2. History of PPD or psychosis
3. Family history of mood disorders
4. Inadequate social support, single parent, young age, low self-esteem
5. Marital discord
6. Intimate partner violence
7. Recent negative, stressful life events (financial problems, job loss, and death)
8. Preterm infant or infant with health problems
9. Multiple births
10. Multiple adverse childhood experiences while growing up (alcoholism, physical/emotional/sexual abuse, and dysfunctional home)

C. CLINICAL PRESENTATION

1. Symptoms of major depression such as depressed mood, tearfulness, mood swings, loss of pleasure in activities/interests, insomnia, fatigue, appetite disturbance, suicidal thoughts, or recurrent thoughts of death.
2. PPD may manifest with anxiety, agitation, restlessness, and impaired concentration as well as obsessive worries about the infant's health and well-being and feelings of inadequacy.
3. Ambivalent or negative feelings toward the infant, guilty feelings, intrusive fears, and thoughts of harming the infant. Angry feelings toward infant, other children, or partner.

D. HISTORY

1. Obtain a depression screen in all patients (see Section VII.G).
2. Assess for risk factors.
3. Determine the onset of symptoms, duration, and course.
4. Determine whether the patient is able to perform usual roles as wife, mother, and employee.
5. Ask about weight loss or gain, intolerance to cold or heat, changes in bowel function, and menstrual pattern.
6. Inquire about support in the home.
7. Ask whether the patient has any thoughts of harming self, infant, or others.

E. PHYSICAL EXAMINATION

1. Check vital signs (no abnormalities are expected).
2. Note general appearance, including affect, response patterns, eye contact with provider, and grooming.
3. Observe interaction with infant, if possible, noting eye contact, tone of voice, appropriateness of expectations, and so on.
4. Perform general physical examination and palpate the thyroid.

F. LABORATORY AND DIAGNOSTIC STUDIES

1. Check CBC (rule out anemia).
2. Check TSH (thyroid-stimulating hormone; rule out thyroid dysfunction).

G. DEPRESSION SCREENING TOOLS

1. Edinburgh Postnatal Depression Scale (EPDS), a 10-item, self-rated questionnaire, is a reliable screening assessment (www.aap.org/en-us/advocacy-and-policy/aap-health-initiatives/practicing-safety/Documents/Post

natal%20Depression%20Scale.pdf). A score of 10 or more requires additional assessment.

2. A three-question version of the EPDS demonstrating excellent sensitivity and predictive value is available (www.nationalperinatal.org/resources/Documents/Position%20Papers/EPDS3.pdf).

3. The two-item Patient Health Questionnaire (PHQ-2) or PHQ-9; the PHQ-2, (cde.drugabuse.gov/instrument/fc216f70-be8e-ac44-e040-bb89ad433387) consists of the following two questions:

a. During the past 2 weeks, have you often been bothered by feeling down, depressed, or hopeless?

b. During the past 2 weeks, have you often been bothered by having little interest or pleasure in doing things?

c. If the PHQ-2 elicits affirmative responses, the PHQ-9 should be used as a confirmatory test (www.drugabuse.gov/sites/default/files/PatientHealthQuestionnaire9.pdf).

4. Other screening tools choices include Beck & Gable's Postpartum Depression Screening Scale (PDSS) and the Beck Depression Inventory II (BDI-II), available commercially.

5. Validation of screening tools by in-depth interview is necessary.

6. Tools should be examined for cultural literacy and appropriateness for the patient population.

H. DIFFERENTIAL DIAGNOSES

1. PPD

2. Postpartum blues—experienced by 85% of women, but symptoms are not as severe and resolve within the first 2 postpartum weeks

3. Postpartum psychosis—dramatic onset with rapidly shifting mood, delusions, hallucinations, and risk of infanticide and suicide. This is an emergency that requires inpatient treatment. Individuals with bipolar and schizoaffective disorders are mostly at risk for postpartum psychosis.

4. Postpartum obsessive-compulsive disorder—obsessive thoughts of harming infant, anxiety, compulsive checking and protectiveness, and depression

5. Thyroid dysfunction

6. Other neuropsychiatric disorder

7. Substance abuse

I. MANAGEMENT

1. Earlier treatment is associated with a better prognosis. See Appendix A for patient education and care resources.

2. Nonpharmacologic treatment strategies, such as cognitive behavioral therapy or interpersonal or group psychotherapy, can be effective for women with mild to moderate PPD. Support groups may also be helpful.

3. Medication may be used along with nonpharmacologic therapies:

a. Selective serotonin reuptake inhibitors (SSRIs) are first-line agents, for example, sertraline (a good choice if nursing), fluoxetine, paroxetine, escitalopram, and citalopram.

b. Serotonin–norepinephrine reuptake inhibitors (SNRIs) are also good choices, for example, venlafaxine or duloxetine.

c. Tricyclic antidepressants, for example, nortriptyline and amitriptyline

d. All psychotropic medications are secreted in small amounts into breast milk. See Chapter 7, Section IV.B.4 for resources to check safety during pregnancy. (For more information, see ACOG Practice Bulletin,

Number 92, "Use of Psychiatric Medications During Pregnancy and Lactation.")

e. Advise patients that prescribed antidepressants may take 4 to 6 weeks for full effect.

f. Continue medication for 6 to 12 months to prevent relapse.

4. Management of sleep disturbances
5. Regular aerobic exercise
6. Massage therapy for mother and infant may help
7. Encourage family support and involvement of patient's partner

J. CONSULTATION/REFERRAL

1. Refer to ED if patient is suicidal or there is evidence of psychosis.
2. Refer patient to psychiatrist, psychologist, social worker, or counselor if depression is severe, no improvement in condition occurs within 2 to 4 weeks, and/or for ongoing care.
3. Refer to postpartum support group if available in one's community.
4. Consult with a psychiatrist as needed to guide care.
5. Inform pediatrician, especially if breastfeeding mother is on medication.

K. FOLLOW-UP

1. Follow up by phone in 48 to 72 hours and office visit in 2 weeks.
2. Provide patient and family with information for crisis line if needed.
3. Initiate home health nursing visit if appropriate.
4. Refer for social services, financial services, and housing assistance as needed.
5. Repeat the depression screen in 4 to 6 weeks to assess improvement; continue ongoing periodic follow-up as indicated by response to treatment.

Bibliography

Adair, F. L. (1935). The American Committee of maternal welfare, Inc: Chairman's address. *Journal of Obstetrics & Gynecology, 30*, 868. https://doi.org/10.1016/S0002-9378(35)90434-3

American College of Obstetricians and Gynecologists. (2006a). Episiotomy (ACOG Practice Bulletin #71, reaffirmed 2015). *Obstetrics & Gynecology, 107*, 957–962. https://doi.org/10.1097/00006250-200604000-00049

American College of Obstetricians and Gynecologists. (2008). Use of psychiatric medications during pregnancy and lactation (ACOG Practice Bulletin #92, reaffirmed 2016). *Obstetrics & Gynecology, 111*, 1001–1020. https://doi.org/10.1097/AOG.0b013e31816fd910

American College of Obstetricians and Gynecologists. (2017). Postpartum hemorrhage (ACOG Practice Bulletin #183). *Obstetrics & Gynecology, 130*(4), e168–e186. https://doi.org/10.1097/AOG.0000000000002351

American College of Obstetricians and Gynecologists. (2018a). Screening for perinatal depression (ACOG Committee Opinion #757). *Obstetrics & Gynecology, 132*(5), e208–e212. https://doi.org/10.1097/AOG.0000000000002927

American College of Obstetricians and Gynecologists. (2018b). Thromboembolism in pregnancy (ACOG Practice Bulletin #2034). *Obstetrics & Gynecology, 131*(1), e1–e17.

Arnett, C., Greenspoon, J. S., & Roman, A. S. (2013). Hematologic disorders in pregnancy. In A. H. DeCherney, L. Nathan, T. M. Goodwin, N. Laufer, & A. S. Roman (Eds.), *Obstetrics & gynecology* (11th ed., pp. 543–554). McGraw Hill.

Association of Women's Health, Obstetric and Neonatal Nurses. (1999). *Mood and anxiety disorders in pregnant and postpartum women. (AWHONN Position Statement, revised, re-titled, and approved 2015).* https://awhonn.org/news-advocacy-and-publications/awhonn-position-statements/

Association of Women's Health, Obstetric and Neonatal Nurses. (2015). Guidelines for oxytocin administration after birth: AWHONN practice brief number 2. *Journal of Obstetric, Gynecologic & Neonatal Nursing, 44*, 161–163. https://doi.org/10.1111/1552-6909.12528

Beck, C. T. (2006). Postpartum depression: It isn't just the blues. *American Journal of Nursing, 106*, 40–50. https://doi.org/10.1097/00000446-200605000-00020

Berens, P., Lockwood, C. J., & Barss, V. A. (2020). *Overview of the postpartum period: Normal physiology and routine maternal care. UpToDate.* http://www.uptodate.com

Bingham, D., & Jones, R. (2012). Maternal death from obstetric hemorrhage. *Journal of Obstetric, Gynecologic & Neonatal Nursing, 41*, 531–539. https://doi.org/10.1111/j.1552-6909.2012.01372.x

Castro, L. C., & Gambone, J. C. (2016). Common medical and surgical conditions complicating pregnancy. In N. F. Hacker, J. C. Gambone, & C. J. Hobel (Eds.), *Essentials of obstetrics and gynecology* (6th ed., pp. 201–223). Elsevier.

Chen, K. T. (2016). *Postpartum endometritis. UpToDate.* http://www.uptodate.com

Cox, J. L., Holden, J. M., & Sagovsky, R. (1987). Detection of postnatal depression: Development of the 10-item Edinburgh postnatal depression scale. *British Journal of Psychiatry, 150*, 782–786. https://doi.org/10.1192/bjp.150.6.782

Dennis, C. L., & Dowswell, T. (2013). Psychosocial and psychological interventions for preventing postpartum depression (review. *Cochrane Database of Systematic Reviews, 2013*(2). https://doi.org/10.1002/14651858.CD001134.pub3

Dixon, J. M., Chagpar, A. B., Sexton, D. J., & Baron, E. L. (2020). *Lactational mastitis. UpToDate.* http://www.uptodate.com.

Douchet, S., Letourneau, N., & Blackmore, E. R. (2012). Support needs of mothers who experience postpartum psychosis and their partners. *Journal of Obstetric, Gynecologic & Neonatal Nursing, 41*, 236–245. https://doi.org/10.1111/j.1552-6909.2011.01329.x

Gabel, K. T., & Weeber, T. A. (2012). Measuring and communicating blood loss during obstetric hemorrhage. *Journal of Obstetric Gynecologic & Neonatal Nursing, 41*, 551–558. https://doi.org/10.1111/j.1552-6909.2012.01375.x

Gilbert, D. N., Eliopoulos, G. M., Chamber, H. F., & Saag, M. S. (2016). *The Sanford guide to antimicrobial therapy 2016* (46th ed.). Antimicrobial Therapy.

Hobel, C. J., & Lamb, A. R. (2016). Obstetric hemorrhage. In N. F. Hacker, J. C. Gambone, & C. J. Hobel (Eds.), *Essentials of obstetrics and gynecology* (6th ed., pp. 136–146). Elsevier.

Joy, S. (2014). *Postpartum depression: Overview.* http://emedicine-.medscape.com/article/271662-overview

Kabir, K., Sheeder, J., & Kelly, L. S. (2008). Identifying postpartum depression: Are 3 questions as good as 10? *Pediatrics, 122*, e696–e702. https://doi.org/10.1542/peds.2007-1759

Mackeen, A. D., Packard, R. E., Ota, E., & Speer, L. (2015). Antibiotic regimens for postpartum endometritis (review. *Cochrane Database of Systematic Reviews, 2015*(2). https://doi.org/10.1002/14651858.CD001067.pub3

MacReady, N. (2014). Postpartum VTE risk highest soon after birth. *Obstetrics & Gynecology, 123*, 987–996. https://doi.org/10.1097/AOG.0000000000000230

Malhotra, A., Weinberger, S. E., Leung, L. K., Lockwood, C. J., Mandel, J., & Finlay, G. (2020). *Deep vein thrombosis in pregnancy: Epidemiology, pathogenesis, and diagnosis. Up To Date.* http://www.uptodate.com.

Petersen, E. E., Davis, N. I., Goodman, D., Cox, S., Mayes, N., Johnston, E., Syverson, C., Seed, K., Shapiro-Mendoza, C. K., Callaghan, W. M., & Barfield, W. (2019). Vital signs: Pregnancy-related deaths, United States, 2011-2015 and strategies for prevention, 13 States 2013–2017. *MMWR, 68*(18), 423–429. https://doi.org/10.15585/mmwr.mm6818e1

Pignone, M. P., Gaynes, B. N., Rushton, J. L., Buchell, C. M., Orleans, C. T., Mulrow, C. D., & Lohr, K. N. (2002). Screening for depression in adults: A summary of the evidence for the U.S. Preventive Services Task Force. *Annals of Internal Medicine, 136*, 765–776. https://doi.org/10.7326/0003-4819-136-10-200205210-00013

Poggi, S. B. (2013). Postpartum hemorrhage & the abnormal puerperium. In A. H. DeCherney, L. Nathan, T. M. Goodwin, N. Laufer, & A. S. Roman (Eds.), *Obstetrics & gynecology* (11th ed., pp. 349–368). McGraw Hill.

Rivlin, M. E. (2019). *Endometritis.* https://emedicine.medscape.com/article/254169-overview

Smith, J. R. (2018). *Postpartum hemorrhage.* http://emedicine.medscape.com/article/275038-overview

Speisman, B. B., Storch, E. A., & Abramowitz, J. S. (2011). Postpartum obsessive-compulsive disorder. *Journal of Obstetric, Gynecologic & Neonatal Nursing, 40*, 680–690. https://doi.org/10.1111/j.1552-6909.2011.01294.x

Spencer, J. (2020). *Common problems of breastfeeding and weaning. UpToDate.* http://www.uptodate.com

Tharpe, N. (2008). Post pregnancy genital tract and wound infections. *Journal of Midwifery & Women's Health, 53*, 236–246. https://doi.org/10.1016/j.jmwh.2008.01.007

Wiener, S. (2006). Diagnosis and management of Candida of the nipple and breast. *Journal of Midwifery & Women's Health, 51*, 125–128. https://doi.org/10.1016/j.jmwh.2005.11.001

Wong, A. W. (2019). *Postpartum infections.* http://emedicine.medscape.com/article/796892-overview

Yellowless, P. (2010). *Accuracy of depression screening tools for identifying postpartum depression among urban mothers.* Medscape Psychiatry Minute Presentation. http://www.medscape.com/viewarticle/724430

Yiadom, M. Y. (2018). *Postpartum hemorrhage in emergency medicine.* http://emedicine.medscape.com/article/796785-overview

III. Guidelines for Management of Common Problems of Pregnancy

9. Oral Health and Oral Health Problems in Pregnancy

NANCY J. CIBULKA | KELLY D. ROSENBERGER

Preventive dental care and timely treatment of oral health problems can halt tooth decay, reverse periodontal disease, and improve both oral health and the overall health of pregnant individuals. Although research is not conclusive, results from several well-designed studies also suggest that maternal periodontitis may be an independent risk factor for preterm birth, low birth weight, and other adverse pregnancy outcomes. Periodontal diseases develop when plaque builds up along the gumline and is not removed by brushing, flossing, or prophylactic cleaning by a dental professional. Periodontal infections are polymicrobial with an average of four to six different bacteria, including anaerobic gram-negative rods and gram-positive cocci, as well as facultative and microaerophilic *Streptococci*. The bacteria adhere to and grow on the surfaces of the teeth. Pregnant women are particularly susceptible to oral health problems because hormonal changes increase the risk of gingivitis, a risk factor of periodontal disease. Other oral health problems related to physiologic changes during pregnancy include benign oral gingival lesions, tooth mobility, tooth erosion, and dental caries (American College of Obstetricians and Gynecologists [ACOG], 2013).

Many patients lack knowledge of the importance of oral health during pregnancy and do not seek dental care during this time. As a result, prenatal care providers often see preventable and treatable dental problems such as tooth pain, dentoalveolar abscess (pus surrounding the teeth), broken or missing teeth, and periodontitis. Dental procedures such as local anesthesia, dental extraction, root canal, restoration (amalgam or composite) of untreated caries, flossing, and scaling/planing of plaque/biofilm are not harmful to the fetus. The American Academy of Periodontology recommends that patients who are pregnant or planning a pregnancy should have an oral health examination, and preventive or therapeutic services should be provided. The ACOG recommends that pregnant patients schedule a checkup with their oral health provider early in pregnancy and continue to brush and floss daily. The American Dental Association (ADA) recommends brushing teeth two or more times daily and flossing teeth at least once daily. Oral health is a lifelong concern that will affect the ongoing health of patients and infants. Therefore, healthcare providers are advised to incorporate oral health screening and education into routine prenatal care.

A. RISK FACTORS FOR PERIODONTAL PROBLEMS

1. Tobacco use
2. High sugar consumption
3. Poor oral hygiene (inadequate brushing and flossing)
4. High levels of stress
5. Substance abuse, especially methamphetamine use
6. Diabetes

7. Infection with HIV and other medical conditions that affect the immune system
8. Low income
9. Poor nutrition
10. Medications that reduce saliva
11. Hormonal changes
12. Genetic susceptibility
13. Poor access to oral health providers, including lack of insurance coverage

B. HISTORY

1. Complaints of toothache, broken tooth, dental pain, gum swelling, loose teeth, sensitive teeth, and/or receding gums
2. Difficulty chewing because of jaw pain
3. Complaints of tender or bleeding gums (a common complaint that needs further evaluation)
4. Reports of heat and cold sensitivity
5. Complaints of bad breath
6. Inquire about the onset, duration, location, and degree of pain, as well as alleviating and aggravating factors.
7. Ask when the patient had last dental checkup.
8. Assess oral hygiene practices (e.g., how often does the patient brush and floss).

C. PHYSICAL EXAMINATION

1. Vital signs: Note whether fever is present.
2. Check weight for possible weight loss resulting from anorexia or mouth pain.
3. Inspect oral cavity, examining gums for bleeding, redness, and swelling; note condition of teeth (e.g., caries, loose, broken, missing, decalcified).
4. Pyogenic granuloma, or "pregnancy tumor" is noted in up to 10% of pregnant individuals; it appears as flat or pedunculated, pink or purplish red growths usually in the upper gum (maxillary) tissue in an inflamed, high-plaque area. More information and a picture are available (emedicine.medscape.com/article/1077040-overview).
5. Palpate neck and submental area for enlarged lymph nodes.
6. Note any halitosis.

D. LABORATORY AND DIAGNOSTIC STUDIES

1. None needed in most cases
2. Complete blood count (CBC) if any indication of severe or systemic infection
3. If x-rays are needed, the maternal abdomen and thyroid should be shielded.

E. DIFFERENTIAL DIAGNOSES

1. Dental abscess
2. Broken and/or missing teeth
3. Pregnancy gingivitis
4. Periodontal disease
5. Pyogenic granuloma
6. Oral cancer

F. MANAGEMENT

1. Patient can apply warm towel or heating pad to face for comfort.
2. Analgesics for pain
    a. Acetaminophen 325 to 500 mg one to two tablets orally every 4 to 6 hours as needed, not to exceed 4,000 mg in 24 hours
    b. Acetaminophen/codeine if needed (use with caution)

3. Advise adequate fluid intake and soft diet as tolerated.
4. Warm saline rinses may reduce mild discomfort (1 teaspoon of salt to 8 oz of warm water).
5. If an abscess is present, give antibiotics while awaiting dental consult.
   a. Penicillin V potassium 500 mg orally twice a day or four times a day for 7 to 10 days (first choice if not allergic to penicillin)
   b. Amoxicillin/clavulanate 500 mg/125 mg or 875 mg/125 mg twice a day for 7 to 10 days
   c. If allergic to penicillin, clindamycin 300 to 450 mg orally four times a day for 7 to 10 days
   d. Erythromycin 250 to 500 mg orally four times a day for 7 to 10 days
6. For dentoalveolar abscesses, surgical drainage may be needed.
7. If periodontitis is present, treatment can include scaling and root planing to remove calculus and bacteria from the tooth surfaces and root. Chlorhexidine 0.12% rinses twice daily may be recommended (risk is low during pregnancy due to minimal systemic absorption).
8. Education: See Appendix A for online patient and provider resources; helpful tips for patients are listed in Box 9.1.
   a. Brush teeth at least twice daily with a fluoridated toothpaste.
   b. Floss once or more daily.
   c. Have regular oral health checkups (every 6–12 months).
   d. Avoid sodas, sweet tea, and other high-sugar drinks and avoid eating sweet snacks.
   e. Avoid tobacco use.
   f. Follow a healthy diet with adequate intake of calcium, protein, and vitamins A, C, and D.
   g. Brush or use an over-the-counter fluoride mouthwash after vomiting to protect teeth.
   h. Engage in regular physical exercise.
   i. Avoid saliva-sharing activities with the infant, such as sharing a spoon or bites of food or by using own saliva to "clean" a pacifier.

G. DENTAL PROCEDURES DURING PREGNANCY

1. Pregnant patients should have checkups and routine dental work.
2. Best time to schedule routine dental work is in the second trimester when fetal organogenesis has been completed, and women often feel better.
3. X-rays can be safely taken with a lead shield placed over the woman's abdomen.
4. Topical and intraoral local anesthetics with vasoconstrictors are safe.
5. If antibiotics are needed, only those that are safe to use during pregnancy should be prescribed; tetracycline should be avoided because it causes staining of the infant's teeth.
6. Emergency services should be provided whenever indicated.

H. COMPLICATIONS OF DENTAL ABSCESS AND/OR PERIODONTITIS

1. Progressive loss of alveolar bone and pocket formation around teeth
2. Loosening and loss of teeth
3. Sepsis from untreated infection
4. Possible facial cellulitis
5. Weight loss from anorexia and/or difficulty chewing
6. Possible increased risk of preterm delivery and low-birth-weight infant
7. Maxillary sinusitis or cavernous sinus thrombosis from spread of infection
8. Increased risk of poor oral health in children

BOX 9.1 ORAL (DENTAL) CARE DURING PREGNANCY

What Is Dental Care?
- Brush twice a day
- Floss daily
- Regular dental checkups

What Are Warming Signs of Poor Oral Health?
- Plaque (a thin film of bacteria on teeth)
- Visible tooth decay
- Tooth abscess
- Red, swollen, and bleeding gums

How Does Oral Health Affect My Pregnancy?
- Serious gum disease (periodontitis) is linked to premature birth and low birth weight.
- Babies born early (<37 weeks) and small (<6 pounds) have more health problems and spend more time in the hospital.

Does Pregnancy Affect Oral Health?
- Your gums might bleed more easily.
- Dental caries might become more serious.

What Are Common Myths About Pregnancy and Oral Health?
- "Lose a tooth for every baby"
- "Calcium will be drawn out of your teeth by the baby" (THESE ARE NOT TRUE! YOU CAN PREVENT PROBLEMS)

How Can I Improve My Dental Health?
- Brush twice a day with fluoride toothpaste.
- Gently brush gumline.
- Floss between teeth daily.
- Schedule a dental checkup early in your pregnancy.

I. CONSULTATION/REFERRAL

1. Provide a written referral to a dentist indicating the nature of the oral health problem, any pregnancy complications or limitations, and whether any medications should be avoided.

2. Advise the patient to keep the appointment, even if the pain resolves.

3. Refer to the ED, if indicated.

4. Refer to a dental specialist such as an endodontist (for root canal) or a periodontist, if needed.

J. FOLLOW-UP

1. Assess whether the patient kept the appointment with the dental provider.

2. Encourage ongoing oral health practices as recommended by the ADA and ACOG.

Bibliography

Alwaeli, H. A., & Al-Jundi, S. H. (2005). Periodontal disease awareness among pregnant women and its relationship with socio-demographic variables. *International Journal of Dental Hygiene, 3*, 74–82. https://doi.org/10.1111/j.1601-5037.2005.00121.x

American Academy of Periodontology. (2004). American Academy of Periodontology statement regarding periodontal management of the pregnant patient. *Journal of Periodontology, 75*, 495. https://doi.org/10.1902/jop.2004.75.3.495

American College of Obstetricians and Gynecologists. (2013). Oral health care during pregnancy and through the lifespan (ACOG Committee Opinion #569, reaffirmed 2015). *Obstetrics & Gynecology, 122,* 417–422. https://doi.org/10.1097/01.AOG.0000433007.16843.10

American College of Obstetricians and Gynecologists. (2015). *Your pregnancy and childbirth: Month to month* (Rev. 6th ed.). Author.

American Dental Association. (2013). *Keeping your mouth healthy during pregnancy.* http://www.ada.org/en/~/media/ADA/Publications/Files/FTDP_Revise

Association of State and Territorial Dental Directors. (2020). *Perinatal oral health policy statement. Association of State and Territorial Dental Directors.* https://www.astdd.org/docs/perinatal-oral-health-policy-statement-2-26-2020.pdf

Bertness, J., & Holt, K (Eds.). (2012). *Oral health care during pregnancy: A resource guide. National Maternal and Child Oral Health Resource Center.* https://www.mchoralhealth.org/PDFs/oralhealthpregnancyresguide.pdf

Cibulka, N. J., Forney, S., Goodwin, K., Lazaroff, P., & Sarabia, R. (2011). Improving oral health in low-income pregnant women with a nurse practitioner directed oral care program. *Journal of the American Academy of Nurse Practitioners, 23,* 249–257. https://doi.org/10.1111/j.1745-7599.2011.00606.x

Eke, C., Mask, A., Reusch, C., Vishnevsky, D., & Quinonez, R. B. (2019). *Coverage brief: Improving access to oral health care in pregnancy.* Children's Dental Health Project. https://www.cdhp.org/resources/384-coverage-brief-improving-access-to-oral-health-care-in-pregnancy

Gould, J. M. (2015). *Dental abscess empiric therapy.* http://emedicine.medscape.com/article/2060395-overview

Hunter, L. P., & Yount, S. M. (2011). Oral health and oral health care practices among low-income pregnant women. *Journal of Midwifery Women's Health, 56,* 103–109. https://doi.org/10.1111/j.1542-2011.2011.00041.x

Jared, H., & Boggess, K. A. (2008). Periodontal diseases and adverse pregnancy outcomes: A review of the evidence and implications for clinical practice. *Journal of Dental Hygiene, 82* (3, Summer Suppl.), 3–21.

Jeffcoat, M. K., Geurs, N. C., Reddy, M. S., Cliver, S. P., Goldenberg, R. L., & Hauth, J. C. (2001). Periodontal infection and preterm birth. *Journal of the American Dental Association, 132,* 875–880. https://doi.org/10.14219/jada.archive.2001.0299

Jeffcoat, M. K., Hauth, J. C., Geurs, N. C., Reddy, M. S., Cliver, S. P., Hodgkins, P. M., & Goldenberg, R. L. (2003). Periodontal disease and preterm birth: Results of a pilot intervention study. *Journal of Periodontology, 74,* 1214–1218. https://doi.org/10.1902/jop.2003.74.8.1214

Kloetzel, M. K. (2011). Referrals for dental care during pregnancy. *Journal of Midwifery Women's Health, 56,* 110–117. https://doi.org/10.1111/j.1542-2011.2010.00022.x

Lorenzo, S., Goodman, H., Stemmler, P., Holt, K., & Barzel, R (Eds.). (2019). *The maternal and child health bureau–funded perinatal and infant oral health quality improvement (PIOHQI) initiative 2013–2019: Final report.* National Maternal and Child Oral Health Resource Center. https://www.mchoralhealth.org/PDFs/piohqi-final-report-2019.pdf

Offenbacher, S., Lieff, S., Boggess, K. A., Murtha, A. P., Madianos, P. N., Champagne, C. M. E., McKaig, R. G., Jared, H. L., Mauriello, S. M., Auten, R. L., Herbert, W. N., & Beck, J. D. (2001). Maternal periodontitis and prematurity. Part I: Obstetric outcome of prematurity and growth restriction. *Annals of Periodontology, 6,* 164–174. https://doi.org/10.1902/annals.2001.6.1.164

Ressler-Maerlender, J., Krishna, R., & Robison, V. (2005). Oral health during pregnancy: Current research. *Journal of Women's Health, 14,* 880–882. https://doi.org/10.1089/jwh.2005.14.880

Svirsky, J. (2014). *Oral pyogenic granuloma.* http://emedicine.medscape.com/article/1077040-overview

U.S. Department of Health and Human Services, National Institutes of Health. (2011). *Oral health in America: A report of the surgeon general.* http://www.nidcr.nih.gov/DataStatistics/SurgeonGeneral

U.S. Department of Health and Human Services, National Institutes of Health. (2020). *Dental caries in permanent (adult) teeth.* https://www.nidcr.nih.gov/research/data-statistics/dental-caries/adults

10. Anemia in Pregnancy

NANCY J. CIBULKA | KELLY D. ROSENBERGER | MICHAEL P. ROSENBERGER

Anemia is a common medical disorder of pregnancy. Two of the most common causes of anemia during pregnancy are iron-deficiency and physiologic anemia caused by blood volume expansion greater than the red blood cell (RBC) mass. However, other inherited and acquired causes of anemia should not be overlooked. Iron requirements increase significantly during pregnancy, and, unfortunately, many individuals start pregnancy without sufficient stores to meet the increased demands. Healthcare providers need to educate individuals about the importance of taking an iron supplement during pregnancy and dietary sources of iron. This chapter addresses the assessment of anemia during pregnancy, management, and patient education.

A. DEFINITION, BACKGROUND, AND PHYSIOLOGIC CHANGES

1. Anemia may be characterized in several ways such as by the causative mechanism, whether inherited or acquired, by a reduction in the number of RBCs or the RBC size (mean corpuscular volume [MCV]), which results in decreased ability to carry oxygen to tissues. In modern practice, automated cell counters and MCV are often utilized to classify anemia.

Microcytic anemia has an MCV <80 fL with the most common cause being late iron deficiency with small RBCs that are pale, or hypochromic. Other microcytic anemias include thalassemias, anemia of chronic disease, sideroblastic anemia, copper deficiency anemia, and anemia associated with lead poisoning. It is important to note an absence of microcytosis does not rule out iron-deficiency anemia.

Normocytic anemia has an MCV between 80 and 100 fL. Common causes of normocytic anemia include hemorrhagic anemia, early iron deficiency, and anemia of chronic disease. Other normocytic anemia causes include anemias associated with bone marrow suppression, chronic renal insufficiency, endocrine dysfunction, hypothyroidism, hypopituitarism, hereditary spherocytosis, paroxysmal nocturnal hemoglobinuria, and autoimmune hemolytic anemia.

Macrocytic anemia has an MCV >100 fL with the most common cause being folic acid deficiency. Other causes associated with macrocytic anemia include: vitamin B12 deficiency, reticulocytosis, liver disease, ethanol abuse, acute myelodysplastic syndrome, and drug-induced hemolytic anemia such as from zidovudine (American College of Obstetricians and Gynecologists [ACOG], 2021).

2. The Centers for Disease Control and Prevention (CDC) and the ACOG define anemia during pregnancy as a hemoglobin (Hgb) level <11 g/dL and a hematocrit (Hct) level of 33% in the first and third trimesters, and <10.5 g/dL and 32% in the second trimester.

3. Anemia is a widespread maternal problem during pregnancy. Most cases are caused by iron deficiency. Iron is one of the building blocks of Hgb and RBCs. Hgb binds oxygen molecules and distributes oxygen throughout the body. A decrease in iron levels leads to decreased Hgb production and decreased oxygen delivery to the tissues throughout the body.

4. During pregnancy, blood volume expands by 50%, and total RBC mass expands by 25% during a singleton gestation. Iron-deficiency anemia is primarily caused by an increased demand for iron, especially in the second half of pregnancy, because of RBC mass expansion and rapid fetal growth.

5. A typical Western diet does not contain sufficient iron to meet the increased requirements of pregnancy, placing a large number of pregnant individuals at risk for anemia. Patients are advised to start taking a prenatal vitamin early in pregnancy because of the beneficial effect of folic acid and other vitamins and minerals. Recommend one that includes 17 mg of iron. Some pregnant individuals prefer "gummy" prenatal vitamins, but many of these do not contain any iron, thereby increasing the risk of anemia by the second trimester.

B. RISK FACTORS FOR IRON-DEFICIENCY ANEMIA

1. Low dietary intake of bioavailable iron
2. Adolescence
3. Pregnancy and breastfeeding
4. Low socioeconomic group
5. Ethnicity: African American, Hispanic, Native American, recent immigrant
6. History of iron-deficiency anemia before pregnancy
7. Underweight before pregnancy
8. Disordered eating
9. Multiparity
10. Short interval between pregnancies (<2 years)
11. Pica
12. Blood loss resulting from complications before or during pregnancy
13. Menorrhagia before pregnancy
14. Frequent blood donation
15. Chronic infectious process, including HIV and parasitic infections
16. Hereditary disorder or malabsorptive disorder
17. Alcohol and/or substance abuse and tobacco use
18. Strict vegetarian diet

C. HISTORY

1. Obtain medical, obstetric, dietary, and family histories.

2. Symptoms may be vague and nonspecific or patient may be asymptomatic.

3. Typical symptoms include fatigue, weakness, headache, palpitations, exercise intolerance, light-headedness or dizziness, irritability, lack of concentration, memory changes, depression, and/or cold intolerance.

4. Ask about pica (ingestion of nonfood substance caused by cravings, such as clay, paper, or laundry starch). Pica can be a symptom of iron-deficiency anemia and contributes to worsening anemia.

D. PHYSICAL EXAMINATION

1. Check vital signs for tachycardia, irregular heartbeat, and orthostatic hypotension.

2. Observe oral cavity, skin, hair, and nails for dryness and pallor; pale nail beds; note brittle and spoon-shaped nails; and brittle hair.

3. Auscultate lungs and observe for dyspnea on exertion and shortness of breath at rest.
4. Auscultate heart for systolic flow murmur.
5. Examine the abdomen for hepatosplenomegaly.
6. Examine lower extremities for temperature, edema, and leg ulcers.

E. LABORATORY AND DIAGNOSTIC STUDIES

1. Confirmatory serum Hgb and Hct

First trimester	<11 g/dL Hgb or 33% Hct
Second trimester	<10.5 g/dL Hgb or 32% Hct
Third trimester	<11 g/dL Hgb or 33% Hct

2. Hgb and Hct levels are lower in Black women compared with Caucasian women; therefore, the Institute of Medicine recommends lowering the cut-off levels by 0.8 g/dL for Hgb and 2% for Hct in this population.
3. Additional complete blood count (CBC) results seen in iron-deficiency anemia:
   a. Low MCV <80 fl
   b. Low mean corpuscular Hgb (MCH) and/or MCH concentration (MCHC)
   c. Low RBC distribution width (RDW)
   d. Peripheral blood smear results: Microcytic and hypochromic RBCs; may show variation in shape and size due to poor erythropoiesis
4. Serum ferritin (iron storage) is the most sensitive test for identifying iron deficiency; levels <10 to 15 mg/L confirm iron-deficiency anemia.
5. Serum iron level: (low if <60 mg/dL)
6. Total iron-binding capacity elevated (>400 mg/dL) and low transferrin saturation (<15%; iron transport)
7. Hgb electrophoresis, if applicable
8. Serum lead level, if applicable
9. Stool for occult blood and/or check emesis for blood, if applicable
10. If MCV is high (>100), check B12 and folate levels. High MCV is associated with vitamin B12 and/or folic acid deficiency and with alcoholism. If patient is poorly nourished, anemia may be caused by multiple deficiencies or may be mixed microcytic–macrocytic.

F. DIFFERENTIAL DIAGNOSES FOR MICROCYTIC ANEMIA

1. Iron-deficiency anemia
2. Hemoglobinopathies, including the thalassemias and sickle cell disease or trait
3. Anemia caused by chronic disease or inflammatory process
4. Anemia caused by lead poisoning or copper deficiency
5. Sideroblastic anemia

G. MANAGEMENT

1. The ACOG recommends screening for iron-deficiency anemia during pregnancy. The Institute of Medicine recommends screening for anemia in each trimester of pregnancy. The U.S. Preventive Services Task Force (USPSTF) and the American Academy of Family Physicians (AAFP) advise that the current evidence is insufficient to assess the balance of benefits and harms of screening all pregnant women for iron-deficiency anemia. Check CBC at initial visit; repeat at 24 to 28 weeks and at 36 weeks, if indicated.
2. The ACOG recommends treating women with iron-deficiency anemia with an iron supplement in addition to prenatal vitamins (which contain a small amount of iron).

3. Give patient information about iron-deficiency anemia, causes, treatment, and prevention (www.uptodate.com/contents/anemia-caused-by-low-iron-beyond-the-basics?source=search_result&search=anemia&selectedTitle=1~46).

4. Advise of need for iron supplements daily with at least 60 mg of elemental iron (about 10% is absorbed)

a. Ferrous sulfate 325 mg (65 mg elemental iron and least expensive form) orally, two to three times daily or

b. Ferrous gluconate 300 mg (34 mg elemental iron) orally, two to three times daily or

c. Ferrous fumarate 325 mg (106 mg elemental iron) orally, two to three times daily

d. Iron supplements are best absorbed on an empty stomach or when given with an iron enhancer (see Section G.4.e)

e. Instruct patient on foods that enhance or block iron absorption. Iron enhancers are orange juice, grapefruit, strawberries, broccoli, and peppers, whereas foods that block iron absorption include milk and other dairy products, or calcium-fortified beverages, soy products, tea, caffeinated drinks, eggs, and bran

f. Antacids, proton pump inhibitors, and certain antibiotics inhibit the absorption of iron and should not be given until 2 hours after iron supplement

g. Sustained-release or enteric-coated capsules may be better tolerated but are less efficient sources of iron

h. About 10% to 20% of patients complain of nausea, constipation, and epigastric distress when taking an iron supplement. To reduce side effects, prescribe a smaller dose of elemental iron, switch from tablet to liquid formulation (advise the patient that liquid iron may stain teeth), titrate slowly from every day, to two or three times a day as tolerated, and/or take iron with meals (but this strategy will reduce absorption).

5. Recommend iron-rich foods such as clams, oysters, beef, shrimp, turkey, enriched cereals, beans, and lentils. Information about a healthy diet and good dietary sources of iron is available in Dietary Guidelines for Americans (health.gov/our-work/food-nutrition/current-dietary-guidelines).

6. Supplemental iron >25 mg may decrease zinc absorption. Zinc is an essential nutrient supporting healthy growth and development and is found in many common foods, such as meat, poultry, dairy products, beans, nuts, whole grains, and fortified cereals. Taking iron supplements between meals will help to decrease its effect on zinc absorption.

H. COMPLICATIONS

1. Potential risks to infant

a. Low birth weight

b. Preterm delivery

c. Perinatal mortality (in severe anemia with maternal Hgb <6 g/dL)

2. Risks to mother

a. Postpartum bleeding and infection

b. Ongoing anemia after delivery

c. Postpartum depression

3. Risk to mother if severe deficiency: congestive heart failure, angina, and myocardial infarction (MI)

I. CONSULTATION/REFERRAL

1. Refer to a dietitian for dietary counseling.
2. Consult with or refer to a physician if Hgb <8.5 dL or Hct <26%.
3. Consult or refer if the patient does not respond to iron therapy (and is compliant). Cause for failure to respond will need to be investigated.
4. Consult with a physician, dietician, and/or pharmacist if the patient cannot tolerate or will not take oral iron supplementation. If anemia is severe (Hgb <6.0) or patient is symptomatic, the patient may be a candidate for transfusion or parenteral iron therapy. (Anaphylactic reactions have been reported in 1% of those receiving IV iron dextran.)
5. Consult or refer patients with anemia other than iron-deficiency anemia.

J. FOLLOW-UP

1. In patients with moderate to severe anemia, an increase in reticulocytes will be noted in 7 to 10 days.
2. Repeat Hgb and reticulocyte count after 2 to 4 weeks of iron therapy (with good compliance, Hgb should increase by 1 g/dL and Hct by 3%; retic count should be elevated).
3. Consider continuation of iron supplement for 3 to 4 months postpartum to replenish maternal stores.

Bibliography

American Academy of Family Physicians. (2015). *Clinical preventive service recommendation: Iron deficiency anemia.* https://www.uspreventiveservicestaskforce.org/uspstf/recommendation/iron-deficiency-anemia-in-pregnant-women-screening-and-supplementation

American College of Obstetricians and Gynecologists. (2021). Anemia in pregnancy (ACOG Practice Bulletin #233). *Obstetrics & Gynecology, 138*(2), e55–64. https://doi.org/10.1097/aog.0000000000004477"10.1097/AOG.0000000000004477

Arnett, C., Greenspoon, J. S., & Roman, A. (2013). Hematologic disorders in pregnancy. In A. H. DeCherney, L. Nathan, T. M. Goodwin, N. Laufer, & A. Roman (Eds.), *Current diagnosis & treatment: Obstetrics & gynecology* (11th ed., pp. 543–554). McGraw-Hill.

Auerbach, M. (2020a). *Causes and diagnosis of iron deficiency and iron deficiency anemia in adults. UpToDate.* http://www.uptodate.com

Auerbach, M. (2020b). *Treatment of iron deficiency anemia in adults. UpToDate.* http://www.uptodate.com

Auerbach, M., & Landy, H. J. (2020). Anemia in pregnancy. *UpToDate.* https://www-uptodate-com.proxy.cc.uic.edu/contents/anemia-in-pregnancy?search=anemia%20in%20pregnancy&source=search_result&selectedTitle=1~150&usage_type=default&display_rank=1#H3444017326

Institute of Medicine. (2011). *Clinical preventive services for women: Closing the gaps.* National Academies Press. http://books.nap.edu/openbook.php?record_id=13181

Killip, S., Bennett, J. M., & Chambers, M. D. (2007). Iron deficiency anemia. *American Family Physician, 75*, 671–678.

Office of Dietary Supplements, National Institutes of Health. (2016). *Zinc: Fact sheet for health professionals.* http://ods.od.nih.gov/factsheets/Zinc-HealthProfessional

Shedd, G. C., & Hays, C. N. (2016). The pregnant patient with asthma: Assessment and management. *Journal for Nurse Practitioners, 12*, 1–6. https://doi.org/10.1016/j.nurpra.2015.10.019

Siu, A. L. (2015). Screening for iron deficiency anemia and iron supplementation in pregnant women to improve maternal health and birth outcomes: U.S. Preventive Services Task Force recommendation statement. *Annals of Internal Medicine, 163*, 529–536. https://doi.og/10.7326/M15-1707.

11. Respiratory Illness During Pregnancy: Upper Respiratory Infection, Influenza, and Asthma

NANCY J. CIBULKA | KELLY D. ROSENBERGER

Acute upper respiratory infections (URIs) and asthma commonly affect pregnant individuals. This chapter reviews assessment and management of common cold, influenza, and asthma during pregnancy. Strategies for prevention of illness and patient education are also addressed. Respiratory illness and other sequelae due to COVID-19 will be addressed in a subsequent chapter.

Upper Respiratory Infection/Nasopharyngitis/Common Cold

A. BACKGROUND

1. URIs are the most common acute illnesses in adults. Nasopharyngitis, or common cold, is typically mild and self-limiting.
2. URIs can be caused by a variety of viruses, including rhinovirus, coronavirus, adenovirus, respiratory syncytial virus, and influenza and parainfluenza viruses.
3. True incidence is unknown, but most adults have two to four episodes per year, although colds occur more frequently in young women, possibly because of increased exposure to children.
4. Person-to-person spread of viruses accounts for the majority of URIs. Either airborne droplets are inhaled or direct contact of secretions occurs by touching an infected person or contaminated surface. Viruses are introduced by touching one's eyes or nose. The incubation period is approximately 1 to 5 days.
5. Initial symptoms include local edema, inflammation of nasal mucosa, and increased mucus production. Thus, symptoms of rhinorrhea, nasal congestion, sneezing, and unproductive cough are characteristic. Viral shedding can continue for up to 2 weeks.
6. Hormonal changes during pregnancy produce hyperemia of the nasal and sinus mucosa and an increase in nasal secretions. These changes may increase the risk of URIs and the intensity of symptoms.
7. Colds can occur year-round in the United States but most commonly occur in fall and winter.

B. HISTORY

1. Assess the patient for the following:
   a. Rhinorrhea with clear mucus production
   b. Nasal congestion and stuffiness, postnasal drainage
   c. Sneezing

   d. Nonproductive cough
   e. Mild sore throat
   f. Low-grade fever
   g. Malaise, fatigue
   h. Watery eyes
   i. Mild headache and/or body aches

2. Ask about the onset, duration, course of illness, home remedies, and over-the-counter treatments.
3. Review history for other respiratory conditions, allergic tendencies, asthma, and smoking, and check whether tobacco is used in the home.
4. Ask about any other complaints or health problems.
5. Assess the following for any signs of evolving pregnancy complications:
   a. Fetal movements
   b. Cramps
   c. Contractions
   d. Leaking fluid from vagina
   e. Severe headache
   f. Swelling

C. PHYSICAL EXAMINATION

1. Check vital signs; may have a low-grade fever.
2. Respiration, blood pressure, and pulse should be within normal limits.
3. Observe the general appearance.
4. Inspect and examine eyes for discharge or conjunctivitis; ears for signs of otitis media and/or eustachian tube dysfunction; nose for erythema, swelling of turbinates, character of secretions, and deviated septum; throat for erythema, size of tonsils, exudate, cobblestoning, petechiae, or lesions on pharyngeal mucosa.
5. Palpate and percuss over sinuses for tenderness, and transilluminate if indicated.
6. Palpate lymph nodes in neck for size and tenderness.
7. Auscultate lung fields bilaterally; auscultate heart.
8. Assess for fetal well-being:
   a. Fundal height
   b. Fetal heart tones

D. LABORATORY AND DIAGNOSTIC STUDIES

1. Diagnostic tests are not indicated for a common cold.
2. If indicated, consider rapid strep test if the patient has symptoms of pharyngitis or a history of exposure.
3. Consider monospot screening test if symptoms have been present for 2 weeks or more.

E. DIFFERENTIAL DIAGNOSES

1. Common cold, also known as *acute nasopharyngitis* or *rhinopharyngitis*
2. Allergic rhinitis
3. Group A streptococcal pharyngitis; if the rapid test is positive
4. Acute sinusitis—symptoms present for more than 1 week, facial pain, thick-colored mucus, sinuses do not transilluminate
5. Influenza (see Section II)
6. Asthma (see Section III)
7. Mononucleosis, if the screening test is positive
8. Bronchitis
9. Pneumonia
10. COVID-19

F. COMMON COLD/NASOPHARYNGITIS MANAGEMENT

1. There is no known cure for the common cold. Advise extra rest, and inform the patient that the symptoms may not resolve for up to 2 weeks.
2. Symptomatic treatment to enhance comfort and mucus flow may include the following:
   a. Increase hydration with water, juice, broth, and warm lemon water with honey to thin secretions; avoid alcohol, sodas, and caffeinated drinks.
   b. Do warm saltwater gargle to relieve sore throat (one fourth to a half teaspoon salt in 8 oz of warm water).
   c. Use saline nasal drops and sprays for nasal stuffiness and congestion as needed.
   d. Chicken soup has been found to reduce cold symptoms, especially congestion.
   e. Prescribe a healthy diet with adequate vitamins; avoid supplementation with excess vitamin C and/or zinc during pregnancy.
   f. Increased humidity with a steamy shower may help with mucus flow. If using a humidifier, change the water daily and clean the unit often.
   g. First-generation antihistamines may provide minor relief of cold symptoms but will not shorten the duration of illness and can cause mouth dryness and drowsiness. Suggest chlorpheniramine 4 mg orally or diphenhydramine 25 mg orally every 4 to 6 hours, which are available without a prescription (risk of fetal harm is low based on human data).
3. Advise acetaminophen 650 mg orally every 4 to 6 hours as needed for fever of ≥100.4 °F or pain. Take acetaminophen only when medically indicated and in consultation with provider. Use the lowest possible dose for the shortest period of time.
4. If necessary, cough preparations with the expectorant guaifenesin and the cough suppressant dextromethorphan may be used. However, cough suppressants are not helpful for the treatment of cough caused by a virus, which accounts for up to 90% of cases, thus are typically discouraged for use in pregnant individuals (Larson & File, 2020).
5. Advise pregnant patients to avoid over-the-counter decongestants, multisystem cold/flu/cough remedies, and herbal remedies unless advised by their provider.
6. Avoid antibiotics; they are ineffective against viruses and will not prevent secondary infections. The Centers for Disease Control and Prevention (CDC) and the American College of Physicians recommend that healthcare providers avoid prescribing unnecessary antibiotics to reduce the risk of future antibiotic-resistant infections. Antibiotic treatment guidelines are available (www.cdc.gov/antibiotic-use/community/materials-references/index.html).
7. Self-treatment guidelines are available (www.cdc.gov/antibiotic-use/community/for-patients/index.html).
8. Encourage smoking-cessation intervention, if needed; advise patients to avoid secondhand smoke; educate about the risks of tobacco exposure during pregnancy.
9. Online resources are listed in Appendix A.

G. PATIENT EDUCATION

1. Wash hands frequently with soap and water or use hand sanitizers.
2. Avoid touching the face, especially around the nose, eyes, and mouth.
3. Do not share drinking glasses or utensils with others.
4. Cover mouth and nose when coughing and sneezing; cough into the elbow; use a hand sanitizer or wash hands following a cough or sneeze.

5. Maintain a healthy diet, get adequate sleep, reduce stress, and get regular exercise.
6. Avoid environmental allergens and irritants such as smoke, dust, or chemicals.
7. Stop smoking completely.

H. POTENTIAL COMPLICATIONS

1. Secondary bacterial infection
2. Infection of adjacent structures resulting in otitis media, bronchitis, bronchiolitis, pneumonia, meningitis, and other infections

I. CONSULTATION/REFERRAL

1. Consult with a physician if URI worsens or is not improving beyond 10 days or if any obstetric complication is detected.
2. Refer to an appropriate specialist if indicated by ongoing and/or worsening symptoms.

J. FOLLOW-UP

1. Advise the patient to return if symptoms of bacterial infection occur (ear pain, facial pain, increasing fever, productive cough with mucopurulent sputum, etc.), the condition worsens, or there is no improvement within 10 days.
2. As recommended for ongoing prenatal care

Influenza During Pregnancy and Postpartum

A. DEFINITIONS AND BACKGROUND

1. Influenza is an infectious, acute, and usually self-limiting illness caused by influenza viruses, types A and B, and is commonly known as the "flu."
2. Person-to-person contact accounts for the majority of influenza cases. Either airborne droplets are inhaled or direct contact with secretions occurs by touching an infected person or contaminated surface. Viruses are introduced by touching one's eyes or nose. Incubation is 1 to 4 days.
3. Influenza affects the upper and lower respiratory tract. Major symptoms are coryza, cough, and sore throat, as well as systemic symptoms of fever, body aches, and headache. Acute illness usually lasts about 1 week.
4. Seasonal outbreaks are typical, occurring every winter with varying degrees of severity.
5. According to the CDC, 5% to 20% of the population are infected with influenza each year in the United States, more than 200,000 people are hospitalized, and about 36,000 die from influenza complications.
6. According to the CDC, influenza pandemic occurs when the virus is a new strain for humans, and there is a global outbreak.
7. Because of the physiologic changes of pregnancy, influenza is more likely to cause severe illness and death in pregnant individuals compared to those who are not pregnant, especially in the second and third trimesters. During the 2009 to 2010 H1N1 pandemic, 5% of all deaths in the United States occurred in pregnant individuals (although they represented only 1% of the population). Of all those hospitalized with influenza, approximately 20% were pregnant individuals needing intensive care, including extracorporeal membrane oxygenation (ECMO).
8. The effect of influenza on the fetus is not well studied. However, some studies have found that influenza increases the risk of miscarriage and congenital abnormalities, preterm delivery, and low-birth-weight infants. No congenital anomalies or fetal risks related to the influenza vaccine have been found; the risk of fetal death is reduced when mothers are vaccinated.

B. HISTORY

1. Assess the patient for the following:
   a. Rapid onset of moderate to high fever (101 °F–103 °F)
   b. Rhinorrhea, nasal stuffiness
   c. Nonproductive cough, dyspnea, shortness of breath
   d. Sore throat
   e. Conjunctivitis, burning sensation, photophobia
   f. Headache
   g. Malaise, fatigue
   h. Muscle and/or joint aches, back pain
   i. Chills
   j. Anorexia
   k. Abdominal pain, nausea, and vomiting (not typical in seasonal influenza)
2. Ask about the onset, duration, course of illness, home remedies, and over-the-counter treatments.
3. Review history for other respiratory conditions, such as asthma or allergic tendencies, and note whether the patient smokes.
4. Review history for other health problems such as preexisting cardiac or immune system problems.
5. Ask about the shortness of breath and any other complaints.
6. Determine whether the patient received a flu vaccine (not 100% effective in prevention).
7. Assess for any signs of evolving pregnancy complications:
   a. Fetal movements
   b. Cramps
   c. Contractions
   d. Leaking fluid from the vagina
   e. Severe headache
   f. Swelling

C. PHYSICAL EXAMINATION

1. Check vital signs; may have fever and tachycardia.
2. Observe general appearance and for signs of dehydration.
3. Inspect and examine eyes for conjunctival erythema and watery or mucopurulent drainage; inspect ears for signs of otitis media and/or eustachian tube dysfunction; inspect nose for erythema, swelling of turbinates, and character of secretions; and inspect throat for erythema, size of tonsils, exudate, and appearance of pharyngeal mucosa.
4. Palpate lymph nodes in the neck for tenderness and size.
5. Auscultate lung fields bilaterally for crackles or rales auscultate heart for rubs, tachycardia, murmurs, or extra sounds.
6. Perform abdominal examination (would expect normal examination).
7. Perform neurological examination; assess the level of consciousness and for signs of meningeal irritation (e.g., nuchal rigidity and Brudzinski's and Kernig's signs).
8. Assess for fetal well-being; check fundal height, fetal heart tones, and fetal movement.

D. LABORATORY AND DIAGNOSTIC STUDIES

1. Symptoms of the flu and COVID-19 are similar, making a diagnosis difficult based on symptoms alone, molecular assays including the reverse transcription polymerase chain reaction (RT-PCR) test and other nucleic acid

amplification tests from nasopharyngeal swab or aspirate are the gold standard for diagnosis of influenza.

2. Rapid influenza diagnostic tests (RIDTs) can be helpful and produce quick results. However, sensitivity and specificity vary according to the manufacturer, and false negatives are fairly common. The Infectious Disease Society of America (IDSA) currently recommends the use of rapid influenza molecular assays (RT-PCR) over RIDTs for detection of influenza in outpatient settings. IDSA recommends RT-PCR or other molecular assays for hospitalized patients (academic.oup.com/cid/advance-article/doi/10.1093/cid/ciy866/5251935).

3. Viral ribonucleic acid (RNA) culture from nasopharyngeal secretions (instead of PCR test); note culture results may take 1 to 3 days. Thus, they do not yield timely results to inform clinical management.

4. Pulse oximetry

5. Complete blood count (CBC) if indicated by severity of illness; may show leukopenia

6. Chest x-ray, if there is evidence of pneumonia or pericarditis

7. Continuous fetal monitoring if indicated by the patient's condition

E. DIFFERENTIAL DIAGNOSES

1. Influenza, type A or B
2. URI, nasopharyngitis, or common cold
3. Infectious mononucleosis
4. Viral or strep pharyngitis
5. Bronchitis
6. Pneumonia
7. COVID-19

F. PREVENTION OF INFLUENZA

1. The CDC Advisory Committee on Immunization Practices (ACIP) recommends that all individuals who are pregnant or will be pregnant during influenza season should receive inactivated influenza vaccine (IIV) or recombinant influenza vaccine (RIV; if age 18 or older) in any trimester (including the first trimester). Vaccine should not be given to individuals with a severe allergy to any vaccine component. Severe reactions are anaphylaxis, high fever, tachycardia, weakness, and altered mental status. Reaction related to egg allergy is believed to be extremely rare. Patients with an egg allergy may receive the vaccine, but it should be given in a setting that is equipped to manage a severe allergic reaction, and the patient should be monitored for 30 minutes. Have the patient review the CDC vaccine information statement prior to administering the vaccine (available at: www.cdc.gov/flu/prevent/keyfacts.htm). Common side effects of the vaccine include sore arm, redness or swelling at the injection site, headache, low-grade fever, and nausea.

2. Influenza vaccine given to the mother during pregnancy protects the infant for up to 6 months after birth. CDC advises that all adults and children older than the age of 6 months should be vaccinated; therefore, the entire family and all caretakers or anyone likely to be in close contact with the mother and infant should receive a flu vaccine yearly, unless it is contraindicated because of serious illness or severe allergic reaction.

3. In the event the pregnant individual was not vaccinated during the antepartum period, the influenza vaccine may be given during the postpartum period.

4. No studies have shown an increased risk of maternal complications or adverse fetal outcomes associated with the IIV during pregnancy.

5. A thimerosal-free formulation of the influenza vaccine is available; however, there is no evidence that thimerosal is harmful when used during pregnancy or is associated with autism.

6. Live, attenuated influenza vaccine (LAIV) administered by nasal spray is not recommended during pregnancy. LAIV is acceptable during the postpartum period but has not been approved for pregnant or breastfeeding women.

7. In addition to the flu vaccine, pregnant individuals should take precautions to reduce or avoid exposure by frequent handwashing and use of hand sanitizers, avoiding contact with infected individuals, avoiding crowds during peak epidemics, and maintaining a healthy lifestyle. See CDC Healthy Habits at www.cdc.gov/flu/prevent/actions-prevent-flu.htm.

8. If significant exposure has occurred, consider antiviral prophylaxis or early treatment as soon as the symptoms of influenza develop (see Section II.G).

9. CDC has specific recommendations addressing the health concerns of pregnant individuals and vaccinations before, during, and after pregnancy, including the influenza vaccine at: (www.cdc.gov/vaccines/pregnancy/index.html?CDC_AA_refVal=https%3A%2F%2Fwww.cdc.gov%2Fvaccines%2Fadults%2Frec-vac%2Fpregnant.html).

10. The CDC ACIP and the Healthcare Infection Control Practices Advisory Committee (HICPAC) recommend all healthcare providers in the United States are vaccinated annually against influenza (www.cdc.gov/flu/professionals/healthcareworkers.htm).

G. MANAGEMENT

1. Advise patients to contact their healthcare provider right away if flu-like symptoms develop. If they have any difficulty in breathing or shortness of breath, new pain or pressure in the chest, are unable to tolerate liquids, or have any signs of dehydration, abnormal mental status, uterine contractions, or decreased fetal movement, recommend that they must go to the hospital immediately. A helpful algorithm for assessment and care published by the American College of Obstetricians and Gynecologists (ACOG) and the Society of Maternal–Fetal Medicine is available: (www.acog.org/programs/immunization-for-women?utm_source=ImmunizationforWomen&utm_medium=Domain&utm_campaign=DomainRedirects).

2. Acetaminophen 650 mg orally every 4 hours is advised as needed for systemic symptoms and to reduce fevers of 101 °F or more. Hyperthermia is a risk factor for adverse pregnancy outcomes.

3. Influenza antiviral treatment is recommended for those at a higher risk of influenza complications, including individuals who are pregnant or within 2 weeks after delivery.

4. Two medications are approved by the Food and Drug Administration (FDA) for outpatient treatment in the United States. Oseltamivir (risk of embryo-fetal toxicity not expected based on available data) and zanamivir (caution advised as there are inadequate human data available to assess risk) are both effective against influenza types A and B. A third medication, peramivir 600 mg, is approved for intravenous use given over 15 to 30 minutes as a single dose.

- **a.** Oseltamivir 75 mg orally twice daily for 5 days
- **b.** Zanamivir 20 mg (two inhalations) twice daily for 5 days; avoid in those with respiratory diseases such as asthma or chronic obstructive pulmonary disease (COPD)

5. The same medications are used for chemoprophylaxis following significant exposure. Antiviral treatment is recommended to be started as early as possible, ideally within 48 hours of symptom onset, but it may still provide some benefit if started later. Do not wait for laboratory confirmation of influenza to start chemoprophylaxis. (Peramivir is not used for prophylaxis.)

a. Oseltamivir 75 mg orally once daily for 7 to 10 days

b. Zanamivir 20 mg (two inhalations) once daily for 7 to 10 days. Avoid in those with respiratory diseases such as asthma or COPD.

6. Healthcare providers are cautioned to review online CDC recommendations often (www.cdc.gov/flu/professionals/index.htm), as resistance to antiviral medications can develop, which will then result in new recommendations for treatment and chemoprophylaxis.

a. Advise measures for symptomatic relief, stressing the need for adequate fluids and plenty of rest as well as preventing spread; self-care tips are available (www.cdc.gov/nonpharmaceutical-interventions)

b. Inform patients of potential complications and ask them to seek immediate care in case of difficulty in breathing or shortness of breath, pain or pressure in the chest or abdomen, dizziness, confusion, severe vomiting, high fever not responding to acetaminophen, decreased fetal movements, vaginal bleeding, and signs of preterm labor or rupture of membranes.

7. Online patient resources for influenza prevention and self-care are available in Appendix A.

H. COMPLICATIONS

1. Pneumonia

2. Respiratory failure

3. Bronchitis

4. Secondary bacterial infection such as otitis media or sinusitis

5. Possible adverse pregnancy outcomes such as miscarriage, congenital defects, low-birth-weight infants, preterm delivery

6. Maternal death (usually from respiratory failure/pneumonia)

I. CONSULTATION/REFERRAL

1. Consult with a physician if severe illness, influenza complications, and/or any obstetric complications are detected.

2. Hospitalization is indicated for severe illness.

J. FOLLOW-UP

1. Advise the patient to return if symptoms of bacterial infection occur (ear pain, facial pain, increasing fever, productive cough with mucopurulent sputum, etc.), if the condition worsens, or there is no improvement within 7 days.

2. As recommended for ongoing prenatal care

Asthma in Pregnancy

A. BACKGROUND

1. Asthma is a common chronic lung disease characterized by the inflammation and narrowing of airways with increased airway reactivity to various triggers. Symptoms are recurrent and include wheezing, chest tightness, coughing, and shortness of breath. During pregnancy, acute exacerbations may occur in 20% to 36% of pregnant individuals.

2. The goal of current therapy is to reduce airway inflammation.

3. Asthma complicates approximately 3% to 8% of pregnancies. Poorly controlled asthma may increase the risk for prematurity, preeclampsia, growth restriction, and other adverse pregnancy outcomes.

4. According to the National Heart, Lung, and Blood Institute's Expert Panel Report 3 (EPR-3), "Guidelines for the Diagnosis and Management of Asthma," asthma is classified by severity in symptoms, nighttime awakening, interference with normal activity, and lung function (www.nhlbi.nih.gov/health-topics/guidelines-for-diagnosis-management-of-asthma). Table 11.1 provides the criteria for the four asthma classes:
   a. Mild intermittent
   b. Mild persistent
   c. Moderate persistent
   d. Severe persistent

5. It is safer for pregnant individuals to be treated with asthma medications than for them to have symptoms and acute exacerbations. Use a stepwise approach to treatment, based on asthma severity classification, as detailed in "Guidelines for the Diagnosis and Management of Asthma" (www.nhlbi.nih.gov/health-topics/guidelines-for-diagnosis-management-of-asthma).

6. The effect of pregnancy on asthma is variable; asthma severity seems to improve in one quarter of cases and worsens in one third, remaining unchanged in the rest.

B. RISK FACTORS

1. Exposure to allergens such as dust, dust mites, animal dander, cockroaches, mold spores, and pollens from trees, grasses, and flowers
2. Exposure to irritants such as smoke, tobacco, air pollution, chemicals, or dust in the workplace; perfumes; air fresheners; cleaning products; and sprays
3. Upper respiratory viral infections or sinusitis
4. Exposure to cold temperatures
5. Physical activity and exercise
6. Sulfites in foods and drinks
7. Gastroesophageal reflux disease (GERD)
8. Abrupt change in weather
9. Overweight, obesity, and/or excessive first-trimester weight gain

TABLE 11.1 CLASSIFICATION OF ASTHMA SEVERITY IN PREGNANT PATIENTS

ASTHMA SEVERITY	SYMPTOM FREQUENCY	NIGHTTIME AWAKENING	INTERFERENCE WITH ACTIVITY	FEV1 OR PEAK FLOW
Intermittent	≤2 days per week	≤2 times per month	None	>80%
Mild persistent	>2 days per week	>2 times per month	Minor limitation	>80%
Moderate persistent	Daily symptoms	More than once per week	Some limitation	60%–80%
Severe persistent	Throughout the day	≥4 times per week	Extremely limited	<60%

FEV1, forced expiratory volume in 1 second.

Source: National Heart Lung and Blood Institute, National Institutes of Health, & U.S. Department of Health and Human Services. (2020a). *What is asthma?* https://www.nhlbi.nih.gov/health/health-topics/topics/asthma/

C. HISTORY

1. Ask about the personal history of asthma and allergies or any allergic disorder, medications used, and usual peak flow measurements.

2. Determine the effect of asthma on any prior pregnancies.

3. Determine whether there is a history of any previous use of oral steroids, hospitalizations, intubations, or ICU admissions; get records if needed.

4. Review family history for allergies and asthma.

5. Assess typical symptoms: wheezing, chest tightness, cough, and shortness of breath. Ask about onset; duration; precipitating, aggravating, and alleviating factors; and course of illness.

6. Ask about recent fever, URI, sinusitis, or GERD.

7. Ask how often symptoms occur, about the frequency of nighttime awakenings, and about any interference with normal activity.

8. If medications were used for symptom treatment, assess their effectiveness.

9. Note whether the patient smokes or whether there is tobacco use in the home.

D. PHYSICAL EXAMINATION

1. Obtain vital signs: Pulse and respirations may be elevated.

2. Inspect eyes for allergic shiners or watery drainage; inspect ears for signs of otitis media and/or eustachian tube dysfunction; inspect nose for erythema, swelling of turbinates, the character of secretions, and nasal polyps; inspect throat for erythema, size of tonsils, exudate, and appearance of pharyngeal mucosa.

3. Inspect chest and thorax for hyper-expansion; auscultate for airflow, wheezes, rales, or other adventitious sounds or prolonged expiration.

4. Auscultate heart for rubs, tachycardia, murmurs, or extra sounds.

5. Inspect the skin for eczema or dermatitis.

6. Assess for fetal well-being: fundal height, fetal heart tones, and movement.

E. LABORATORY AND DIAGNOSTIC STUDIES

1. Measure peak expiratory flow rate (PEFR) using flow meter reading. Record the best of three attempts at each prenatal visit. The "personal best" varies according to age and height, but expected values may range between 380 and 500 L/min for pregnant individuals with well-controlled asthma.

2. Spirometry if needed to confirm the diagnosis or to assess forced vital capacity (FVC) and forced expiratory volume in 1 second (FEV1) in moderate or severe persistent asthma

3. May assess response to therapy by measuring PEFR or FEV1 before and after the patient inhales a short-acting beta-adrenergic medication

4. Chest x-ray and CBC are needed only if necessary to exclude other diagnoses or infection

5. Pulse oximetry if indicated

6. Continuous fetal monitoring if indicated by the patient's condition

F. DIFFERENTIAL DIAGNOSES

1. Asthma

2. Other allergic disorders

3. URI

4. Bronchitis

5. Cough caused by post-viral syndrome, environmental irritants, tobacco use or exposure, side effect to medication (angiotensin-converting enzyme [ACE] inhibitors), or stress

6. Pneumonia
7. GERD
8. COPD
9. Pulmonary emboli
10. Congestive heart failure (CHF)
11. Benign dyspnea of pregnancy
12. Panic or anxiety
13. COVID-19

G. MANAGEMENT

1. Education is the key to good asthma control during pregnancy. Information for patients is available (www.uptodate.com/contents/asthma-and-pregnancy-beyond-the-basics). Additional online resources for patients are listed in Appendix A.
2. Advise patients to avoid asthma triggers and unnecessary exposures to allergens and to review environmental controls. More information for patients is available (www.uptodate.com/contents/trigger-avoidance-in-asthma-beyond-the-basics).
3. Educate patients that short-acting beta 2-agonists (SABA), such as albuterol, are used for "rescue" when acute symptoms develop. Use up to a maximum of 12 puffs in 24 hours. Long-acting beta 2-agonists (LABA) and inhaled corticosteroids (ICSs) are maintenance medications and should be used on a daily basis as prescribed.
4. Asthma medications are generally safe to use during pregnancy. Risk of teratogenicity is low for ICS, SABA, and LABA agents and for montelukast based on animal and/or human data. Less is known about their safety during breastfeeding. Management guidelines are based on asthma severity classification:
   a. Mild intermittent—SABA, albuterol is preferred, one to two puffs every 4 to 6 hours as needed for acute symptoms.
   b. Mild persistent—low-dose ICSs, such as budesonide, two puffs twice daily. SABA as needed for acute symptoms; double the ICS for self-limiting conditions such as allergen exposure or URI.
   c. Moderate persistent—medium-dose ICSs or medium-dose ICS and LABA such as salmeterol 50 mcg/actuation dry powder inhalation or formoterol 4.5 mcg per actuation in combination with ICS such as budesonide, one puff twice daily. SABA as needed for acute symptoms.
   d. Severe persistent—high-dose ICSs and either LABA or montelukast if no relief with salmeterol or formoterol and, if needed, oral corticosteroids (prednisone)
   e. Alternative regimens may include montelukast and/or zafirlukast with recent limited but reassuring accumulated evidence. The clinical utilization of theophylline during pregnancy has the potential for altered metabolism, need to monitor drug levels, and the potential for fetal tachycardia and/or irritability; thus, this drug is not often used. Cromolyn availability varies, and one study reported fetal musculoskeletal abnormalities after maternal use; thus, this drug is not widely utilized.
5. Develop an asthma action plan with the patient. Templates are available online at: (www.cdc.gov/asthma/actionplan.html?CDC_AA_refVal=https%3A%2F%2Fwww.cdc.gov%2Fasthma%2Ftools_for_control.htm).
6. Teach patients how to use a peak flow meter and encourage them to check peak flows daily and bring the results to visits. Directions and a video for using a peak flow meter are available: (www.lung.org/lung-health-diseases/

lung-disease-lookup/asthma/living-with-asthma/managing-asthma/measuring-your-peak-flow-rate).

7. Review patient instructions for the use of inhalers and spacers, which are available with videos and other resources at: (www.lung.org/lung-health-diseases/lung-disease-lookup/asthma/patient-resources-and-videos).

8. The use of SABA more than twice a week indicates that asthma is not well controlled, and therapy may need to be stepped up to the next level.

9. Inhaled albuterol is the first choice for rescue therapy during pregnancy. Patients may take up to two treatments (two to six puffs) of inhaled albuterol or nebulized albuterol at 20-minute intervals for mild to moderate symptoms. Counsel patients to start the rescue treatment at home when an exacerbation occurs. If symptoms resolve and PEFR is 80% or better than personal best, the patient can continue normal activity. If symptoms persist or do not resolve adequately, seek medical attention immediately.

10. Oral corticosteroids may be prescribed for an acute exacerbation, for example, prednisone 40 to 60 mg orally in a single or divided dose for 3 to 10 days. Use with caution because of the risk of intrauterine growth retardation based on human data and risk of teratogenicity based on animal data. However, benefit may exceed risk.

11. Serial growth scans by ultrasound starting at 32 weeks' gestation and twice-a-week nonstress tests are advised for pregnant individuals with moderate or severe persistent asthma, poorly controlled asthma, or after a severe exacerbation.

12. Daily fetal movements (kick counts) are recommended for all pregnant individuals (see Appendix A).

13. Pregnant individuals with asthma should receive trivalent or quadrivalent IIV in any trimester; the pneumococcal vaccine is recommended for adults with asthma but not during pregnancy or while breastfeeding as safety has not been confirmed.

14. Smoking-cessation counseling and a smoke-free environment are essential.

H. COMPLICATIONS

1. Acute asthma exacerbation
2. Respiratory failure
3. Adverse pregnancy outcome: prematurity, preeclampsia, growth restriction
4. Status asthmaticus
5. Maternal death

I. CONSULTATION/REFERRAL

1. Consult with a physician and refer for care if there is moderate or severe persistent asthma or if any obstetric complication is detected.
2. Consult with the physician if the patient has a history of frequent ED visits, hospitalization, intubation, and/or ICU admissions for asthma.
3. Consult with the physician if mild asthma is not responding to treatment.
4. Refer to ED for acute, severe exacerbations or if PEFR is 70% or less than baseline or if asthma symptoms are unresponsive to treatment.
5. Refer to an asthma specialist as needed for poorly controlled asthma and/or specialized testing and management.

J. FOLLOW-UP

1. Follow up with the patient within 2 to 5 days after treatment for an acute asthma exacerbation. Patients discharged after an acute asthma exacerbation should continue SABA two to four puffs every 3 to 4 hours as needed and continue prednisone and/or ICS as ordered.
2. Follow up with the patient 2 weeks after initiating treatment for mild or moderate persistent asthma.
3. Follow up with patients as soon as possible if they are experiencing persistent and/or worsening symptoms.
4. Follow up as recommended for ongoing prenatal care.

Bibliography

Ali, Z., Nilas, L., & Ulrik, C. S. (2018). Excessive gestational weight gain in first trimester is a risk factor for exacerbation of asthma during pregnancy: A prospective study of 1283 pregnancies. *The Journal of Allergy and Clinical Immunology, 141,* 761–767. https://doi.org/10.1016/j.jaci.2017.03.040

American College of Obstetricians and Gynecologists. (2008). Asthma in pregnancy (ACOG Practice Bulletin #90, and reaffirmed 2016). *Obstetrics & Gynecology, 111,* 457–464. https://doi.org/10.1097/AOG.0b013e3181665ff4

American College of Obstetricians and Gynecologists. (2013). Ethical issues in pandemic influenza planning concerning pregnant women (Committee Opinion No. 563, and reaffirmed 2016). *Obstetrics & Gynecology, 121,* 1138–1143. https://doi.org/10.1097/01.AOG.0000429660.31589.6a

Barclay, L. (2008). *New guidelines issued for management of asthma during pregnancy.* http://www.medscape.org/viewarticle/569862

Centers for Disease Control and Prevention. (2020a). *Be antibiotics aware.* https://www.cdc.gov/antibiotic-use/index.html

Centers for Disease Control and Prevention. (2020b). *Flu and nonpharmaceutical interventions.* http://www.cdc.gov/nonpharmaceutical-interventions

Centers for Disease Control and Prevention. (2020c). *Nonspecific upper respiratory tract infection—Fact sheet.* http://www.cdc.gov/getsmart/community/materials-references/print-materials/hcp/adult-tract-infection.pdf

Centers for Disease Control and Prevention. (2020d). *Pregnant women & influenza (flu).* http://www.cdc.gov/flu/protect/vaccine/pregnant.htm

Centers for Disease Control and Prevention. (2020e). *Seasonal influenza (flu).* http://www.cdc.gov/flu

Gerald, L. B., & Carr, T. F. (2020). *Patient education: How to use a peak flow meter (beyond the basics).* http://www.uptodate.com/contents/how-to-use-a-peak-flow-meter-beyond-the-basics

Gerald, L. B., & Dhand, R. (2020). *Patient education: Asthma inhaler techniques in adults (beyond the basics).* http://www.uptodate.com/contents/asthma-inhaler-techniques-in-adults-beyond-the-basics

Harris, A. M., Hicks, L. A., & Qaseem, A. (2016). High value care task force of the American College of Physicians and for the Centers for Disease Control and Prevention. Appropriate antibiotic use for acute respiratory tract infection in adults: Advice for high value from the American College of Physicians and for the Centers for Disease Control and Prevention. *Annals of Internal Medicine, 164*(6), 425–435. https://doi.org/10.7326/M15-1840

Jamieson, D. J., & Rasmussen, S. A. (2016). *Influenza and pregnancy.* http://www.uptodate.com

Larson, L., & File, T. M. (2020). *Treatment of respiratory infections in pregnant women.* http://www.uptodate.com

Little, M. (2106). *Asthma in pregnancy.* http://emedicine.medscape.com/article/796274-overview

Mayo Clinic Staff. (2021). *Cold remedies: What works, what doesn't, what can't hurt.* https://www.mayoclinic.org/diseases-conditions/common-cold/in-depth/cold-remedies/art-20046403

Meneghetti, A. (2020). *Upper respiratory tract infection.* http://emedicine.medscape.com/article/302460-overview

Miller, R. L. (2020). *Patient education: Trigger avoidance in asthma (beyond the basics).* http://www.uptodate.com/contents/trigger-avoidance-in-asthma-beyond-the-basics

Murphy, V. E., Jensen, M. E., Powell, H., & Gibson, P. G. (2017). Influence of maternal body mass index and macrophage activation on asthma exacerbations in pregnancy. *The Journal of Allergy and Clinical Immunology, 5,* 981–987. https://doi.org/10.1016/j.jaip.2017.03.040

National Heart Lung and Blood Institute, National Institutes of Health, & U.S. Department of Health and Human Services. (2020a). *What is asthma?* http://www.nhlbi.nih.gov/health/health-topics/topics/asthma/

National Heart Lung and Blood Institute, National Institutes of Health, & U.S. Department of Health and Human Services. (2020b). *2020 focused updates to the Asthma Management Guidelines: A report from the National Asthma Education and Prevention Program Coordinating Committee Expert Panel Working Group* .Retrieved from: https://www.nhlbi.nih.gov/health-topics/all-publications-and-resources/2020-focused-updates-asthma-management-guidelines

Schatz, M., & Weinberger, S. E. (2020). *Management of asthma during pregnancy*. http://www.uptodate.com

Shedd, G. C. (2016). The pregnant patient with asthma: Assessment and management. *Journal for Nurse Practitioners, 12*, 1–8. https://doi.org/10.1016/j.nurpra.2015.10.019

Weinberger, S. E., Schatz, M., & Dombrowski, M. P. (2020). *Patient education: Asthma and pregnancy (beyond the basics)*. http://www.uptodate.com/contents/asthma-and-pregnancy-beyond-the-basics

Weinberger, S. E., & Schatz, M. (2020). *Asthma in pregnancy: Clinical course and physiologic changes*. http://www.uptodate.com

12. Asymptomatic Bacteriuria and Urinary Tract Infection in Pregnancy

MARY LEE BARRON | KELLY D. ROSENBERGER | AMY M. SEIBERT

Urinary Tract Infections in Pregnancy

A. DEFINITION

1. Asymptomatic bacteriuria (ASB) is a microbiologic diagnosis that indicates the presence of a positive urine culture in an asymptomatic person. In the literature, bacteriuria may be defined as a single organism identified in the urine in any amount, but more specifically at a colony count of equal to or greater than 10^5 (100,000) colony-forming units per milliliter (CFU/mL).

2. Urinary tract infection (UTI) is defined as either a lower tract (acute cystitis) or upper tract (acute pyelonephritis) infection. Cystitis is bacteriuria in the presence of urinary symptoms.

B. ETIOLOGY

1. The smooth muscle relaxation caused by progesterone and subsequent ureteral dilatation (occurring in about 90% of pregnant women) that accompany pregnancy may facilitate the ascent of bacteria from the bladder to the kidney. Decreased bladder and ureteral tone contribute to urinary stasis, allowing bacteria to proliferate. Mechanical compression from the enlarging uterus may lead to hydroureter and hydronephrosis. Pregnancy-induced glycosuria and proteinuria also may facilitate bacterial growth. As a result, bacteriuria has up to a 40% greater likelihood of progressing to pyelonephritis in pregnant individuals than in nonpregnant individuals.

2. *Escherichia coli* is the most commonly identified causative organism, responsible for up to 80% of positive urine cultures during pregnancy. Other culprits include *Klebsiella*, *Enterobacter*, *Proteus*, *Pseudomonas*, and less common gram-negative organisms (Glaser & Schaeffer, 2015.)

3. Group B Streptococcus (GBS), a gram-positive organism, is responsible for up to 10% of ASB cases during pregnancy and is a notable leading cause of newborn infection. Traditionally, GBS-positive bacteriuria has been treated at any identified colony count due to the perceived risk of newborn infection and questionable evidence that GBS is associated with increased rates of pyelonephritis and preterm birth. Updated research has shown no significant increased risk due to GBS compared to any other source of bacteriuria (Rosenberger, Seibert, & Hormig, 2020).

C. EPIDEMIOLOGY

1. Bacteriuria occurs in 2% to 10% of pregnancies. Bacteriuria often develops in the first month of pregnancy and is often associated with a reduction in the ability to concentrate urine, suggesting the involvement of the kidney.

2. Bacteriuria has been associated with an increased risk of pyelonephritis. The associations of ASB with preterm birth, low birth weight, and perinatal mortality that were noted in earlier studies are questionable due to the poor methodological quality of the studies and lack of adjustment for demographic and social factors (Matuszkiewicz-Rowińska et al., 2015).

3. Untreated ASB in pregnancy can progress to overt cystitis, UTI, or acute pyelonephritis in up to 40% of pregnant individuals with a positive urine culture.

4. Cystitis occurs in 1% to 4% of pregnant individuals, a similar rate in the nonpregnant population.

5. Acute pyelonephritis is one of the most common medical complications of pregnancy and is the primary nonobstetric reason for hospitalization. It occurs in 1% of pregnant individuals. Before routine screening for ASB became the standard of care, pyelonephritis had an incidence of 4% or higher during pregnancy (Glaser & Schaeffer, 2015). Up to 90% of cases are reported to occur in the second and third trimesters. Pyelonephritis may result in significant maternal morbidity as well as fetal morbidity and mortality and is the leading cause of septic shock during pregnancy (Gomi, et al., 2015). It is also an independent risk factor for preterm birth.

D. RISK FACTORS

1. History of UTI
2. Urinary tract anomalies
3. Low socioeconomic status
4. Sexual activity
5. Young age
6. Sickle cell disease or trait
7. Diabetes mellitus, pregestational
8. Catheterization
9. Multiparity (for ASB) or nulliparity (for pyelonephritis)
10. Smoking

Asymptomatic Bacteriuria

A. HISTORY

1. No symptoms

B. PHYSICAL EXAMINATION

1. Within normal limits

C. LABORATORY AND DIAGNOSTIC STUDIES

1. Screening should be performed at the first prenatal visit or at 12 to 16 weeks' gestation. According to Moore et al. (2018), a patient's preference regarding antibiotic treatment for ASB should be considered in determining if to perform the urine culture at all.

2. Rescreening is not performed in low-risk individuals but can be considered in those at high risk (urinary tract anomalies, hemoglobin S, or preterm labor).

3. Urine dipstick may be positive for protein, leukocyte esterase, nitrites, and/or blood.

4. Microscopic analysis may show white blood cells (WBCs), red blood cells (RBCs), or bacteria.

5. Gram stain of uncentrifuged urine may show gram-negative bacilli or gram-positive cocci.

6. Urine culture on clean-catch midstream-voided specimen shows the growth of single bacterial strain at a colony count ≥10^5 CFU/mL. For the most accurate diagnosis, urine culture on two consecutive urine specimens with isolation of the same bacteria strain ≥10 CFU/mL or a single catheterized specimen with one bacterial species at 10^2 is the gold standard. However, according to the U.S. Preventative Services Task Force and American College of Obstetricians and Gynecologists (ACOG), a single voided urine specimen with a positive culture is sufficient to initiate antibiotic treatment.

7. GBS bacteriuria is treated no differently than bacteriuria from any other source, with antibiotics prescribed only for colony counts ≥10^5 CFU/mL, or in the presence of urinary symptoms. GBS bacteriuria always indicates genital colonization and is an indication for prophylactic antibiotic treatment during labor to prevent vertical transmission from mother to newborn during delivery (ACOG, 2020). A rectovaginal swab between 36 and 37 6/7 weeks gestational age is not necessary for individuals who have GBS isolated in the urine during pregnancy.

D. TREATMENT

Generally, penicillins and cephalosporins (Food and Drug Administration [FDA]) are safe in pregnancy. However, drugs with very high protein binding, such as ceftriaxone, may be inappropriate the day before parturition because of the possibility of bilirubin displacement and subsequent kernicterus. Nitrofurantoin and sulfonamides have been associated with birth defects. Therefore, it is prudent to avoid using nitrofurantoin in the first trimester if a safe and effective antibiotic is available. Nitrofurantoin has also been reported to cause hemolytic anemia in the mother and fetus with glucose-6-phosphate-dehydrogenase deficiency, a risk estimated in <0.01% of cases, and its use should be avoided near term for this reason. Sulfonamides inhibit folate synthesis and should be avoided during the first trimester due to possible teratogenesis, as well as in the last days before delivery because of their association with neonatal hyperbilirubinemia (Glaser & Schaeffer, 2015). Trimethoprim is also avoided in the first trimester because of a possible association with birth defects. Again, as long as another antibiotic is available, it is prudent to avoid its use.

Concerns regarding the teratogenicity of fluoroquinolones have resulted in their restricted use during gestation. Quinolone use has been associated with birth defects in animal studies, but similar effects have not been seen in humans. Because of the relatively higher cost of these agents and the concern about the emergence of antibiotic-resistant pathogens with frequent use, fluoroquinolones are not prescribed as first-line agents in uncomplicated UTIs. In cases of infections with resistant micropathogens or complicated UTIs during pregnancy, the benefits of fluoroquinolone use outweigh the risks to the fetus.

Widmer, Lopez, Gülmezoglu, Mignini, and Roganti (2015), in a systematic evidence-based review, assessed the effects of different durations of treatment for ASB in pregnancy. Based on high-quality evidence, a 4- to 7-day regimen of antibiotics was shown to have a high cure rate and less incidence of low birth weight than a single dose treatment. The authors concluded that ASB in pregnancy should be treated with a 3- to 7-day regimen of antibiotics until more data become available. The authors did note a longer treatment duration had the drawback of nonadherence for lower income patients. In low-resource settings where compliance is an issue, a single treatment that can be administered onsite should be considered. In 2016, the World Health Organization (WHO) issued recommendations for a 7-day antibiotic regimen for all pregnant individuals with ASB to prevent persistent bacteriuria, preterm birth, and low birth weight.

1. The duration of antimicrobial therapy should be 3 to 7 days, except for Fosfomycin.

2. Fluoroquinolones should be avoided if alternatives are available narrow-spectrum antibiotics should be prescribed based on the specific sensitivities when possible.

3. Periodic screening for recurrent bacteriuria should be undertaken after therapy if daily prophylactic therapy is not instituted.

4. No recommendation can be made for or against the routine repeated screening of culture-negative patients in the later phase of pregnancy.

5. If organism is susceptible and gestation week is appropriate, recommended regimens to minimize the risk of adverse events are the following:

- **a.** Amoxicillin (500 mg orally every 12 hours for 3–7 days) first-line therapy
- **b.** Amoxicillin–clavulanate (500 mg orally every 12 hours for 3–7 days)
- **c.** Cephalexin (500 mg orally every 12 hours for 3–7 days) first-line therapy
- **d.** Nitrofurantoin (Macrobid®; 100 mg orally every 12 hours for 5 days) avoid first trimester
- **e.** Fosfomycin (3 g orally as a single dose)
- **f.** Cefuroxime (250 mg orally every 12 hours for 3–7 days)

E. FOLLOW-UP

1. A urine culture may be obtained a week after completion of the antibiotic therapy; as many as 30% of pregnant individuals persist with bacteriuria after a short course of therapy.

2. Persistent bacteriuria is present if a follow-up culture is positive with the same species of bacteria. In this case, another course of antibiotics selected based on susceptibility data should be administered: either the same antibiotic in a longer course (e.g., 7 days, if a 3-day regimen was used previously) or a different antibiotic in a standard regimen.

3. If the repeat culture shows a different causative organism, the antibiotic regimen should be given according to susceptibility data; this is not persistent bacteriuria.

F. SUPPRESSIVE THERAPY

1. Suppressive therapy may be appropriate with bacteriuria that persists after two or more courses of therapy. Administering nitrofurantoin (50–100 mg orally at bedtime) for the duration of pregnancy may be used if the organism is susceptible. Monthly cultures are not necessary if suppressive therapy is administered; however, breakthrough bacteriuria can occur during suppressive therapy, so at least one later culture, such as at the start of the third trimester, should be performed to ensure suppression is working.

2. If a follow-up culture is positive ($\geq 10^5$ CFU/mL), another course of antimicrobial therapy based on susceptibility data should be prescribed. The suppressive regimen should be reassessed and adjusted if needed.

G. HISTORY OF RECURRENT UTI PRIOR TO PREGNANCY

1. For those individuals with a history of UTI related to sexual intercourse prior to pregnancy, a postcoital regimen of either cephalexin (250 mg) or nitrofurantoin (50 mg) may be prescribed.

Cystitis

A. HISTORY

1. Dysuria
2. Urinary frequency and/or urgency
3. Hematuria
4. Suprapubic pain or discomfort
5. Medical history may include:
   a. Kidney stones
   b. Prior cystitis
   c. Pyelonephritis
   d. Sickle cell trait or disease

B. PHYSICAL EXAMINATION

1. Vital signs: Afebrile
2. Abdominal exam: Suprapubic pain
3. Back exam: No costovertebral angle (CVA) tenderness

C. LABORATORY AND DIAGNOSTIC STUDIES

1. Urine dipstick may be positive for protein, leukocyte esterase, nitrites, and/or blood.
2. Urinalysis
   a. Microscopic analysis may show WBCs, RBCs, or bacteria.
   b. Detection of pyuria by dipstick or microscope has a sensitivity of 80% to 90% and a specificity of 50% for predicting UTI.
3. Urine culture and sensitivity with clean-catch urine sample
   a. Consider catheterized urine sample if unable to obtain clean catch or if specimen has multiple organisms consistent with contamination. If the urine is not collected in a sterile manner, the urine sample may be contaminated by bacteria that originate from the skin or genital area and not from the urinary tract. This is often described by the clinical laboratory as "mixed growth bacteria" and may include two or more microorganisms. A contaminated sample may lead to a false-positive urine culture result. In a noncontaminated specimen, only a single strain of bacterial growth is identified.
4. Complete blood count (CBC) with differential
   a. May show an increased WBC with a left shift differential

D. TREATMENT: SEE SECTION II.D

E. FOLLOW-UP: SEE SECTION II.E

1. A follow-up culture for the test of cure should be obtained a week after completion of therapy.
2. Repeat cultures periodically until delivery to evaluate for persistent or recurrent bacteriuria (Glaser & Schaeffer, 2015).

Pyelonephritis

A. HISTORY

1. Fever generally above 100.4°F/38°C
2. Shaking chills
3. Nausea or loss of appetite, vomiting
4. Myalgias
5. Dysuria, frequency, urgency if cystitis is also present

6. Low back pain/flank pain
7. Abdominal pain and/or suprapubic pain
8. Contractions
9. Preterm labor
10. ASB, previous episodes of pyelonephritis, immunosuppression
11. Young age and/or nulliparity

B. PHYSICAL EXAMINATION

1. Vital signs: Fever, maternal tachycardia
2. Fetal tachycardia
3. Back exam: CVA tenderness to palpation
4. Pelvic exam: May reveal cervical dilatation if preterm labor is occurring

C. LABORATORY AND DIAGNOSTIC STUDIES

1. Urinalysis
2. Urine culture and sensitivity
   a. Catheterized urine sample if unable to obtain a clean catch
3. Strain urine for calculi (as indicated by presentation)
4. CBC with differential
5. Chemistry panel
6. Renal ultrasound (as indicated by presentation, not required for diagnosis)
   a. Hydronephrosis may be present with renal calculi
   b. No evidence for routine blood cultures

D. TREATMENT

May require inpatient hospitalization for intravenous (IV) antibiotic therapy, hydration, and possible tocolysis for the initial 48 hours. Young healthy patients before 24 weeks' gestational age with less severe symptoms may be treated on an outpatient basis follow-up medical care is attainable.

1. Initial empiric treatment for mild to moderate infection with IV antibiotics for 48 hours or until resolution of fever:
   a. Amoxicillin–clavulanic acid 1.2 g every 12 hours
   b. Cefepime 1 g every 24 hours
   c. Ceftriaxone 1 g every 24 hours
   d. Aztreonam 1 g every 8 to 12 hours
2. If severe infection:
   a. Piperacillin with tazobactam 3.375 g every 6 hours
   b. Meropenem 0.5 g every 8 hours.

   Follow up with well-established oral antibiotics and limit the use of newer antibiotics of potential concern in cases in which no safer alternative exists for a total of 10 to 14 days:
      i. Amoxicillin–clavulanate 875 mg orally, twice a day for 14 days
      ii. Nitrofurantoin (risk of newborn hemolysis after 38 weeks) Initial: 100 mg orally, four times a day for 14 days
      iii. Cephalexin 250 mg orally, four times a day for 14 days
      iv. Suppressive therapy should be initiated following treatment

E. CONSULTATION/REFERRAL

1. Consult with a collaborating physician for management.

F. FOLLOW-UP

1. Recurrent pyelonephritis during pregnancy occurs in 6% to 8% of patients; therefore, suppressive therapy is indicated until delivery: nitrofurantoin (50–100 mg/daily at bedtime) or cephalexin (250–500 mg orally at bedtime).
2. A follow-up culture for the test of cure should be obtained a week after completion of therapy.
3. Repeat cultures monthly until delivery to evaluate for persistent or recurrent bacteriuria.
4. Repeat urine culture at 6 to 8 weeks postpartum.

Bibliography

American College of Obstetricians and Gynecologists. (2020). Prevention of group B streptococcal early-onset disease in newborns. ACOG committee opinion no. 797. *Obstetrics & Gynecology, 135*(2), e51–e72. https://doi.org/10.1097/AOG.0000000000003668

American College of Obstetricians and Gynecologists Committee on Obstetric Practice. (2011). American College of Obstetricians and Gynecologists, committee opinion no. 494 (Reaffirmed 2015): Sulfonamides, nitrofurantoin, and risk of birth defects (Committee Opinion No. 494, reaffirmed 2015). *Obstetrics & Gynecology, 117*(6), 1484–1485. https://doi.org/10.1097/AOG.0b013e3182238c57

Curtiss, N., Meththananda, I., & Duckett, J. (2017). Urinary tract infection in obstetrics and gynaecology. *Obstetrics, Gynaecology and Reproductive Medicine, 27*(9), 261–265. https://doi.org/10.1016/j.ogrm.2017.06.006

Farkash, E., Weintraub, A., Sergienko, R., Wiznitzer, A., Zlotnik, A., & Sheiner, E. (2012). Acute antepartum pyelonephritis in pregnancy: A critical analysis of risk factors and outcomes. *European Journal of Obstetrics & Gynecology and Reproductive Biology, 162*(1), 24–27. https://doi.org/10.1016/j.ejogrb.2012.01.024

Glaser, A. P., & Schaeffer, A. J. (2015). Urinary tract infection and bacteriuria in pregnancy. *Urologic Clinics of North America*, 42, 547–560. https://doi.org/10.1016/j.ucl.2015.05.004

Glaser, A. P., & Schaeffer, A. J. (2015). Urinary tract infection and bacteriuria in pregnancy. *Urologic Clinics of North America, 42*, 547–560. https://doi.org/10.1016/j.ucl.2015.05.004

Gomi, H., Goto, Y., Laopaiboon, M., Usui, R., Mori, R., & Mori, R. (2015). Routine blood cultures in the management of pyelonephritis in pregnancy for improving outcomes. *Cochrane Database of Systematic Reviews, 2015*(2). https://doi.org/10.1002/14651858.CD009216.pub2

Hill, J. B., Sheffield, J. S., McIntire, D. D., & Wendel, G. D. (2005). Acute pyelonephritis in pregnancy. *Obstetrics & Gynecology, 150*, 18–23. https://doi.org/10.1097/01.AOG.0000149154.96285.a0

Matuszkiewicz-Rowińska, J., Małyszko, J., & Wieliczko, M. (2015). Urinary tract infections in pregnancy: Old and new unresolved diagnostic and therapeutic problems. *Archives of Medical Science, 11*(1), 67–77. https://doi.org/10.5114/aoms.2013.39202

Moore, A., Doull, M., Grad, R., Groulx, S., Pottie, K., Tonelli, M., Courage, S., Garcia, A. J., & Thombs, B. D. (2018). Recommendations on screening for asymptomatic bacteriuria in pregnancy. *Canadian Medical Association journal, 190*(27), E823–E830. https://doi.org/10.1503/cmaj.171325

Nicolle, L. E. (2015). Management of asymptomatic bacteriuria in pregnant women. *The Lancet Infectious Diseases, 15*, 1252–1254. https://doi.org/10.1016/S1473-3099(15)00145-0

Rosenberger, K., Seibert, A., & Hormig, S. (2020). Asymptomatic GBS bacteriuria during antenatal visits: To treat or not to treat? *The Nurse Practitioner, 45*(7), 18–25. https://doi.org/10.1097/01.NPR.0000669112.69022.aa

Smaill, F. M., & Vazquez, J. C. (2015). Antibiotics of asymptomatic bacteriuria in pregnancy. *Cochrane Database of Systematic Reviews, 8*, CD000490. https://doi.org/10.1002/14651858.CD000490.pub3

Widmer, M., Lopez, I., Gülmezoglu, A. M., Mignini, L., & Roganti, A. (2015). Duration of treatment for asymptomatic bacteriuria during pregnancy. *Cochrane Database of Systematic Reviews, 11*, CD000491. https://doi.org/10.1002/14651858.CD000491.pub3

World Health Organization. (2016). *WHO recommendation on antibiotics for asymptomatic bacteriuria.* https://apps.who.int/iris/bitstream/handle/10665/250796/9789241549912-eng.pdf;jsessionid=ED6F2789886B44A3902191BA11FEE561?sequence=1

13. Vaginitis and Sexually Transmitted Infections

KELLY D. ROSENBERGER | MARY LEE BARRON | AMY M. SEIBERT

Vaginitis and Vaginosis

A. DEFINITION AND BACKGROUND

1. Vaginitis or vaginosis in pregnancy is not uncommon. The offending organisms are *Hemophilus vaginalis, Candida albicans,* and *Trichomonas vaginalis.* The most common causes of vaginal symptoms in patients are bacterial vaginosis (BV; 40%–45%), vaginal candidiasis (20%–25%), and trichomoniasis (15%–20%); yet 7% to 72% of patients with a vaginal infection may remain undiagnosed. Many patients mistake physiologic leukorrhea for a vaginal infection. Normal physiologic leukorrhea is increased during pregnancy formed by mucoid secretions in combination with sloughing epithelial cells. The nurse practitioner (NP) must first differentiate leukorrhea from other infections, diagnose the type of vaginal infection (which can be elusive), treat it as appropriate, and educate the patient.

2. Chapter 23 in Fantasia and colleagues' 12th edition of *Guidelines for Nurse Practitioners in Gynecologic Settings* (2020) has a comprehensive presentation on vaginal conditions, including sexually transmitted infections (STIs). The reader is referred to that chapter for complete information. Presented here is the information on vaginal conditions and STIs during pregnancy.

B. HISTORY

1. Patients with vaginitis almost always present with a chief complaint of abnormal vaginal discharge (see Table 13.1). Ascertain the following attributes of discharge:

- **a.** Quantity
- **b.** Duration
- **c.** Color
- **d.** Consistency
- **e.** Odor

2. Previous similar episodes
3. STI risk or known exposure
4. Sexual activities
5. Douching practice
6. Antibiotic use
7. Systemic symptoms (e.g., lower abdominal pain, fever, chills, nausea, and vomiting)

TABLE 13.1 CHARACTERISTIC CLINICAL MANIFESTATIONS OF VAGINITIS/VAGINOSIS

CONDITION	SYMPTOMS	CHARACTERISTICS OF DISCHARGE	VAGINAL DISTRIBUTION	VAGINAL PH/OTHER
Physiologic leukorrhea	None	White, thick	Dependent	4.0–4.5
BV	"Fishy" malodor, irritation	Gray, thin, homogenous	Adherent, that is, coats the vaginal walls	>4.5
Candidiasis	Pruritus, irritation, erythema, pustules, vulvar edema	"Curd-like" white, thick discharge	Adherent, that is, coats the vaginal walls	4.0–4.5 Pain with urination as the urine passes over the irritated vulvar tissue
Trichomoniasis	Malodor, irritation, pruritus, dysuria, frequency; postcoital bleeding may occur	Gray-yellow to green, thin, homogenous (10%–30% of women), frothy appearance	Adherent, that is, coats the vaginal walls	5.0–6.0 Cervix may have "strawberry" appearance, erythema of the vaginal walls

BV, bacterial vaginosis.

8. Ask questions to exclude the possibility of a foreign body in the vagina. Foreign bodies in the vagina result in a persistent, foul-smelling, serosanguineous discharge.

9. Chemical irritation (e.g., recent bubble baths, washing hair with shampoo while bathing, use of feminine hygiene sprays)

10. Latex condom use

11. Semen exposure

12. Mechanical irritation

13. Poor hygiene

14. Contact dermatitis from unusual exposures

15. Cigarette smoking

16. Other symptoms: pruritis, burning, irritation, erythema, dyspareunia, spotting, and/or dysuria

C. PHYSICAL EXAMINATION

1. Vital signs: Blood pressure, pulse, respiration, and temperature

2. Abdominal examination: Costovertebral angle tenderness (CVAT) assessment

3. Inguinal lymph nodes

4. External genitalia: Note lesions, sores, rash, genital warts, condition of the urethra, Bartholin's and Skene's glands

5. Vaginal speculum examination

- **a.** Inspect vaginal walls noting the character of discharge, lesions, tears
- **b.** Inspect cervix noting friability (a pregnant cervix bleeds more readily), ectropion, discharge from os (there should be a mucus plug), tenderness, color
- **c.** Bimanual examination: Not indicated for evaluation of vaginal discharge unless pelvic pain, dyspareunia, or concerns about labor are present. If performing, note cervical position, tenderness, dilation, and uterine size and position.

D. LABORATORY AND DIAGNOSTIC STUDIES (AS INDICATED BY FINDINGS)

1. Saline wet preparation
   a. (Amsel criteria for BV) requires any three of the following:
      i. Homogenous, thin, white, or gray discharge coating the vaginal walls
      ii. Presence of >20% clue cells on wet mount microscopy on vaginal saline preparation. Clue cells are vaginal epithelial cells infected by coccobacilli.
      iii. pH is greater than 4.5 on nitrazine paper (*most sensitive for BV*).
      iv. False elevations in pH may be caused by:
         a) Cervical mucus
         b) Blood
         c) Semen
         d) Recent medication
         e) Intercourse within last 24 hours
         f) Lubricants (KY-Jelly)
         g) Leakage of amniotic fluid
   b. Positive whiff test, that is, fishy odor with the addition of 10% potassium hydroxide (KOH). A positive whiff test is most specific for BV.
   c. Visualization of motile parasite has 65% sensitivity for *T. vaginalis*. Samples should be visualized within 10 minutes of collection.
2. KOH wet preparation: Positive for hyphae, pseudohyphae, spores, or buds in the presence of candidiasis
3. QuickVue Advance pH and amines test
4. QuickVue Advance *Gardnerella vaginalis* test
5. BD Affirm VPIII microbial identification test
6. Culture (if possible): A culture of *T. vaginalis* has near 100% specificity but requires rapid transport to the laboratory.
7. Nucleic acid amplification testing (NAAT): NAATs are the most sensitive tests available for *T. vaginalis* and can be used with urine, vaginal, or cervical swabs.
8. Gram stain is rarely necessary and increases the cost of the visit.

E. DIFFERENTIAL DIAGNOSES

1. Physiologic leukorrhea
2. BV
3. Vulvovaginal candidiasis
4. Trichomoniasis
5. Chlamydial cervicitis
6. Gonococcal cervicitis
7. Herpes simplex
8. Urinary tract infection (UTI)
9. Ureaplasma or mycoplasma genitalium

F. MANAGEMENT OF BACTERIAL VAGINOSIS

1. Pharmacologic treatment: For pregnant individuals *with symptoms*, treat with any one of the three following regimens:
   a. Metronidazole 500 mg orally twice daily for 7 days
   b. Clindamycin 300 mg orally twice daily for 7 days
   c. Vaginal metronidazole or clindamycin: Oral therapy has not been shown to be superior to topical therapy for treating symptomatic BV in effecting cure; symptomatic pregnant individuals can be treated with either of the oral or vaginal regimens recommended for nonpregnant individuals (Centers for Disease Control and Prevention [CDC], 2021).

i. Topical therapy is not recommended for treatment of BV to avoid adverse pregnancy outcomes in individuals *at risk for preterm birth* (Yudin & Money, 2017).

d. Tinidazole is not approved for use in pregnancy.

2. Follow-up
   a. As indicated by the gestational age
   b. If symptomatic, retest 1 month after treatment
3. Consultation/referral
   a. Consider for multiple infections in 1 year. May consider testing for ureaplasma and mycoplasma genitalium in the presence of recurrent BV and BV-like symptoms. Motomura et al. (2020) reviewed intra-amniotic infections in mothers of preterm infants, noting a significant prevalence of ureaplasma infections caused a heightened inflammatory response leading to adverse perinatal outcomes, including preterm birth, chorioamnionitis, and newborn infection.
4. Patient education
   a. If treated with oral metronidazole, reinforce the need for abstinence from alcohol (patient should be abstaining anyway during pregnancy) for 24 hours after completion of metronidazole.
   b. Stress the importance of finishing the medication.
   c. May use mints to counteract the "tin taste" that many patients experience
   d. No treatment is necessary for the partner.
   e. Discontinue douching (pregnant individuals should be advised to avoid douching regardless).
   f. Patient did not develop BV from exposure to toilet seats, swimming pools, or hot tubs.
   g. Vaginal hygiene
      i. Wipe the genital area from front to back.
      ii. Wash with warm water only.
      iii. Avoid scented soaps and feminine hygiene products.
      iv. Wear cotton underwear.
      v. Avoid constricting, tight-fitting clothing.
   h. Advise patients to review updated information on the CDC website regarding BV at: www.cdc.gov/std/bv/stdfact-bacterial-vaginosis.htm.

G. MANAGEMENT OF CANDIDIASIS

1. Do not treat *Candida* identified by culture or PAP in the absence of symptoms; up to 20% of individuals harbor *Candida* sp. and other yeasts in the vagina at all times, and a positive culture or *Candida* noted on PAP does not indicate a yeast infection. Pharmacologic treatment for symptomatic candidiasis:
   a. Because of their efficacy, topical azole antifungals are the recommended treatments during pregnancy for at least 7 days. Treatment for up to 14 days and/or repeat treatments may be required for the resolution of symptoms during pregnancy.
      i. Clotrimazole (Gyne-Lotrimin, Lotrimin) 1% cream 5 g intravaginally for 7 to 14 days
      ii. Clotrimazole 100-mg vaginal tablet for 7 days
      iii. Miconazole (Monistat) 100-mg vaginal suppository; one suppository or full applicator each day for 7 days
      iv. Terconazole 0.4% cream 5 g intravaginally for 7 days
   b. It is prudent to avoid the use of oral fluconazole (Diflucan) during pregnancy. Large studies and more research are necessary, but there is evidence of an association with statistically significant increased risk of

spontaneous abortion compared with risk among unexposed individuals and those with topical azole exposure in pregnancy (Mølgaard-Nielsen et al., 2016). In addition, associations between fluconazole and both cleft lip with cleft palate and d-transposition of the great arteries are consistent with earlier published case reports, but rare use of the drug limited the findings in later epidemiologic studies (Howley et al., 2016).

c. Nystatin 100,000-unit vaginal tablet for 14 days (poor vaginal absorption)

i. Consider a topical steroid for those with vulvar erythema, edema, excoriation, and/or fissuring.

2. Follow-up

a. As indicated by the gestational age

3. Consultation/referral

a. Persistent or recurrent (>4/year) fungal infections because other comorbidities may be present

4. Patient education

a. Abstain from intercourse until symptoms subside.

b. Stress the importance of finishing the medication.

c. Review vaginal hygiene

i. Wipe the genital area from front to back.

ii. Wash with warm water only.

iii. Avoid scented soaps and feminine hygiene products.

iv. Wear cotton underwear.

v. Sleep without underwear.

vi. Avoid constricting, tight-fitting clothing.

d. Advise patients to review updated information on the CDC website regarding candidiasis at: www.cdc.gov/fungal/diseases/candidiasis/genital/index.html

H. MANAGEMENT OF TRICHOMONIASIS

1. *Trichomonas vaginalis* infection is usually asymptomatic and has been associated with adverse pregnancy outcomes. The prevalence of trichomoniasis increases with age and is twice as high in individuals with HIV. Pharmacologic treatment has not been shown to reduce adverse perinatal outcomes, although vaginal trichomoniasis has been associated with the premature rupture of membranes (PROM), preterm delivery, and low birth weight.

a. Metronidazole 500 mg orally twice daily for 7 days (recommended regimen)

b. Metronidazole 2 g orally in a single dose (more gastrointestinal [GI] side effects in individuals who may already have problems with nausea and vomiting)

c. Tinidazole therapy in pregnancy has not been evaluated and is not recommended.

d. The option of therapy deferral until after 37 weeks should be discussed in asymptomatic pregnant individuals.

2. Trichomoniasis is the most common nonviral, STI. The partner should be treated. Patients should abstain from intercourse until both partners have completed treatment and symptoms have disappeared.

3. Follow up

a. As indicated by the gestational age

4. Consultation/referral

a. Refractory cases

5. Advise patients to review updated information on the CDC website regarding trichomonas at: www.cdc.gov/std/trichomonas/STDFact-Trichomoniasis.htm

A. ACUTE CERVICITIS (CAUSED BY GONORRHEA OR CHLAMYDIA)

1. Definition and etiology: Inflammation of the uterine cervix, primarily affecting the columnar epithelial cells of the endocervix. It may affect the squamous epithelium. The etiology may be infectious or noninfectious, and the condition may be acute or chronic. Acute cervicitis results from infection from chlamydia or gonorrhea, whereas chronic infection is usually noninfectious (may be caused by mechanical or chemical irritation). *T. vaginalis* also accounts for some cases, but far fewer than chlamydia and gonorrhea. The condition is clinically important because in pregnant individuals it may cause maternal and/or neonatal complications as a result of infection of the fetus, placenta, amniotic fluid, decidua, or membranes.

2. Almost half of individuals infected with *Chlamydia trachomatis* (CT) are coinfected with *Neisseria gonorrhoeae* (GC). Since 2014, in the United States, STIs caused by gonorrhea have increased by 56% (CDC, 2019), and STIs caused by chlamydia have increased by 19% (CDC, 2019). The most recent CDC vital statistics demonstrated the rates of chlamydia and gonorrhea increased by 2% and 16%, respectively, in pregnant individuals from 2016 to 2019. Risk factors for chlamydia and gonorrhea infection:

- **a.** Patients with a history of gonorrhea infection, HIV positive, and/or other STIs
- **b.** Age younger than 25 years
- **c.** New, multiple sexual partners, or sex partner with multiple concurrent sex partners
- **d.** Inconsistent condom use
- **e.** Sex workers
- **f.** Drug users
- **g.** People living in a community with a higher prevalence of gonorrhea (correctional facility or juvenile detention center)
- **h.** Single marital status
- **i.** Low educational or socioeconomic status

3. Screening during pregnancy

- **a.** CDC and U.S. Preventative Services Task Force (USPSTF) recommend screening for chlamydia and gonorrhea in all pregnant individuals ages 24 and younger, and pregnant individuals of all ages with risk factors, at the first prenatal visit.
- **b.** All pregnant individuals who test positive for CT or GC at any time during pregnancy should be retested within 1 to 3 months.
- **c.** Pregnant individuals with risk factors and those ages 24 and younger should be tested during the third trimester, regardless of previous negative screen.

4. History

- **a.** *Chlamydia trachomatis*
  - **i.** Most pregnant individuals are asymptomatic, but 30% present with urethral syndrome
    - **a)** Dysuria, dyspareunia
    - **b)** Labial pain (Bartholin gland inflammation)
  - **ii.** Change in vaginal discharge
  - **iii.** Mucopurulent cervical discharge
  - **iv.** Postcoital bleeding
- **b.** *Neisseria gonorrhoeae*
  - **i.** Most are asymptomatic.
  - **ii.** In most pregnant individuals, gonococcal infection is limited to the lower genital tract: cervix, urethra, periurethral, and vestibular glands.

iii. May complain of increased vaginal discharge
iv. May complain of dysuria
v. Labial pain (Bartholin gland inflammation)
vi. At higher risk for ectopic pregnancy, but acute salpingitis is rare in pregnancy
vii. Pregnant individuals account for disproportionate numbers of disseminated gonococcal infection (rare complication), which presents as arthritis affecting medium-size joints or as a diffuse violet skin rash and may include:
a) Body ache
b) Dull headache
c) Fever
d) Lack of appetite

5. Physical examination
   a. Vital signs: Temperature, blood pressure, pulse
   b. Abdominal examination: Check for guarding, referred pain, rebound tenderness.
   c. External genitalia: Observe perineum for edema, lesions, sores, enlarged tender Bartholin's gland, Skene's gland.
   d. Speculum examination: Inspect the vaginal walls, character of discharge, cervix (friability).
   e. Bimanual examination: Cervical motion tenderness, adnexal fullness (if before 12 weeks), tender uterus, salpingitis (though rare in pregnancy)
6. Laboratory and diagnostic studies (as indicated by findings) sensitivities and specificities of laboratory tests vary:
   a. Endocervical culture (only 100% specific test for *N. gonorrhoeae*)
   b. NAAT testing (more sensitive than culture for *N. gonorrhoeae*). First void urine and vaginal swabs can be self-collected and may be preferred by individuals due to being less invasive.
   c. DNA probe (not as sensitive as NAAT)
   d. Direct fluorescent antibody (DFA) testing: Secretions are fixed on a slide and stained with monoclonal antibody solution specific for chlamydial antigens.
   e. Rapid test with endocervical swab or brush; wait 30 minutes for results
   f. Enzyme-linked immunosorbent assay (ELISA) and enzyme-linked immune assay (EIA) to detect chlamydial antigens
   g. Saline wet preparation: Too numerous to count white blood cells (WBCs); this is only supportive data and is associated with cervicitis.
7. Treatment in pregnancy: In late 2020, the CDC published new guidelines regarding the treatment for gonorrhea and chlamydia, as there is evidence of increasing resistance to azithromycin, and prudent practice of antimicrobial stewardship supports limiting its use. Dual therapy is no longer recommended, and the CDC now recommends monotherapy for the treatment of gonorrhea at a higher dose and includes treatment dose adjusted for obese individuals.
   a. Ceftriaxone 500 mg intramuscularly (IM) in a single dose is now recommended for uncomplicated urogenital, rectal, or pharyngeal **gonorrhea**. For persons weighing ≥150 kg (300 pounds), a single 1 g (1,000 mg) dose of ceftriaxone is recommended.
   b. Alternative therapy if unable to tolerate cephalosporin
   c. When cephalosporin allergy or other considerations preclude treatment with this regimen and spectinomycin (2 g IM) is not available, consultation with an infectious disease specialist is recommended.

d. Azithromycin, 1 g orally as single dose, or amoxicillin, 500 mg orally three times a day for 7 days, are recommended for presumptive or diagnosed urogenital, rectal, or pharyngeal **chlamydia** infection. Alternatives, if allergic, include erythromycin base 500 mg orally four times a day for 7 days or at lower dose of 250 mg orally four times a day for 14 days if GI tolerance is an issue.

e. Infected patients and their partners should both receive treatment and abstain from intercourse until 1 week after treatment is complete.

f. Treatment for **+chlamydia in first trimester with amoxicillin 500 mg three times per day for 7 days** is advised due to recent studies identifying associations of macrolide antibiotics (azithromycin, erythromycin, and clarithromycin) with birth defects such as cardiovascular malformations and genital malformations.

8. Complications
- **a.** Septic spontaneous abortion
- **b.** Preterm delivery
- **c.** PROM
- **d.** Chorioamnionitis
- **e.** Disseminated gonococcal infection
- **f.** Ophthalmia neonatorum in infants of infected pregnant individuals
- **g.** Postpartum endometritis

9. Consultation/referral
- **a.** If no response to treatment
- **b.** If complications develop

10. Follow up

a. As indicated by the gestational age, see Section E.3.

b. Per the past CDC guidelines, test of cure to detect therapeutic failure (i.e., repeat testing 3–4 weeks after completing therapy) was not advised for nonpregnant persons treated with the recommended or alterative regimens, unless therapeutic adherence is in question, symptoms persist, or reinfection is suspected. Moreover, the use of chlamydial NAATs at less than 3 weeks after completion of therapy is not recommended because the continued presence of nonviable organisms can lead to false-positive results. Similarly, the limits of a rescreening method according to laboratory requirements specific to that test. For example, a DNA probe cannot be repeated until 3 weeks after the infection is treated. Culture is 100% specific for gonorrhea. The CDC recommends test-of-cure to document chlamydial eradication by NAAT 3 to 4 weeks after completion of therapy since severe sequelae is possible in mothers and neonates with persistent infection and advises all pregnant individuals should be retested within 3 months after treatment. Those with increased risk should also be rescreened during the third trimester to prevent maternal postnatal and neonatal complications.

c. Serology test for syphilis

d. HIV testing (see Chapter 20)

e. Disease reporting varies by state regulations—contact your local county health department.

B. HUMAN PAPILLOMAVIRUS (*CONDYLOMATA ACUMINATA* AKA GENITAL WARTS)

1. Definition: A contagious projecting warty growth on the external genitals or at the anus, consisting of fibrous overgrowths covered by thickened epithelium showing koilocytosis, which are caused by sexual contact with someone infected with human papillomavirus (HPV); genital warts are usually benign, although malignant change has been reported and is associated with particular types of the virus.

2. Background: HPV is the most common symptomatic STI. The seroprevalence in pregnancy is about 30%, although not all individuals are symptomatic because of the variance of effect in more than 100 strains of HPV. Ninety percent of genital warts are caused by HPV types 6 and 11. The incubation period is 1 to 6 months or even longer. Up to 70% regress spontaneously. For reasons that are not clear, genital warts frequently increase in number and size during pregnancy. Viral replication, accelerated by the physiologic changes during pregnancy, may explain some of the growth. Some of the growth is so severe that the vagina is filled, making vaginal delivery difficult.
3. Risk factors
   a. History of multiple sexual partners
   b. Presence of another STI
4. History
   a. "Bump" or "bumps" in the vulvar area
   b. Change in vaginal discharge
   c. Itching, burning, pain in the vulvar area
   d. Slight bleeding
5. Physical examination
   a. External genitalia
      i. Small flesh-colored, soft, raised "warty" lesions or growths present anywhere on the external genitalia. If located in a hair-bearing area, may have a keratotic appearance.
      ii. Signs of secondary infection of lesions (from scratching)
   b. Vaginal examination (speculum examination)
      i. Inspect vaginal walls for the presence of warts.
      ii. Inspect cervix, although it may not be readily visible.
6. Laboratory examination and diagnostic findings
   a. Diagnosis of genital warts is usually clinical and made by visual inspection. Application of acetic acid (vinegar) will turn the warty tissue white but is not a specific test for HPV infection. The routine use of this procedure for screening to detect mucosal changes attributed to HPV infection is not recommended.
   b. Genital warts are usually asymptomatic, but depending on the size and anatomic location, they might be painful or pruritic. The use of HPV DNA testing for genital wart diagnosis is not recommended, because test results would not alter clinical management of the condition.
   c. Genital warts can be confirmed by biopsy, which might be indicated if:
      i. Diagnosis is uncertain.
      ii. Lesions do not respond to standard therapy.
      iii. Disease worsens during therapy.
      iv. Lesion is atypical.
      v. Patient has compromised immunity.
      vi. Warts are pigmented, indurated, fixed, bleeding, or ulcerated
7. Differential diagnoses
   a. Condylomata lata (associated with syphilis)
   b. *Molluscum contagiosum*
   c. Nevi
   d. Seborrheic keratoses
   e. Psoriatic plaques
   f. Benign lesion such as lipoma, fibroma, or adenoma

g. Cancerous lesion
h. Herpes simplex
i. Angiokeratoma

8. Treatment
   a. Defer until the postpartum period. Genital warts often regress after delivery and may disappear. The primary reason for treating genital warts is the amelioration of symptoms (including relieving the cosmetic concerns) and, ultimately, removal of warts. Although removal of warts during pregnancy can be considered, resolution might be incomplete or poor until pregnancy is complete. If left untreated, visible genital warts can resolve on their own, remain unchanged, or increase in size or number. Available therapies for genital warts likely reduce the infection but do not eradicate HPV infection. The reduction in HPV viral DNA resulting from treatment reduces future transmission; however, this treatment remains unclear. No evidence indicates that the presence of genital warts or their treatment is associated with the development of cervical cancer.
   b. Cryotherapy with liquid nitrogen
   c. Trichloroacetic acid (TCA) or bichloroacetic acid (BCA) 80% to 90% is applied to warts. Only a small amount should be applied to warts and allowed to dry, at which time a white frosting develops. Petroleum jelly can be applied to the surrounding area with a cotton-tipped swab to prevent an excess amount of acid being applied to unaffected skin; this should be done very precisely so as not to coat the warty tissue.
   d. The treated area should be powdered with sodium bicarbonate or liquid soap applied to remove unreacted acid. This treatment can be repeated weekly, if necessary.
   e. Imiquimod, sinecatechins, podophyllin, and podofilox should not be used during pregnancy.
   f. Cesarean delivery is indicated for pregnant individuals with genital warts only if the pelvic outlet is obstructed or if vaginal delivery would result in excessive bleeding.
9. Complications
   a. Respiratory papillomatosis in the infant: It is unclear whether cesarean section prevents respiratory papillomatosis in infants and children. Therefore, cesarean delivery should *not* be performed solely to prevent transmission of HPV infection to the newborn. Pregnant individuals with genital warts should be counseled concerning the low risk for warts on the larynx (recurrent respiratory papillomatosis) in their infants or children.
   b. Low-grade cervical changes
   c. High-grade cervical lesions, cervical neoplasia
10. Consultation/referral
   a. Consult an obstetrician if vaginal or cervical warts are present
   b. Warts in large clusters
   c. Wart >2 cm in size
   d. Abnormal cervical cytology: High-grade lesion
11. Follow-up
   a. As indicated by the gestational age or by treatment
   b. Partner would benefit from counseling and education
12. Patient education
   a. Available at: www.cdc.gov/std/hpv/default.htm

C. HERPES SIMPLEX VIRUS

1. Definition and background: Genital herpes caused by the herpes simplex virus (HSV) is a chronic viral infection of the skin and mucous membranes

that is transmitted through direct bodily contact. There are two strains: HSV-1 and HSV-2. In the past, HSV-2 caused the majority of genital infections, but presently, HSV-1 is estimated to cause 30% to 50% of new genital HSV infections. Infections are classified by timing and antibody presence.

a. A primary infection refers to an infection in a patient without preexisting antibodies to either HSV-1 or HSV-2. Type-specific antibodies to HSV generally develop within the first 12 weeks after infection.

b. A nonprimary first-episode genital infection refers to the acquisition of genital HSV-2 in a patient with preexisting antibodies to HSV-1; or acquisition of genital HSV-1 in a patient with preexisting antibodies to HSV-2.

c. A recurrent infection refers to the reactivation of genital HSV in a seropositive person; in this case, the HSV type recovered in the lesion is the same type as that identified by serologic testing.

2. Epidemiology: Overall, national HSV-2 prevalence remains high (15.1%), is more common in women than men (20.3% vs. 10.6% in 14–49-year-olds), and the disease continues to disproportionately burden African Americans (41.2% prevalence). Most persons with HSV-2 have *not* received a diagnosis. Seroprevalence studies indicate that <10% of seropositive individuals report a history of genital herpes.

3. Screening in pregnancy: Evidence does not support routine HSV-2 serologic screening among asymptomatic pregnant individuals. However, type-specific serologic tests might be useful for identifying pregnant individuals at risk for HSV infection and guide counseling regarding the risk for acquiring genital herpes during pregnancy (CDC, 2021).

4. Transmission

a. HSV is rarely transmitted in utero (0.5%). However, this infection is one of the most common STIs.

b. Intrauterine viral transmission is high in the first 20 weeks of gestation and leads to spontaneous abortion, stillbirth, and congenital anomalies. The perinatal mortality is 50%.

c. Neonatal transmission occurs via three routes: Intrauterine (5%), intrapartum (85%), or postnatal (10%; Cunningham et al., 2014). The fetus becomes infected by virus shed from contact with virus-infected maternal mucosa during labor or delivery. The virus either invades the uterus following membrane rupture or is transmitted by contact with the fetus at delivery. The rate of transmission is 1 in 3,200 to 1 in 30,000 births, depending on the population studied (Cunningham et al., 2014). The most critical determinant of neonatal infection is primary genital HSV infection nearing delivery. However, transmission and infection are most likely with viral shedding during labor, invasive fetal monitoring, and premature delivery.

5. History

a. Genital herpes prior to pregnancy

b. Primary infection: It occurs after an incubation period of 2 to 20 days and lasts up to 21 days

i. Painful grouped vesicular genital lesions
ii. Myalgia
iii. Headache
iv. Arthralgia
v. Malaise
vi. Fever
vii. Lymphadenopathy
viii. Dysuria
ix. Pain with urination if urine passes over lesions

c. Nonprimary infection
   i. Symptoms are less severe than primary infection
   ii. Lesions less painful
   iii. Fewer or no systemic symptoms
   Recurrent infection
      a) Prodrome frequently present
      b) Pruritus
      c) Tingling or burning at the site of previous lesions
      d) Grouped vesicular lesions in the same site as previous infection are less painful with primary infection
d. Risk factors for recurrence
   i. Prolonged exposure to ultraviolet light, that is, sun exposure
   ii. Excessive friction to the genital area
   iii. Compromise of the immune system
   iv. Stress

6. Physical examination
   a. Vital signs: Temperature, blood pressure
   b. Genital examination: Grouped vesicular lesions on an erythematous base are filled with cloudy fluid. When the vesicles break, coalescence usually occurs, leading to an ulcerative lesion with irregular borders and maceration.
   c. Speculum examination may or may not be possible depending on the location of the lesions.
   d. Lymphadenopathy may be present in the groin.
   e. Bladder distention may occur because of difficulty urinating.

7. Clinical presentation guides the choice of testing. The presence of viral shedding is a key issue. If active genital lesions are present, the vesicle may be unroofed for sampling of vesicular fluid for viral culture. The overall sensitivity of viral culture of genital lesions is low, at only approximately 80% during primary HSV and 35% during recurrent disease. Although viral culture determines HSV-1 or HSV-2, polymerase chain reaction (PCR) assays for HSV DNA are more likely to detect viral shedding and are two to four times more sensitive. PCR assays are increasingly used in many settings. Failure to detect HSV by culture or PCR does not indicate the absence of HSV infection because viral shedding is intermittent. Laboratory examination and diagnostic studies include:
   a. Viral culture
   b. PCR
   c. DFA testing
   d. Type-specific serologic tests
      i. Both type-specific and non–type-specific antibodies to HSV develop during the first several weeks after infection and persist indefinitely. Both laboratory-based assays and point-of-care tests that provide results for HSV-2 antibodies from capillary blood or serum during a clinic visit are available. The sensitivities of these glycoprotein G type-specific tests for the detection of HSV-2 antibody vary from 80% to 98%, and false-negative results might be more frequent at early stages of infection. The specificities of these assays are 96%. False-positive results can occur, especially in patients with a low likelihood of HSV infection. Repeat or confirmatory testing might be indicated in some settings, especially if recent acquisition of genital herpes is suspected. Immunoglobulin M (IgM) testing for HSV is not useful, because the IgM tests are not type specific and might be positive during recurrent episodes of herpes.

ii. Detection of HSV-2 antibodies is diagnostic for genital HSV infection. Detection of HSV-1 antibodies could indicate orolabial or genital infection.

8. Differential diagnoses
 a. Syphilis
 b. Chancroid
 c. Lymphogranuloma inguinale
 d. Granuloma inguinale

9. Management of genital herpes during pregnancy
 a. Pharmacologic treatment is dependent on whether the infection is primary or recurrent.
  i. Therapy is always offered to patients with a primary infection.
  ii. Suppressive therapy is offered from 36 weeks until delivery for patients with recurrent genital herpes to reduce the incidence of recurrence at term and, therefore, the risk of cesarean delivery. Asymptomatic viral shedding is markedly reduced using this approach, although it is not completely eliminated (Table 13.2).
 b. Comfort measures adapted from CDC
  i. Keep the genital area clean and dry; use of hairdryer on a cool setting to dry the area is less likely to irritate than towel drying.
  ii. Take sitz baths with baking soda or Domeboro solution.
  iii. Apply cold, wet compresses to the affected area.
  iv. Wrapped pads containing glycerin and witch hazel may provide temporary relief.

TABLE 13.2 ANTIVIRAL MEDICATIONS FOR HERPES SIMPLEX IN PREGNANCY

Primary episode	Acyclovir	400 mg three times daily	7–10 d
	Valacyclovir	1 g orally twice daily	7–10 d
	Famciclovir	250 mg three times daily	7–10 d*
Recurrent infection	Acyclovir	400 mg three times daily	5 d
	Acyclovir	800 mg twice daily	5 d
	Acyclovir	800 mg three times daily	2 d
	Valacyclovir	500 mg orally twice daily	3 d
	Valacyclovir	1 g orally twice daily	5 d
	Famciclovir	125 mg twice daily	5 d
	Famciclovir	1 g orally twice daily	1 d
	Famciclovir	500 mg orally once, followed by 250 mg twice daily for 2 days	
Suppressive therapy	Acyclovir	400 mg three times daily	From 36 wk to delivery
	Valacyclovir	500 mg orally twice daily	From 36 wk to delivery

*Treatment can be extended if healing is incomplete after 10 days of therapy.

Note: There is sufficient data to support the safety of acyclovir during pregnancy. The safety of valacyclovir and famciclovir therapy in pregnant individuals has not been definitively established. The current available data do not indicate an increased risk for major birth defects compared with the general population in patients treated with these medications during the first trimester.

v. Apply local anesthetic cream, such as lidocaine, especially if there is pain with urination.
vi. Wear loose cotton clothing, including white cotton underwear.
c. Hygiene measures
i. Use a different towel for the affected area to avoid spreading the infection to another part of the body.
ii. Wash hands with soap and water if there has been direct contact with the sores.
iii. Avoid intercourse during the prodromal period and/or during an outbreak.
iv. Do not use scented soaps, feminine deodorants, or douches, as these can irritate the skin.

10. Complications
a. Most primary and first-episode infections in early pregnancy are not associated with spontaneous abortion or stillbirth. A primary infection in late pregnancy may be associated with preterm labor.
b. Perinatal mortality for fetus/neonate is 50%.
c. Operative delivery
d. Secondary infection of lesions
e. Abortion
f. Stillbirth
g. Disseminated herpes infection
h. Meningitis
i. Encephalitis
j. Pneumonitis
k. Hepatitis
l. Liver failure
m. Death

11. Consultation/referral
a. Primary infection
b. Secondary infections
c. Urinary retention/difficulty voiding
d. Suspected ocular episode
e. Symptoms associated with complications, such as nausea and vomiting, upper right quadrant pain, headache, shortness of breath, chest pain

12. Follow-up
a. As indicated by condition and gestational age
b. Sex partners can benefit from evaluation and counseling.

13. Patient education
a. www.uptodate.com/contents/genital-herpes-beyond-the-basics?source=search_result&search=herpes%20and%20pregnancy&selectedTitle=1~4
b. www.cdc.gov/std/herpes/default.htm Pregnant individuals without known genital herpes should be counseled to abstain from vaginal intercourse during the third trimester with partners known or suspected of having genital herpes. In addition, pregnant individuals without known orolabial herpes should be advised to abstain from receptive oral sex during the third trimester with partners known or suspected of having orolabial herpes. Type-specific serologic tests may be useful for identifying pregnant individuals at risk for HSV infection and for guiding counseling regarding the risk for acquiring genital herpes during pregnancy. For example, such testing could be offered to individuals with no history of genital herpes whose sex partner has HSV infection. Routine

HSV-2 serologic screening of pregnant individuals is not recommended (CDC, 2021).

c. Pregnant individuals with known HSV infection diagnosed either prior to or during pregnancy should be counseled that a cesarean delivery is indicated if there are active genital lesions or prodromal symptoms. A cesarean delivery should be performed promptly in the presence of prelabor rupture of membranes and active genital HSV lesions (ACOG, 2020).

D. PEDICULOSIS PUBIS

1. Definition and background: Pubic lice (pediculosis pubis), also known as *crab lice* or *crabs*, are lice (a type of wingless, bloodsucking insect) that can live and multiply (infest) on skin that grows pubic hair. This infestation has been increasing, and it is estimated that three million cases are treated each year in the United States. The incubation period of pediculosis is 30 days. The female lays approximately 40 eggs per day, which attach to the shaft of the hair near the root. Seven days later, a nymph is hatched. Sexual maturity occurs in pubic lice in 3 to 4 weeks.

2. Epidemiology: Acquisition is nearly always through sexual contact, but pubic lice can be spread on fomites. Pediculosis pubis is the most contagious STI, with a transmission rate of 95%. The infection is most common in 15- to 19-year-olds. Current worldwide prevalence has been estimated at approximately 2% of the human population.

3. History

a. Irritation

b. Intense pruritus

c. Patient may state that a crab louse or lice was noted moving over the skin.

d. Mild fever

e. Malaise

f. Irritability

4. Physical examination

a. External genital examination: Visualization of the lice, larvae, and nits with the use of a magnifying glass is diagnostic.

5. Treatment

a. Pharmacologic

i. Permethrin 1% cream, rinse the affected areas and apply; wash off after 10 minutes

ii. Pyrethrins with piperonyl butoxide applied to the affected area and washed off after 10 minutes

iii. Alternatively, prescribe ivermectin 250 mcg/kg orally, repeated in 2 weeks. Ivermectin may not prevent recurrence from eggs present at time of treatment, therefore repeat in 14 days. When taken with food, the bioavailability is increased. Because no teratogenicity or toxicity attributable to ivermectin has been observed in human pregnancy, ivermectin is classified as "human data suggest low risk" in pregnancy and is probably compatible with breastfeeding (CDC, 2015).

iv. Lindane is no longer recommended and is contraindicated in pregnancy.

v. Resistance to pediculicides is increasing and has become widespread.

vi. Retreatment is indicated after 7 days if lice are found or eggs are observed at the hair–skin junction.

b. Hygiene

i. Clothing and bed linen that may have been contaminated should be machine washed and machine dried on a hot cycle or dry cleaned or removed from body contact for at least 72 hours. If this cannot be done, placing blankets and other clothing in plastic bags and storing them can kill the lice. Without blood, the lice cannot live for more than 24 hours.

ii. All sexual contacts, family members, and close contacts must be treated at the same time, even if asymptomatic.

6. Follow-up

a. Reevaluate in 1 week if symptoms persist.

b. If no response to treatment, an alternative should be tried.

c. To rule out persistent disease, abstain from sexual contact until reevaluation has occurred.

7. Patient education

a. www.cdc.gov/std/tg2015/ectoparasitic.htm#pubiclice

E. SYPHILIS

1. Definition and background: Syphilis is a sexually transmitted systemic infection caused by the spirochete bacterium *Treponema pallidum*. The primary route of transmission is through sexual contact; it may also be transmitted from mother to fetus during pregnancy or at birth, resulting in congenital syphilis. In the United States, since 2014, the rates of both primary and secondary syphilis have increased by 74% and congenital syphilis has increased by 279% (CDC, 2019). The 2019 STD Surveillance Report highlighted an alarming increase of newborn deaths from syphilis. The most recent CDC vital statistics demonstrated in 2019, there were 128 congenital syphilis-related deaths (94 stillbirths and 34 infant deaths), and an increase of 36.2% from 2018 (94 to 128 deaths) and of 255.6% from 2015 (36 to 128 deaths).

2. Epidemiology: Eighty percent of women with syphilis are in the childbearing age group and, therefore, are at risk for transmitting syphilis to the fetus. Approximately 30% to 60% of those exposed to primary or secondary syphilis will get the disease. Syphilis can lead to serious, long-term sequelae, including cardiac and neurologic manifestations.

a. Risk factors associated with syphilis in pregnancy

i. Lack of health insurance

ii. Poverty

iii. Sex worker

iv. Use of illicit drugs

v. Infection with other STIs, particularly HIV

vi. Living in an area with a high prevalence of syphilis

vii. Previous incarceration

3. Screening during pregnancy: Universal screening of pregnant individuals for syphilis at the first prenatal visit is recommended (CDC, 2021). Patients at high risk should undergo repeat serologic testing at 28 to 32 weeks gestation and at delivery. Most states have laws requiring antenatal syphilis testing. A list of syphilis screening requirements by state can be found at www.cdc.gov/std/treatment/syphilis-screenings-2018.htm. Up to Date has a new algorithm available for the screening and diagnosis of syphilis in pregnant individuals without prior history of syphilis. (www-uptodate-com.proxy.cc.uic.edu/contents/syphilis-in-pregnancy?search=syphilis%20in%20pregnancy&source=search_result&selectedTitle=1~150&usage_type=default&display_rank=1)

4. Diagnosis: Diagnosis relies upon either direct visualization of the organism (dark-field examination) or serologic testing. Pregnant individuals with titered positive nontreponemal screening tests (rapid plasma reagin [RPR] or VDRL), should have confirmatory testing with treponemal tests (*Treponema pallidum* particle agglutination assay [TP-PA] or fluorescent treponemal antibody absorption [FTA-ABS]). The TP-PA is a more sensitive test than the FTA-ABS. Nontreponemal tests do not result as positive until 7 to 10 days after the appearance of the chancre. These tests are designed to detect the presence of nonspecific antibodies and are fast, relatively inexpensive, very sensitive, and moderately nonspecific. The false-positive rate for pregnant individuals is 1% to 2%. A high titer (>1:16) usually indicates an active disease. A low titer (<1:8) indicates biologic false-positive test in 90% of the cases or occasionally may be the result of late or late latent syphilis. Prior to treatment, quantitation is always performed. A fourfold drop in the titer indicates a response to therapy. Treatment of primary syphilis usually causes a progressive decline (i.e., low titers) to a negative VDRL titer within 2 years. In secondary, late, or latent syphilis, low titers persist in approximately 50% of the cases after 2 years despite a fall in the titer. This does not indicate treatment failure or reinfection and these patients are likely to remain positive even if retreated. Titer response

TABLE 13.3 SUMMARY OF THE STAGES OF SYPHILIS INFECTION

STAGE/TIME AFTER EXPOSURE	CLINICAL FINDINGS	LABORATORY CHANGES
Primary		
10–90 d (average is 3 wk)	Infectious chancre: painless lesion at site of entry	Dark-field positive
4 wk	Lymphadenopathy: inguinal or trochlear	Serology often negative or rising titers VDRL and RPR
Secondary		
4–10 wk after chancre appearance	Infectious skin lesions: maculopapular rash on soles and palms; patchy alopecia, condylomata lata; generalized nontender lymphadenopathy; symptoms of systemic illness	Dark-field exam positive; peak antibody titers Seroconversion: FTA-ABS or TP-PA test positive
Latent		
Early: 3–12 mo Late > 12 mo	May have asymptomatic secondary lesions None in late latent	CSF: VDRL or RPR negative
		Falling VDRL or RPR titers
Tertiary	Cutaneous, cardiac, and/or neurosyphilis	CSF: VDRL positive or increased cells and protein
Stage/Time After Exposure	**Clinical Findings**	**Laboratory Changes**
Usually, >4 y and as long as 25–30 y	Asymptomatic or symptomatic CNS disease: apathy, seizures, dementia, tabes dorsalis	Serum treponemal test positive; nontreponemal test positive or negative; VDRL remains positive indefinitely with declining titer

CNS, central nervous system; CSF, cerebral spinal fluid; FTA-ABS, fluorescent treponemal antibody absorption; RPR, rapid plasma reagin; TP-PA, treponema pallidum particle agglutination assay.

is unpredictable in late or latent syphilis. Rising titer (four times) indicates relapse, reinfection, or treatment failure. See Table 13.3 for information on the various stages and presentation.

5. Treatment
   - **a.** Penicillin G Benzathine 2.4 million units IM usually administered as 1.2 million units in each buttock. Therapy regimen should be appropriate to the stage of infection. Parenteral (IM or intravenous [IV]) Penicillin G is the only therapy with documented safety and efficacy for both the mother and fetus during pregnancy. IV therapy is indicated for neurosyphilis.
   - **b.** The CDC (2021) suggests that additional therapy can be beneficial for pregnant individuals in some settings (e.g., a second dose of benzathine penicillin 2.4 million units IM administered 7–9 days after the initial dose). When syphilis is diagnosed during the second half of pregnancy, management should include a sonographic fetal evaluation for congenital syphilis, but this evaluation should not delay the therapy. Sonographic signs of fetal or placental syphilis (i.e., hepatomegaly, ascites, hydrops, fetal anemia, or a thickened placenta) indicate a greater risk for fetal treatment failure; such cases should be managed in consultation with obstetric specialists.
   - **c.** Pregnant individuals who have a history of penicillin allergy should be desensitized and treated with penicillin. Oral stepwise penicillin dose challenge or skin testing might be helpful in identifying patients at risk for acute allergic reactions.
   - **d.** Partners should be treated. Intercourse should be avoided until both partners are treated, and, if lesions were present, they should be healed.
   - **e.** The disease is reportable (usually done through laboratory).
6. Complications
   - **a.** Lack of prenatal care is associated with congenital syphilis. Detection and treatment of maternal syphilis should occur as early as possible to prevent congenital syphilis. Research has consistently shown that increased rates of syphilis screening during the first trimester leads to decreased incidence of congenital syphilis and related adverse outcomes (Norwitz & Hicks, 2020).
   - **b.** Congenital syphilis occurs in 50% to 80% of untreated primary, secondary, or early latent maternal syphilis cases. The risk of congenital syphilis is much lower, approximately 10%, for untreated late latent maternal syphilis (Adhikari, 2020).
   - **c.** Maternal syphilis is associated with increased risk for stillbirth (21%), preterm delivery (6%), and neonatal death (9%)
   - **d.** Low birth weight
   - **e.** Congenital anomalies
   - **f.** Long-term sequelae such as deafness and neurologic impairment
7. Consultation/referral
   - **a.** Consult with perinatologist with a positive diagnosis of the disease.
   - **b.** Consultation needed if elevated titers persist (if possible, consult with an infectious disease specialist).
8. Follow-up
   - **a.** All persons who have syphilis should be tested for HIV infection.
   - **b.** A fourfold decrease in the nontreponemal test titer within 6 to 12 months is expected with treatment success. However, greater than 15% of patients with early syphilis treated with the recommended therapy will not achieve the two dilution declines in nontreponemal titer used to

define response at 1 year after treatment. The person who persists with an elevated titer should be tested for HIV.

c. Quantitative nontreponemal serologic tests should be repeated at 6, 12, and 24 months. A cerebral spinal fluid (CSF) examination should be performed if

i. Titers increase fourfold

ii. An initially high titer (>1:32) fails to decline at least fourfold (i.e., two dilutions) within 12 to 24 months of therapy.

iii. Signs or symptoms attributable to syphilis develop.

d. For retreatment, weekly injections of benzathine penicillin G 2.4 million units IM for 3 weeks is recommended unless CSF examination indicates that neurosyphilis is present.

9. Patient education

a. www.cdc.gov/std/syphilis/syphilis-factsheet.pdf

Bibliography

Adhikari, E. H. (2020). Syphilis in pregnancy. *Obstetrics & gynecology, 135*(5), 1121–1135. https://doi.org/10.1097/AOG.0000000000003788

American College of Obstetricians and Gynecologists. (2020). Management of herpes in pregnancy (ACOG practice bulletin no. 220). *Obstetrics & Gynecology, 135*(5), e193–e202. https://doi.org/10.1097/AOG.0000000000003840

BD Diagnostic Systems. (n.d). *BD affirm™ VPIII microbial identification system*. http://www.bd.com/ds/productCenter/MD-AffirmVPIII.asp

Brown, H., Fuller, D., Jasper, L., Davis, T., & Wright, J. (2004). Clinical evaluation of affirm VPIII in the detection and identification of *Trichomonas vaginalis, Gardnerella vaginalis*, and Candida species in vaginitis/vaginosis. *Infectious Diseases in Obstetrics and Gynecology, 12*(1), 17–21. https://doi.org/10.1080/10647440420002103 75

Centers for Disease Control and Prevention. (n.d.-a). *Bacterial vaginosis—CDC fact sheet*. http://www.cdc.gov/std/bv/stdfact-bacterial-vaginosis.htm

Centers for Disease Control and Prevention. (n.d.-b). *STDs during pregnancy—CDC fact sheet*. http://www.cdc.gov/std/pregnancy/STDfact-Pregnancy.htm

Centers for Disease Control and Prevention. (2019). *2019 Sexually transmitted disease surveillance report*. U.S. Department of Health and Human Services. https://www.cdc.gov/std/statistics/2019/default.htm

Centers for Disease Control and Prevention. (2021). *2021 Sexually transmitted infections treatment guidelines*. https://www.cdc.gov/std/treatment-guidelines/toc.htm

Cunningham, F. G., Leveno, K. J., Bloom, S. L., Spong, C. Y., Dashe, J. S., Hoffman, B. L., Casey, B. M., & Sheffield, J. S. (2014). *William's obstetrics* (24th ed.). McGraw-Hill.

Curry, K. (2018). Screening for syphilis infection in pregnant women: US Preventive Services Task Force reaffirmation recommendation statement. *JAMA: The Journal of the American Medical Association, 320*(9), 911–917. https://doi.org/10.1001/jama.2018.11785

DynaMed. (2016, February 15). *Gonococcal cervicitis*. EBSCO Publishing. http://www.dynamed.com/topics/dmp~AN~T113822/Gonococcal-cervicitis

DynaMed. (2016, April 27). *Vulvovaginal candidiasis*. EBSCO Publishing. http://www.dynamed.com/topics/dmp~AN~T116590#anc-1826900482

DynaMed. (2016, May 10). *Trichomoniasis*. EBSCO Publishing. http://www.dynamed.com/topics/dmp~AN~T116226/Trichomoniasis

Fantasia, H. C., Harris, A. L., & Fontenot, H. B. (2020). *Guidelines for nurse practitioners in gynecologic settings* (12th ed.). Springer Publishing Company.

Fyle-Thorpe, O. (2019). Chlamydia and gonorrhea: An update. *Journal for Nurse Practitioners, 15*(6), 424–428. https://doi.org/10.1016/j.nurpra.2018.12.027

Howley, M. M., Carter, T. C., Browne, M. L., Romitti, P. A., Cunniff, C. M., & Druschel, C. M. (2016). Fluconazole use and birth defects in the National Birth Defects Prevention Study. *American Journal of Obstetrics & Gynecology, 214*(5), 657.e1–657.e9. https://doi.org/10.1016/j.ajog.2015.11.022

Jensen, J. S., Cusini, M., Gomberg, M., & Moi, H. (2016). 2016 European guideline on Mycoplasma genitalium infections. *Journal of the European Academy of Dermatology and Venereology: JEADV, 30*(10), 1650–1656. https://doi.org/10.1111/jdv.13849

Kayem, D. (2018). Antibiotics for amniotic-fluid colonization by Ureaplasma and/or Mycoplasma spp. to prevent preterm birth: A randomized trial. *PloS One, 13*(11), e0206290. https://doi.org/10.1371/journal.pone.0206290

Lee, N. (2016). Sexually transmitted infections: Recommendations from the U.S. Preventive Services Task Force. *American Family Physician, 94*(11), 907–915.

Mølgaard-Nielsen, D., Svanström, H., Melbye, M., Hviid, A., & Pasternak, B. (2016). Association between use of oral fluconazole during pregnancy and risk of spontaneous abortion and stillbirth. *Journal of the American Medical Association, 15*(1), 58–67. https://doi.org/10.1001/jama.2015.17844

Money, S. (2017). 208-Guidelines for the management of herpes simplex virus in pregnancy. *Journal of Obstetrics and Gynaecology Canada, 39*(8), e199–e205. https://doi.org/10.1016/j.jogc.2017.04.016

Motomura, K., Romero, R., Xu, Y., Theis, K. R., Galaz, J., Winters, A. D., Slutsky, R., Garcia Flores, V., Zou, C., Levenson, D., Para, R., Ahmad, M. M., Miller, D., Hsu, C. D., & Gomez-Lopez, N. (2020). Intra-amniotic infection with *Ureaplasma parvum* causes preterm birth and neonatal mortality that are prevented by treatment with clarithromycin. *mBio, 11*(3), e00797-20–. https://doi.org/10.1128/mBio.00797-20

Norwitz, E. R., & Hicks, C. B. (2020). *Syphilis in pregnancy. UpToDate.* https://www-uptodate-com.proxy.cc.uic.edu/contents/syphilis-in-pregnancy?search=syphilis%20in%20pregnancy&source=search_result&selectedTitle=1~150&usage_type=default&display_rank=1

Olaleye, B. (2020). Sexually transmitted infections in pregnancy – An update on Chlamydia trachomatis and Neisseria gonorrhoeae. *European Journal of Obstetrics & Gynecology and Reproductive Biology, 255*, 1–12. https://doi.org/10.1016/j.ejogrb.2020.10.002

Rac, R. (2016). Syphilis during pregnancy: A preventable threat to maternal-fetal health. *American Journal of Obstetrics and Gynecology, 216*(4), 352–363. https://doi.org/10.1016/j.ajog.2016.11.1052

Sobel, J. (2012). *Trichomonas vaginalis. UpToDate.* . www.uptodate.com

Soong, D., & Einarson, A. (2009). Vaginal yeast infections during pregnancy. *Canadian Family Physician, 55*(3), 255–256.

Straface, G., Selmin, A., Zanardo, V., De Santis, M., Ercoli, A., & Scambia, G. (2012). Herpes simplex virus infection in pregnancy. *Infectious Diseases in Obstetrics & Gynecology, 2012*, 385697. https://doi.org/10.1155/2012/385697

Tsai, S. (2019). Syphilis in pregnancy. *Obstetrical & Gynecological Survey, 74*(9), 557–564. https://doi.org/10.1097/ogx.0000000000000713

van Schalkwyk, Y. (2015). Vulvovaginitis: Screening for and management of trichomoniasis, vulvovaginal candidiasis, and bacterial vaginosis. *Journal of Obstetrics and Gynaecology Canada, 37*(3), 266–274. https://doi.org/10.1016/S1701-2163(15)30316-9

Williamson, M. A., & Snyder, L. M. (2014). *Wallach's interpretation of diagnostic tests* (10th ed.). Lippincott Williams & Wilkins.

Workowski, K. A., & Bolan, G. A. (2015). Sexually transmitted diseases treatment guidelines. *MMWR Recommendations & Reports, 64*(3), 1–134.

Young, G. L., & Jewell, D. (2013). Topical treatment for vaginal candidiasis (thrush) in pregnancy. *Cochrane Database of Systematic Reviews, 2013*(4). https://doi.org/10.1002/14651858.CD000225

Yudin, M., & Money, D. M. (2017). 211-Screening and management of bacterial vaginosis in pregnancy. *Journal of Obstetrics and Gynaecology Canada, 39*(8), e184–e191. https://doi.org/10.1016/j.jogc.2017.04.018

14. Dermatoses of Pregnancy

NANCY J. CIBULKA | KELLY D. ROSENBERGER

The skin is the largest and most visible organ of the body and undergoes changes during pregnancy that may be distressing for patients. Although many skin changes, such as hyperpigmentation, striae gravidarum, vascular changes, increase in sweat gland activity, and rashes, may be benign, pregnant individuals with complaints involving the skin need to be thoroughly assessed. Pruritus (itching) is a common complaint during pregnancy and, although often related to normal skin changes, in some instances, it may indicate a serious health concern.

This chapter reviews assessment and management of four dermatoses that cause severe itching during pregnancy: pruritic urticarial plaques and papules (PUPPP), atopic eruption, pemphigoid gestationis (PG), and intrahepatic cholestasis of pregnancy (ICP). Although ICP is actually a disease of the liver, it presents with intense itching, and so it is often classified as a pregnancy dermatosis. ICP and PG carry significant risk to the fetus.

Pruritic Urticarial Plaques and Papules of Pregnancy or Polymorphic Eruption of Pregnancy

A. BACKGROUND

1. Polymorphic eruption of pregnancy (PEP) is the most common dermatosis of pregnancy and is characterized by pruritic papules and urticarial plaques that start on the abdomen within striae and then may spread to thighs, buttocks, back, and extremities. The face, palms, soles of the feet, and umbilicus are usually spared. The lesions form urticarial plaques. Itching is extreme.

2. Typically begins in the third trimester or immediate postpartum period.

3. Average age of onset is 25 years; about 40% of cases occur in primigravidas, 30% in individuals who are pregnant for the second time, and 15% in individuals who are pregnant for the third time (Habif et al., 2011).

4. PUPPP is associated with excessive stretching of the abdomen; thus it is seen more often with large weight gain resulting in abdominal distension and with multifetal pregnancies.

5. The condition is self-limited and generally resolves by 15 days postpartum. There are no associated complications during pregnancy and delivery and no known risks to the fetus.

6. Itching can affect sleep and quality of life as well as cause or exacerbate depression.

B. HISTORY

1. Assess the patient for the following:

a. Number of weeks gestation and any prior pregnancy-related health problems

b. Changes in skin: Dryness, pruritus, lesions, and color
c. Temporal sequence and location: Time and site of symptom onset, progression of rash or lesions in skinfolds or surface areas
d. Symptoms and associated symptoms: Itching, pain, bleeding, color change, fever, nausea, vomiting, and diarrhea
e. Recent exposure to drugs, irritants, toxins or chemicals, travel, or anyone else with similar symptoms

2. Ask about presence of skin problems before pregnancy and effect of pregnancy on any preexisting conditions.
3. Ask about home remedies and over-the-counter treatments.
4. Ask about any other complaints or health problems.
5. Assess for any signs of evolving pregnancy complications:
   a. Fetal movements
   b. Cramps
   c. Contractions
   d. Leaking fluid from the vagina
   e. Swelling/edema

C. PHYSICAL EXAMINATION

1. Check vital signs: Blood pressure, pulse, respiration, and temperature should be within normal limits.
2. Observe the general appearance.
3. Inspect rash and location of lesions. Lesions typically begin as red papules surrounded by a pale halo, quickly increase in number, and often coalesce into plaques. Lesions may also appear target-like (see www.uptodate.com, Google Images, or a dermatology text for pictures).
4. Lesions start on the abdomen, often in or around the striae, then spread in a symmetric fashion to cover the buttocks, legs, arms, and back of the hands.

D. LABORATORY AND DIAGNOSTIC STUDIES

1. Diagnosed by clinical observation
2. Biopsy and labs are not indicated

E. DIFFERENTIAL DIAGNOSES

1. PUPPP
2. PG
3. Erythema multiforme
4. Any atopic eruption during pregnancy (urticarial, drug eruption, eczema, contact dermatitis, drug eruption, insect bites, etc.)
5. Viral exanthem
6. Scabies

F. MANAGEMENT

1. Low- to mid-potency topical corticosteroids (groups IV–VI) applied to affected areas
2. Antipruritic lotions or emollients
3. Cool baths or cool, wet dressings
4. Diphenhydramine 25 to 50 mg every 4 to 6 hours or hydroxyzine 25 mg every 6 to 8 hours as needed, or nonsedating antihistamines such as loratadine or cetirizine 10 mg once daily may be used after the first trimester. Chlorpheniramine may be used during pregnancy when a first-generation antihistamine is needed with the lowest effective dose used. Hydroxyzine 25 mg every 6 to 8 hours may be used in the second and third trimesters but

should not be used during or prior to labor due to increased seizure risk in infants, decreased fetal heart rate, and increased side effects when combined with narcotics.

5. Prednisone 30 to 40 mg per day may be required if itching is severe and unrelieved by other measures

G. CONSULTATION/REFERRAL

1. Consult with a physician if symptoms are unrelieved with treatment or if any obstetric complication is detected.

2. Refer to a dermatologist if indicated by ongoing and/or worsening symptoms.

H. FOLLOW-UP

1. Typically resolves shortly after delivery, and recurrence is not usual in future pregnancy

Atopic Eruption During Pregnancy

A. BACKGROUND

1. Patients may present at any stage of pregnancy with exacerbation of preexisting or new-onset atopic dermatitis.

2. Eczema or atopic dermatitis is pruritic, recurrent, and often occurs in flexural areas of the body. Other areas, such as face, neck, breast cleavage, and extremities, can also be affected. This disorder generally begins early in life and is characterized by periods of remission and exacerbation.

3. Prurigo of pregnancy is an atopic eruption of erythematous or excoriated nodules or papules on extensor surfaces beginning in the second or third trimester and resolving in the immediate postpartum period (Pomeranz, 2020). Lesions may be crusted and are grouped, appearing on the abdomen and extremities.

4. Pruritic folliculitis is a noninfectious eruption of pruritic, follicular lesions that may appear pustule-like. This disorder begins in the second or third trimester and occurs on the trunk and extremities. It usually resolves within 2 weeks postpartum.

5. Atopic disorders are associated with personal or family history of eczema, asthma, or hay fever.

6. Itching can affect sleep and quality of life as well as cause or exacerbate depression.

7. There are no associated complications during pregnancy and delivery and no known risks to the fetus.

B. HISTORY

1. Assess the patient for the following:

- **a.** Number of weeks gestation and any prior pregnancy-related health problems
- **b.** Changes in skin: Dryness, pruritus, lesions, and color
- **c.** Temporal sequence and location: Time and site of symptom onset, progression of rash or lesions in skinfolds or surface areas
- **d.** Symptoms and associated symptoms: Itching, pain, bleeding, color change, fever, nausea, vomiting, and diarrhea
- **e.** Recent exposure to drugs, irritants, toxins or chemicals, excessive heat and sweating, travel, anyone else with similar symptoms

2. Ask about personal and/or family history of asthma, allergic rhinitis or conjunctivitis, and/or atopic dermatitis.

3. Ask about home remedies and over-the-counter treatments.
4. Ask about any other complaints or health problems.
5. Assess for any signs of evolving pregnancy complications:
   a. Fetal movements
   b. Cramps
   c. Contractions
   d. Leaking fluid from the vagina
   e. Swelling/edema

C. PHYSICAL EXAMINATION

1. Check vital signs; blood pressure, pulse, respiration, and temperature should be within normal limits.
2. Observe the general appearance.
3. Inspect rash and location of lesions; excoriation may be present from scratching (see www.uptodate.com, Google Images, or a dermatology text for pictures).
4. The most common atopic disorder is eczema. Acute lesions may be oozing and vesicular, whereas older lesions are often scaly and crusted; chronic lesions may be dull red and lichenified (Habif et al., 2011). In adults, flexural surfaces are commonly involved, hand dermatitis may be present, and dermatitis of the upper eyelid is common.

D. LABORATORY AND DIAGNOSTIC STUDIES

1. Diagnosed by clinical observation
2. Biopsy and labs are not indicated unless bacterial superinfection is suspected. If so, culture and sensitivity testing should be done.
3. Pustule-appearing nodules (present in pruritic folliculitis) should be cultured to rule out infection.

E. DIFFERENTIAL DIAGNOSES

1. Atopic eruption of pregnancy
2. PUPPP
3. PG
4. Viral exanthem
5. Scabies
6. Tinea

F. MANAGEMENT

1. Eliminate or reduce exposure to aggravating external exposures.
2. Apply low- to mid-potency topical corticosteroids (groups IV–VI) applied twice daily for 10 to 21 days.
3. Antipruritic lotions or emollients
4. Soft, light clothing and cool environment
5. Diphenhydramine 25 to 50 mg every 4 to 6 hours or nonsedating antihistamines such as loratadine or cetirizine 10 mg once daily may be used after the first trimester. Chlorpheniramine may be used during pregnancy when a first-generation antihistamine is needed with the lowest effective dose used. Hydroxyzine 25 mg every 6 to 8 hours may be used in the second and third trimesters, but should not be used during or prior to labor due to increased seizure risk in infants, decreased fetal heart rate, and increased side effects when combined with narcotics.
6. A short course of oral corticosteroids may be indicated to reduce inflammation but is rarely needed.
7. Stress reduction may be helpful.

G. COMPLICATIONS

1. Secondary infection with *Staphylococcus aureus* or other bacteria
2. Increased risk of viral infections, such as herpes simplex or fungal infections
3. Hypopigmentation or hyperpigmentation from chronic inflammation

H. CONSULTATION/REFERRAL

1. Consult with a physician if symptoms are unrelieved with treatment or if any obstetric complication is detected.
2. Refer to a dermatologist if indicated by ongoing and/or worsening symptoms, severe or refractory disease.

I. FOLLOW-UP

1. Examine at each prenatal visit and postpartum.

Pemphigoid Gestationis

A. BACKGROUND

1. PG is a rare, autoimmune disorder that usually appears late in pregnancy and is associated with fetal risk.
2. PG is characterized by blistering lesions; as a result, it was originally named *herpes gestationis.* However, this disorder is not related to the herpes virus.
3. Initial symptom is intense itching around the umbilical area followed by a papulo-urticarial rash with erythematous plaques in the periumbilical region. Plaques turn dark red in 1 to 3 weeks as vesicles and fluid-filled bullae begin to develop.
4. Lesions spread rapidly, extending to the trunk, back, buttocks, and extremities, including palms and soles, but rarely occur on the face or mucous membranes (Pomeranz, 2020).
5. Although the etiology is multifactorial, it is thought that an immune response during pregnancy may trigger this condition.
6. PG may flare up postpartum; however, most cases resolve spontaneously, but this may take several weeks; breastfeeding is not contraindicated.

B. HISTORY

1. Assess the patient for the following:
   - a. Number of weeks gestation and any prior pregnancy-related health problems
   - b. Changes in skin: Dryness, pruritus, lesions, and color
   - c. Temporal sequence and location: Time and site of symptom onset, progression of rash or lesions in skinfolds or surface areas
   - d. Symptoms and associated symptoms: Itching, pain, bleeding, color change, fever, nausea, vomiting, and diarrhea
   - e. Recent exposure to drugs, irritants, toxins or chemicals, travel, anyone else with similar symptoms
2. Ask about presence of skin problems before pregnancy or in a previous pregnancy.
3. Ask about home remedies and over-the-counter treatments.
4. Ask about any other complaints or health problems.
5. Assess for any signs of evolving pregnancy complications:
   - a. Fetal movements
   - b. Cramps

c. Contractions
d. Leaking fluid from the vagina
e. Swelling/edema

C. PHYSICAL EXAMINATION

1. Check vital signs; blood pressure, pulse, respirations, and temperature should be within normal limits.
2. Observe the general appearance.
3. Inspect rash and location of lesions. Rash begins as extremely pruritic around the umbilicus followed by papulo-urticarial rash with erythematous plaques. Plaques turn dark red in 1 to 3 weeks as vesicles and fluid-filled bullae begin to develop.
4. Lesions start in the periumbilical area, and then extend to trunk, back, buttocks, and extremities; they rarely spread to the face (Phillips & Boyd, 2015; see www.uptodate.com, Google Images, or a dermatology text for pictures).

D. LABORATORY AND DIAGNOSTIC STUDIES

1. Diagnosis is made by skin biopsy.

E. DIFFERENTIAL DIAGNOSES

1. PG
2. Herpes viral infection
3. Allergic contact dermatitis
4. PUPPP
5. Viral exanthem
6. Erythema multiforme

F. MANAGEMENT

1. A dermatologist and obstetrician should coordinate care for a patient with PG.
2. Treatment is mid- to high-potency topical corticosteroids (groups II–IV) applied two or three times daily.
3. Cool baths or cool, wet compresses and emollients may help.
4. Nonsedating antihistamines may help; consider diphenhydramine or hydroxyzine 25 to 50 mg at bedtime.
5. In severe cases, treatment with oral steroids is advised (prednisone 0.5 mg/kg/d).

G. COMPLICATIONS

1. Increased risk for placental insufficiency, intrauterine growth restriction (IUGR), prematurity, and stillbirth
2. A small number of newborns will have a mild blistering rash that can persist for 6 weeks but will resolve spontaneously.
3. PG often reoccurs with subsequent pregnancies and may be worse each time.

H. CONSULTATION/REFERRAL

1. Refer patient to an obstetrician and a dermatologist for care.
2. Patients are at risk for recurrence with menstruation and use of oral contraceptives and at risk for developing other autoimmune diseases; therefore, follow-up with their primary provider is recommended after pregnancy.

I. FOLLOW-UP

1. PG typically resolves within days or weeks after delivery.

Intrahepatic Cholestasis

A. BACKGROUND

1. ICP is a liver disorder that affects individuals in the second or third trimester of pregnancy. This disorder presents with intense itching and elevation in serum bile acid concentrations. Itching is usually generalized but most intense on the palms of the hands and soles of the feet. It is worse at night.

2. No rash or lesions are associated with ICP.

3. Etiology is not completely understood but thought to occur in genetically predisposed pregnant individuals. Hormonal and environmental factors are also involved (Holley, 2013).

4. Other risk factors include multiple gestation, maternal age older than 35 years, family or personal history of ICP, assisted reproduction therapy, and preeclampsia; the risk of recurrence is 60% to 70% in future pregnancies.

5. ICP is associated with the risk of poor outcome to the fetus, including preterm birth, intrauterine death, and an increased risk for neonatal respiratory distress syndrome associated with bile acids entering fetal lungs (Lindor & Lee, 2020).

6. ICP is not a contraindication for breastfeeding.

B. HISTORY

1. Assess the patient for the following:

a. Number of weeks gestation and any pregnancy-related health problems

b. Changes in skin: Rash, dryness, pruritus, lesions, and color

c. Temporal sequence and location: Time and site of symptom onset

d. Symptoms and associated symptoms: Itching, pain, bleeding, color change, fever, nausea, vomiting, and diarrhea

e. Recent exposure to drugs, irritants, toxins or chemicals, travel, anyone else with similar symptoms

2. Presence of skin problems before pregnancy

3. History of itching or ICP in a prior pregnancy

4. Ask about home remedies and over-the-counter treatments.

5. Ask about any other complaints or health problems

a. Patients with ICP have an increased risk for urinary tract infection.

b. Fatigue may be present as a result of sleep deprivation related to itching at night.

6. Assess for any signs of evolving pregnancy complications:

a. Fetal movements

b. Cramps

c. Contractions

d. Leaking fluid from the vagina

e. Swelling/edema

C. PHYSICAL EXAMINATION

1. Check vital signs; blood pressure, pulse, respiration, and temperature should be within normal limits.

2. Observe the general appearance

3. Inspect the skin for any lesions or rash or excoriations from itching.

4. Inspect the color of skin (jaundice may occur around 10% of the time).

D. LABORATORY AND DIAGNOSTIC STUDIES

1. Check total serum bile acids (most sensitive marker for ICP, confirms diagnosis if >10 µmol/L).

2. Check liver transaminases: Alanine aminotransferase (ALT), aspartate aminotransferase (AST), and gamma glutamyl transferase (GGT).
3. Other labs: Cholic acid, chenodeoxycholic acid, total bilirubin, prothrombin time (PT), and partial prothromboplastin time (PPT)
4. Consider liver ultrasound to rule out biliary obstruction.

E. DIFFERENTIAL DIAGNOSES

1. ICP
2. Preeclampsia or early HELLP (hemolysis/elevated liver enzymes/low platelet count) syndrome
3. Cholelithiasis
4. Hepatitis
5. Acute fatty liver
6. Dermatitis

F. MANAGEMENT

1. Ursodeoxycholic acid (UDCA) improves symptoms and liver parameters and is the drug of choice for ICP. Although the optimal dose has not been determined, start with 3,500 mg twice daily or 300 mg three times a day; increase further to a maximum of 15 to 20 mg/kg/d if needed (Lindor & Lee, 2020; Rigby, 2016).
2. Cool baths or compresses and emollients may help with itching.
3. Antihistamines, such as chlorpheniramine or hydroxyzine, are often given along with UDCA to relieve pruritus and help treat insomnia.
4. Antenatal testing is recommended, including umbilical artery Doppler studies, biophysical profile, and nonstress testing; however, the predictive value is uncertain because the mechanism for fetal demise is unknown and not thought to be the result of placental insufficiency. Daily fetal kick counts are also advised.
5. Delivery at 36 to 37 weeks is associated with a low risk of adverse outcomes; however, as the risk of fetal demise appears to increase with higher bile acid levels, some providers are waiting until 38 to 39 weeks if pruritus has resolved with treatment and bile acids are not significantly elevated. The Society for Maternal-Fetal Medicine recommends the timing of delivery should be based on the total bile acid level, and American College of Obstetricians and Gynecologists (ACOG) endorses the recommendations:
   a. Total bile acid levels ≥100 micromol/L, delivery is offered at 36 0/7ths weeks GA
   b. Total bile acid levels <100 micromol/L, delivery is offered at 36 0/7ths to 39 0/7ths weeks GA, with the timing individualized toward the later end of this time range for patients with bile acid levels <40 micromol/L and toward the earlier end of this time range for patients with total bile acid levels ≥40 micromol/L.

G. COMPLICATIONS

1. Increased risk for prematurity
2. Increased risk for sudden fetal death
3. Increased risk for meconium in amniotic fluid and for neonatal respiratory distress
4. Increased risk for maternal cholestasis

H. CONSULTATION/REFERRAL

1. Refer the patient to an obstetrician for care or comanage care.

2. Refer the patient to the primary care provider or to a specialist if symptoms persist and/or bile acid levels and liver function tests remain elevated 3 to 6 months postpartum.

I. FOLLOW-UP

1. Serum bile acid levels and liver function tests should be checked at 6 to 8 weeks postpartum. If levels remain elevated, refer to primary care provider or to a specialist for further evaluation.

2. Maternal prognosis is good, and itching usually resolves in the first few days after birth. Patients may be at risk for cholestasis in the future.

3. Patients with a history of ICP should be cautioned to use hormonal contraception with care, as there is a 10% chance of developing hepatic impairment or cholestasis. Use the lowest possible dose and monitor liver function tests periodically.

Bibliography

Freiman, A. (2015). *Pemphigoid gestationis.* http://emedicine.medscape.com/article/1063499-overview

Habif, T. P., Campbell, J. L., Chapman, M. S., Dinulos, J. G. H., & Zug, K. A. (2011). *Skin disease* (3rd ed.). Elsevier Mosby.

Holley, S. L. (2013). Intrahepatic cholestasis of pregnancy. *Journal for Nurse Practitioners, 9*(6), 398–399. https://doi.org/10.1016/j.nurpra.2013.02.024

Kar, S., Krishnan, A., Preetha, K., & Mohankar, A. (2012). A review of antihistamines used during pregnancy. *Journal of Pharmacology & Pharmacotherapeutics,* 3(2), 105–108. https://doi.org/ 10.4103/0976-500X.95503

Lee, R. H., Greenberg, M., Metz, T. D., & Pettker, C. M. (2020). *Society for maternal-fetal medicine consult series #53: Intrahepatic cholestasis of pregnancy (Replaces consult #13).* https://www-sciencedirect-com.proxy.cc.uic.edu/science/article/pii/S0002937820312849?via%3Dihub

Lindor, K. D., & Lee, R. H. (2020). *Intrahepatic cholestasis of pregnancy.* http://www.uptodate.com

Phillips, C., & Boyd, M. (2015). Intrahepatic cholestasis of pregnancy. *Nursing for Women's Health, 19*(1), 46–57. https://doi.org/10.1111/1751-486X.12175

Pierson, J. C. (2016). *Polymorphic eruption of pregnancy.* http://emedicine.medscape.com/article/1123725-overview

Pomeranz, M. K. (2020). *Dermatoses of pregnancy.* http://www.uptodate.com

Rigby, F. B. (2016). *Intrahepatic cholestasis of pregnancy.* http://emedicine.medscape.com/article/1562288-overview

IV. Guidelines for Management of Selected Complications of Pregnancy

15. Bleeding and Pregnancy Loss

MARY LEE BARRON | KELLY D. ROSENBERGER

First-trimester vaginal bleeding occurs in up to 20% to 40% of pregnant individuals. Approximately half of these bleeding episodes precede miscarriage. Causes of first-trimester bleeding range from life-threatening to minor complaints. Causes include implantation bleeding, miscarriage, ectopic pregnancy, gestational trophoblastic disease (GTD), cervicitis, cervical polyps, postcoital bleeding, clotting disorder, and/or sexual assault. *Second and third trimester vaginal bleeding*, because of abruptio placentae or placenta previa, may result in hemorrhage. Hemorrhage during pregnancy is one of the leading causes of maternal death in the United States (Creanga et al., 2015).

Implantation Bleeding

A. DEFINITION

1. This is typically defined as bleeding that occurs 10 to 14 days after conception; duration is short: 1 to 2 days and is usually lighter than a menstrual period.
2. Patient may confuse this with a normal menstrual period, making dating the pregnancy more complex.
3. No treatment is necessary as it stops spontaneously.

Miscarriage (Early Pregnancy Loss)

A. DEFINITION

1. Miscarriage, formerly known as *spontaneous abortion*, is defined as a pregnancy that ends spontaneously before the fetus has reached the age of viability (typically at 20–22 weeks gestation). Although the term "fetus" is used, this also applies to the embryo (<8 weeks gestation). The change in terminology has been recommended by the American College of Obstetricians and Gynecologists (ACOG; 2015) as being more sensitive to what patients experience in pregnancy loss. Abortion describes both elective and spontaneous processes, but the term *abortion* is politically charged. In 2018, ACOG changed the terminology to early pregnancy loss in its practice bulletins.

B. INCIDENCE

1. Most common complication of early pregnancy
2. 8% to 30% of clinically recognized pregnancies will be spontaneously miscarried; 80% of these will occur in the first 12 weeks. 50% of pregnant individuals with first-trimester bleeding will have a spontaneous miscarriage; the other 50% will continue with the pregnancy.

3. The frequency of miscarriage decreases with gestational age (GA); loss rates are higher at the extremes of childbearing age with the lowest loss rates in pregnant individuals in their 20s.

4. African American pregnant individuals have a higher loss rate in nearly every age group when compared with Caucasian and Asian American pregnant individuals (Cunningham et al., 2014; Wyatt et al., 2005).

C. RISK FACTORS

1. Age: Advanced maternal age is the most important risk factor; the loss rate by age:
  - **a.** 20 to 30 years—9% to 17%
  - **b.** 35 years—20%
  - **c.** 40 years—40%
  - **d.** 45 years—80%

2. Miscarriage occurs in only about 5% of individuals in their first pregnancy and in those who had a previous pregnancy that was successful. But in those who have experienced a miscarriage, the risk of recurrence rate is:
  - **a.** 20% after one miscarriage
  - **b.** 28% after two consecutive miscarriages
  - **c.** 43% after three or more consecutive miscarriages

3. Previous elective abortion

4. Gravidity: Repeated miscarriage results in higher gravidity or short interconception interval in multigravida individuals.

5. Uterine abnormalities
  - **a.** Congenital
  - **b.** Adhesions
  - **c.** Fibroids

6. Prolonged time to achieving pregnancy

7. Low serum levels of progesterone

8. Chromosomal and/or congenital anomalies

9. Celiac disease (untreated); once treated, the risk is about the same as the normal population.

10. Polycystic ovarian syndrome (PCOS)
  - **a.** Mechanism unknown (may be the result of the effects of abnormal ovulation on the hormonal milieu)
  - **b.** Rate is 20% to 40%

11. Maternal endocrinopathies
  - **a.** Thyroid dysfunction
  - **b.** Cushing's syndrome

12. Antiphospholipid syndrome and other thrombophilias such as systemic lupus erythematosus

13. Maternal infection (large number of organisms such as *Listeria monocytogenes, Toxoplasma gondii*, parvovirus B19, rubella, herpes simplex, cytomegalic virus, etc.)

14. Fever >100°F (37.8°C) *may* increase risk (studies are contradictory)

15. Trauma from invasive intrauterine procedures such as chorionic villus biopsy or amniocentesis

16. Maternal body mass index (BMI) <18.5 or >25 kg/m^2

17. Smoking (both maternal and paternal) up to 3.4 relative risk (when taken together)

18. Alcohol (moderate to high consumption)

19. Cocaine

20. Medications
  - **a.** Nonsteroidal anti-inflammatory drugs (NSAIDs); may be associated if used around the time of conception

b. Prostaglandin inhibitors interfere with implantation, which leads to abnormal implantation and subsequent miscarriage

c. Misoprostol (Cytotec)

d. Retinoids

e. Methotrexate

21. High caffeine intake (possible): There are multiple limitations in the research methodology and inconsistent outcomes; variations exist in caffeine metabolism; may be related to GA-specific exposure. Prudent practice is to recommend less than 200 mg/d. The Center for Science in the Public Interest (2021) provides a caffeine chart containing approximate content in foods and beverages:

a. Coffee (6-oz cup): drip, 175; percolated, 132; instant regular, 64; decaffeinated, 3; A 20-ounce coffee may contain up to 398 mg.

b. Cola drinks (12 oz): Coca-Cola Classic, 46; Coke Free, 0; Pepsi, 43; Pepsi Free, 0 to 2; Dr Pepper, 38; Mountain Dew, 52; Tab, 50; Jolt, 71; 44-oz "cup" of Coke/Pepsi, 169/158

c. Tea (5-minute brew, 6 oz), 24 to 60. A 16-ounce iced or regular tea may contain up 98 mg.

d. Varied sizes of caffeinated shakes and waters range from 30 to 100 mg.

e. Cocoa and chocolate: cocoa beverage (water mix, 6 oz), 18. Milk-chocolate candy bar (8 oz) 48; baking chocolate (1 oz), 35. Assorted sizes of chocolate candy/drinks range from 2 to 600 mg

f. A 16-ounce energy drink may contain up to 300 mg and indeterminate amounts of herbal stimulants

g. Over-the-counter weight loss supplements and medications range from 64 to 300 mg

22. Toxins: arsenic, lead, ethylene glycol, carbon disulfide, polyurethane, heavy metals, and organic solvents

D. TERMINOLOGY AND CLINICAL MANIFESTATIONS

1. Threatened miscarriage: Bleeding through a closed cervical os in the first half of pregnancy with the absence of passing/passed tissue; bleeding may be painless or accompanied by pain that is not very intense. The bleeding is rarely severe. Diffuse uterine and/or adnexal tenderness may be present.

2. Inevitable miscarriage: Imminent; bleeding increases, tissue may be present, painful uterine cramps/contractions reach peak intensity, and the cervix is dilated

3. Complete miscarriage: Occurs before 12 weeks gestation, common for the entire contents of the uterus to be expelled. The patient may present with a history of bleeding, abdominal pain, and tissue passage. By the time the miscarriage is complete, bleeding and pain usually subside.

4. Incomplete miscarriage: The contents of the uterus are not completely expelled. After 12 weeks, the membranes rupture and the fetus is expelled, but the placental tissue may be retained. The cervical os is open, the uterine size may be smaller than GA but not well contracted (because of the interference of retained placenta). Vaginal bleeding may be intense and accompanied by abdominal pain.

5. Missed miscarriage: In utero death of the embryo or fetus before the 20th week of gestation, with retention of the pregnancy for a prolonged period of time. The patient may report that symptoms associated with early pregnancy (e.g., nausea and breast tenderness) have abated and "not feeling pregnant" anymore; vaginal bleeding may occur.

6. Septic abortion: Miscarriage or induced abortion associated with bacterial infection (as by *Escherichia coli, Staphylococcus aureus*, beta-hemolytic streptococci, or *Clostridium perfringens*). The infection leads to salpingitis, generalized peritonitis, and septicemia. The patient may present with fever, chills, malaise, abdominal pain, vaginal bleeding, and discharge, which is often sanguinopurulent. The patient may also be tachycardic, tachypneic, complain of lower abdominal tenderness, and a have a boggy, tender uterus with dilated cervix.

E. HISTORY

1. Date of last menstrual period (LMP)
2. Estimated length of gestation
3. Ultrasound results if previously done
4. Previous miscarriage or induced abortions
5. Bleeding disorders history or familial history
6. Character and duration of vaginal bleeding
   a. Presence of blood clots or tissue
   b. Number of pads or tampons used
7. Presence and location of pain or cramps
   a. Pain may be suprapubic or abdominal
   b. May radiate to lower back, genitalia, and perineum
8. Gush of fluid
9. Fever
10. Medication use

F. PHYSICAL EXAMINATION

1. Vital signs: Should be within normal limits for pregnancy unless the infection is present or hemorrhage has caused hypovolemia.
2. Abdominal examination
   a. Tenderness
   b. Guarding
   c. Bowel sounds
   d. Distension
3. Pelvic examination should focus on the source of the bleeding
   a. Blood from the cervical os
   b. Intensity of bleeding
   c. Presence of clots or tissue fragments
   d. Cervical motion tenderness (presence increases suspicion for ectopic pregnancy)
   e. Status of internal cervical os: Closed cervical os indicates threatened miscarriage; open indicates inevitable or possibly incomplete miscarriage, but this is not reliable for distinguishing between incomplete and complete miscarriage
   f. Uterine size and tenderness as well as adnexal tenderness or masses

G. LABORATORY AND DIAGNOSTIC STUDIES

1. Qualitative urine pregnancy test to confirm pregnancy if the patient is <6 weeks from LMP
2. Complete blood count (CBC) with differential
3. Potassium hydroxide and "wet prep" microscopy of any vaginal discharge
4. Gonorrhea and chlamydia testing, if not already obtained, should be considered
5. Blood type and Rh factor
   a. Blood type must be documented for every pregnant individual with vaginal bleeding.

b. If Rh negative, facilitate the administration of RhoGAM® to prevent hemolytic disease of the newborn in this pregnancy and subsequent pregnancies.

6. Quantitative beta-human chorionic gonadotropin (β-HCG)

a. The discriminatory level of serum β-HCG levels that correlates with the size and GA in normal embryonic growth is approximately 1,500 mIU/mL above which there should be sonographic evidence of early intrauterine pregnancy, if present.

b. Serum β-HCG levels that correlate with the size and GA in normal embryonic growth doubles approximately every 48 hours for 85% of intrauterine pregnancies. The remaining 15% may rise with a different slope or have plateaued.

c. A higher likelihood of ectopic pregnancy or subsequent miscarriage exists if β-HCG levels that correlate with the size and GA in normal embryonic growth blood are lower than predicted by estimated GA based on the LMP.

d. The possibility of molar pregnancy exists if β-HCG is very high and out of proportion to predicted GA.

7. Progesterone level

a. A value >25 ng/mL has been associated with healthy pregnancy, and therefore ectopic can be excluded. A level <5 ng/mL indicates a nonviable pregnancy.

8. Factor XIII and fibrinogen, if indicated per history

9. Ultrasound is the most accurate diagnostic modality in the confirmation of a viable pregnancy during the first trimester. A high-resolution vaginal ultrasound probe can detect pregnancy at 3 to 4 weeks' gestation and embryonic heart activity at 5.5 weeks. The presence of embryonic cardiac activity in patients with bleeding in early pregnancy has a sensitivity of 97% and a specificity of 98% for fetal survival to the 20th week of pregnancy. However, maternal age makes a difference. At 5 to 6 weeks' gestation, in patients younger than 36 years of age, the risk of subsequent miscarriage was 4.5%; risk increased to 10% in patients aged 36 to 39 years, and to 29% in patients 40 years of age or older. In individuals with recurrent pregnancy loss, the risk of miscarriage after the observation of embryonic heart activity is about 22% (UpToDate, 2020).

10. Sonographic signs suggestive of a nonviable pregnancy or impending loss include the following:

a. Irregular gestational sac (i.e., gestational sac >25 mm mean sac diameter [MSD] on transabdominal sonogram; >16 mm MSD on transvaginal sonogram without a detectable embryo)

b. Slow heart rate: Embryonic heart rate <100 bpm at 5 to 7 weeks' gestation is slow, survival is 62%; <70 bpm, survival is zero.

c. Nonliving embryo (embryo without a heartbeat)

d. Presence of abnormal hyperechoic material within the uterine cavity

e. Subchorionic hematoma is a risk factor; a large hematoma (>25% of the volume of the gestational sac) is cause for concern. Pregnancy outcome depends on the location of the hematoma, with worse outcomes for retroplacental than marginal hematomas.

H. DIFFERENTIAL DIAGNOSES

1. Miscarriage (early pregnancy loss)

2. Cervical abnormalities (e.g., excessive friability, malignancy, polyps, and trauma)

3. Ectopic pregnancy

4. Idiopathic bleeding in a viable pregnancy
5. Dysfunctional uterine bleeding
6. Infection of the vagina or cervix
7. Molar pregnancy
8. Subchorionic hemorrhage
9. Vaginitis
10. Pregnancy, urinary tract infection
11. Vaginal trauma

I. MANAGEMENT

If the patient was hemodynamically stable, historically, management was dependent on what type of miscarriage was diagnosed. Newer studies have revealed expectant, medical, and surgical management of early pregnancy loss all result in the complete evacuation of pregnancy tissue in most patients, with serious complications being rare and comparable across treatment types. Thus, treatment plan options for early pregnancy loss include expectant, medical, or surgical management, and individuals without medical complications or symptoms requiring urgent surgical treatment may be offered the choice of treatment plan. In most practices, the nurse practitioner (NP) would collaborate and/or refer a patient who was diagnosed with inevitable, incomplete, or missed miscarriage or septic abortion.

1. For threatened miscarriage, management is expectant until symptoms resolve, a diagnosis of nonviable pregnancy is made, or there is progression to inevitable, incomplete, or complete miscarriage.
   a. Bed rest: There is no evidence to support this practice, although it was commonly recommended in the past. Bed rest is not currently recommended.
   b. Abstinence from sexual intercourse: No data to support this practice but is also often recommended; this is an intuitive rather than evidence-based recommendation.
   c. Use of progesterone: The rate of miscarriage is reduced when compared with placebo or no treatment (Wasabi et al., 2011). However, the protocol for progesterone therapy is emerging, not standardized, and varies regionally and institutionally. This may include oral, vaginal, and/or intramuscular injection dosing. A 2008 Cochrane review found no benefit of progesterone use in reducing early pregnancy loss. While the use of progesterone is controversial and evidence is lacking, in 2018 ACOG suggested in patients with at least three prior pregnancy losses, the use of progesterone therapy may be beneficial.
2. For complete miscarriage
   a. Maintain pelvic rest, that is, nothing in the vagina, until 2 weeks after evacuation and/or passage of the products of conception. Tampon use and sexual intercourse may be resumed at that time.
   b. Light vaginal bleeding typically persists for approximately 2 weeks; menses typically resumes within 6 weeks in patients who were regularly cycling before pregnancy. This may take longer in a patient who has irregular cycling or oligomenorrhea from conditions such as PCOS.
   c. Serum HCG values typically return to prepregnancy levels within 2 to 4 weeks following the miscarriage. Follow-up HCG testing is unnecessary if normal menstrual cycles resume.
   d. Avoiding pregnancy for two to three cycles is the customary advice.
   e. Family planning should be discussed; assess the plans for pregnancy in the future.

f. Preconception counseling is indicated for those who plan to become pregnant when advisable; maintain use of prenatal vitamins.

g. Anticipatory guidance may be helpful regarding risk recurrence of miscarriage, especially if there are reversible risk factors present. A recent multicenter trial post hoc analysis supports the use of low-dose aspirin prior to conception for individuals who have experienced a prior pregnancy loss (Naimi et al., 2021).

3. Protocol for the Medical Management of Early Pregnancy Loss utilized as Interprofessional Teams collaborating and coordinating care for the patient desiring medical management:

a. Misoprostol 800 mcg vaginally, with 1 repeat dose no sooner than 3 hours or later than 7 days with no response to the first dose

b. If available, a dose of mifepristone (200 mg orally) may be given 24 hours before misoprostol.

c. Prescriptions for pain management should be provided.

d. Patients who are Rh(D) negative and unsensitized should receive Rh(D)-immune globulin within 72 hours of first misoprostol dose.

e. Ultrasound performed after 7 to 14 days to document complete passage of tissue. Serial β-HCG may be used when ultrasound is not available and are typically followed weekly until <5.

f. If medical management fails, the patient may be offered more time for expectant management, if clinically stable, or surgical management with suction curettage.

Ectopic Pregnancy

A. DEFINITION

1. Pregnancy that occurs somewhere other than in the uterus.

B. EPIDEMIOLOGY

1. The incidence of ectopic pregnancy is reported most commonly as the number of ectopic pregnancies per 1,000 conceptions. Since 1970, when the reported rate in the United States was 4.5 cases per 1,000 pregnancies, the frequency of ectopic pregnancy has increased sixfold, with ectopic pregnancies now accounting for approximately 1% to 2% of all pregnancies. These data are based on the Centers for Disease Control and Prevention's (CDC) analyses of hospitalization rates. Since outpatient medical treatment has been used, it is more difficult to assess; however, the rate seems to be staying at about 2% of pregnancies. Approximately 85% to 90% of ectopic pregnancies occur in multigravid individuals. In the United States, rates of ectopic pregnancy and associated mortality are nearly twice as high for pregnant individuals of other races compared with Caucasian individuals. From 1991 to 1999, ectopic pregnancy was the cause of 8% of all pregnancy-related deaths among African American pregnant individuals, compared with 4% among Caucasian individuals (Chang et al., 2003).

C. ETIOLOGY

1. Requires fertilization of the ovum and abnormal implantation

2. Multiple factors contribute to risk. Anything that impairs the migration of the blastocyst to the endometrial cavity can predispose to ectopic pregnancy.

D. RISK FACTORS

1. Previous genital tract infections; pelvic inflammatory disease (PID)

2. Infertility (history of 2 or more years, treated or not)

3. Use of fertility drugs or assisted reproductive technology
4. Altered tubal motility (the result of hormonal contraception); progestin-only contraception and progestin intrauterine device (IUD)
5. Current or past smoker (damage to the ciliated cells in the fallopian tubes)
6. Previous ectopic pregnancy
7. History of multiple sexual partners
8. Increasing maternal age (highest rate occurs in women age 35–44 years)
9. Salpingitis isthmica nodosum: Also known as *diverticulosis of the fallopian tube*, it is a nodular thickening of the narrow (isthmic) portion of the tube caused by inflammation; when severe, it may lead to complete obliteration of the tube
10. Sterilization
11. Previous abortion
12. Tubal surgery history and conception after tubal ligation
13. In utero diethylstilbestrol (DES) exposure (these patients should have aged out of childbearing years as the last should be age >50 now)
14. Anatomic abnormalities of the uterus such as bicornuate uterus or fibroids
15. Previous pelvic/abdominal surgeries or appendectomy
16. Age of first intercourse <18 years
17. Vaginal douching

E. HISTORY

1. Date of LMP
2. History of ectopic, discrepant HCG level for estimated GA
3. Pain
4. Amenorrhea
5. Vaginal bleeding
6. Other symptoms of early pregnancy may include the following:
    a. Nausea and vomiting
    b. Breast fullness
    c. Fatigue
7. Heavy cramping
8. Shoulder pain (reflective on peritoneal irritation)
9. Recent dyspareunia
10. Dizziness or weakness
11. Syncope
12. Fever

F. PHYSICAL EXAMINATION

1. Vital signs: Should be within normal limits for pregnancy unless infection is present or hemorrhage has caused hypovolemia
2. Abdominal examination
    a. Auscultate bowel sounds (may be diminished with appendicitis).
    b. Auscultate fetal heart sounds if greater than 10 weeks' gestation.
    c. Fundal height
    d. Tenderness: Direct and rebound
    e. Guarding
    f. Bowel sounds
    g. Distension
    h. Costovertebral angle (CVA) tenderness (may be pyelonephritis with referred pain)

3. Pelvic examination
   a. Screen for cervicitis and vaginitis if not already done.
   b. Observe cervical os for dilation, blood, and clots.
   c. Bimanual examination for uterine size, adnexal masses (typically unilateral adnexal mass if in the fallopian tube), and cervical motion tenderness

G. LABORATORY AND DIAGNOSTIC STUDIES

1. CBC with differential
2. Blood type and Rh, antibody screen
3. Urine pregnancy test
4. Serum quantitative β-HCG
5. In a normal pregnancy, the β-HCG level doubles every 48 to 72 hours until it reaches 10,000 to 20,000 international units/L (IU/L). In ectopic pregnancies, β-HCG levels usually increase less rapidly. Even though ectopic pregnancies have been established to have lower mean serum β-HCG levels than healthy pregnancies, no single serum β-HCG level is diagnostic of an ectopic pregnancy. Serial serum β-HCG levels are necessary to differentiate between normal and abnormal pregnancies and to monitor the resolution of ectopic pregnancy once therapy has been initiated. The discriminatory zone of β-HCG is the level above which a normal intrauterine pregnancy is reliably visualized on ultrasound but depends on the type of ultrasound performed. Once the β-HCG has reached a level of 2,000 IU/L, a gestational sac should be seen within the uterus on **transvaginal** ultrasonographic images by an experienced ultrasonographer. However, the discriminatory zone threshold may vary by institution, experience of the sonographer, and type of scan (transvaginal or abdominal) and is not absolute proof of ectopic pregnancy. If an **abdominal** ultrasound scan is done, a gestational sac should be visualized within the uterus once the β-HCG has reached a level of 6,000 IU/L. Many institutions recommend setting the discriminatory zone at 3,500 IU/L to minimize the risk of interfering with an early viable intrauterine pregnancy. The lack of an intrauterine pregnancy when the β-HCG level is above the discriminatory zone represents an ectopic pregnancy or a recent miscarriage (Sepilian, Wood, & Rivlin, 2012). Drawbacks to β-HCG testing with suspicion of an ectopic pregnancy are the delay in the results and the altered levels associated with multiple gestations and/or pregnancies resulting from assisted reproductive therapy.
6. Progesterone level
   a. An ectopic pregnancy can be excluded if the value is >25 ng/mL; a level <5 ng/mL indicates a nonviable pregnancy
7. Transvaginal ultrasonography has become the cornerstone for the evaluation of early bleeding during pregnancy.

H. MANAGEMENT

1. Refer for medical or surgical management once the ectopic pregnancy is confirmed on an emergent basis, especially if the patient is not hemodynamically stable.

I. FOLLOW-UP

As appropriate to treatment

1. See the section "Grief Following a Pregnancy Loss" at the end of this chapter.

Gestational Trophoblastic Disease: Hydatidiform Mole

A. DEFINITION

1. A vesicular or polycystic placental mass resulting from the proliferation of the trophoblast and the hydropic degeneration and avascularity of the chorionic villi, usually indicative of an abnormal pregnancy. The embryo is usually absent or dead. In a partial hydatidiform mole, the pregnancy has chromosomal abnormalities that result from two sperm having fertilized a single egg. In the resulting molar pregnancy, an embryo may develop in the uterus but with an abnormal, overgrown placenta. These pregnancies are not viable; the chromosomal abnormalities are not compatible with life.

B. EPIDEMIOLOGY

1. Occurring in 1 in 1,200 pregnancies; patients older than 35 have a two-fold increase and patients older than 40 have a five- to tenfold increase. Parity does not affect the risk.

C. HISTORY

1. Vaginal bleeding (may occur in the first or second trimester)
2. Hyperemesis: Excessive nausea and vomiting
3. Hyperthyroidism symptoms (caused by stimulation of the thyroid gland by high levels of HCG or by thyrotropin produced by the trophoblasts)

D. PHYSICAL EXAMINATION

1. Vital signs: Should be within normal limits for pregnancy unless infection is present; if thyroid symptoms are present, tachycardia may occur. Preeclampsia may occur with elevated blood pressure (BP).
2. Abdomen
   a. Absence of fetal heart tones
   b. Fundal height
   c. Tenderness
   d. Guarding
   e. Bowel sounds
   f. Distension
3. Pelvic examination
4. Discrepancy between GA and uterine size; size greater than expected is a classic sign of complete mole
5. Presence of dark fluid at the cervical os

E. LABORATORY AND DIAGNOSTIC STUDIES

1. β-HCG: Levels may be normal to greater than 100,000.
2. CBC with differential, including platelet count; anemia could be present and coagulopathy can occur.
3. Vaginal ultrasonography—diffuse echogenic pattern described as a "snowstorm or grape-like" vessels in the uterus
4. Depending on the condition of the patient:
   a. Clotting function
   b. Liver function tests
   c. Blood urea nitrogen (BUN) and serum creatinine
   d. Thyroxine

F. TREATMENT/REFERRAL

1. Refer to collaborating physician for treatment.

G. FOLLOW-UP

1. Dependent on diagnosis

Cervicitis

A. See Chapter 13

Cervical Polyps

A. DEFINITION

1. Growths originating from the surface of the cervix or endocervical canal. These small, fragile growths hang from a stalk and protrude through the cervical opening (the os).

B. ETIOLOGY

1. Etiology is unclear; most are benign; the incidence of malignancy is 1:1,000.

C. HISTORY

1. During pregnancy, the patient may present with the following:
   a. Postcoital bleeding
   b. Bleeding not related to intercourse
   c. No symptoms

D. PHYSICAL EXAMINATION

1. Incidental finding on pelvic examination
2. Manipulating the lesion with a swab away from the cervical canal in four directions helps to differentiate a polyp from a polypoid irregularity of the cervix.

E. LABORATORY AND DIAGNOSTIC STUDIES

1. Ultrasound imaging may be indicated if bleeding is recurrent and unexplained.

F. DIFFERENTIAL DIAGNOSES

1. Cervical polyps
2. Cervical mass
3. Cervicitis

G. TREATMENT

1. There are no management guidelines available for pregnancy.
2. Expectant management is most often the choice of obstetricians and removal after delivery as needed.

H. CONSULTATION/REFFERAL

1. Refer to the collaborating physician if active management is planned.

I. PATIENT EDUCATION

1. Educate the patient regarding the need for further evaluation, what to do, and when to call if experiences heavy bleeding.

Postcoital Bleeding

A. DEFINITION

1. Bleeding after sexual intercourse (may occur at any time during gestation)

B. ETIOLOGY

1. Postcoital bleeding, which can arise from the cervix or other genital area, may be of benign or malignant etiology. Cervical ectropion occurs when eversion of the endocervix exposes columnar epithelium to the vaginal milieu. This is a common occurrence in pregnant individuals because of the physiologic hyperemia of the cervix resulting from the hormonal changes during pregnancy. The cervical epithelium associated with cervical intraepithelial neoplasia (CIN) and invasive cancer (most commonly of the squamous type) is thin and friable and readily detaches from the cervix. In patients with postcoital bleeding, CIN is found in 7% to 10% and cervical, vaginal, or endometrial cancer in less than 1%. Some patients with postcoital bleeding may have pathologic lesions identifiable by colposcopy and biopsy that are missed by cervical cytology alone.

C. HISTORY

1. Painless vaginal spotting or bleeding occurs after intercourse.
2. Resolves spontaneously in 1 to 2 days

D. PHYSICAL EXAMINATION

1. Abdominal Exam
   a. Tenderness
   b. Guarding
   c. Bowel sounds
   d. Distension
   e. Assess fetal heart tones if beyond 10 weeks' gestation
2. Pelvic Exam
   a. External genitalia: Observe perineum for trauma.
   b. Assess the presence of hemorrhoids.
   c. Observe cervix for ectropion or erosion, lesions, and polyps.
   d. Observe cervical os for dilation, blood, and clots.
   e. Screen for cervicitis and vaginitis if not already done.
   f. Screen with cervical cytology if not already done.
   g. Observe vagina for remnant bleeding/dark brown vaginal secretions.
   h. Observe vaginal walls for lesions or evidence of trauma.
   i. Evaluate the amount and the type of bleeding.
   j. Perform a bimanual examination assessing uterine size, adnexal masses, cervical motion tenderness, and pain on examination.
3. Rectovaginal examination as indicated: Pain and/or bleeding

E. LABORATORY AND DIAGNOSTIC STUDIES

1. Depends on history and assessment; if postcoital bleeding and screening for cervicitis and cervical lesions are already performed, then no testing is required

F. DIFFERENTIAL DIAGNOSES

1. Cervicitis
2. Cervical polyps
3. Sexual assault

G. TREATMENT

1. Treatment is rarely required except for excessive mucus discharge or bothersome spotting.

H. CONSULTATION/REFERRAL

1. Patients with unexplained postcoital bleeding should be referred to a colposcopist for a colposcopic examination.

Placenta Previa

A. DEFINITION

Placenta previa classically presents as painless vaginal bleeding in the third trimester secondary to an abnormal placentation near or covering the internal cervical os. However, because of ultrasonography improvements, the diagnosis of placenta previa is often made earlier in pregnancy. Recently, definitions of previa have been consolidated as complete and marginal previa.

1. A *complete previa* is defined as complete coverage of the cervical os by the placenta.
2. If the edge of the placenta is <2 cm from the internal os but does not fully cover the cervical opening, this is considered a *marginal previa*. However, early diagnosis of "low-lying placenta" may not prove problematic as 90% of those present on early ultrasound are no longer present in the third trimester.

B. ETIOLOGY/RISK FACTORS

The etiology of placenta previa is unknown. Hemorrhaging is often associated with cervical dilation, thereby disrupting the placental implantation from the cervix and lower uterine segment. The lower uterine segment does not contract sufficiently to constrict the vessels, which leads to continued bleeding. Placenta previa is frequently reported to occur in 0.5% of all U.S. pregnancies. The condition may be multifactorial and is likely related to the following risk factors:

1. Multiparity (5% in grand multiparous patients)
2. Multiple gestation
3. Advancing maternal age (>35 years: 2%; >40 years: 5%)
4. Short interpregnancy interval
5. Infertility treatment
6. Previous uterine surgery; uterine injury or insult
   a. Previous cesarean delivery, including the first subsequent pregnancy (risk increases with each cesarean, with a rate of 1% after one cesarean delivery, 2.8% after three cesarean deliveries, and as high as 3.7% after five cesarean deliveries (Marshall, Fu, & Guise, 2011)
7. Previous spontaneous or induced abortions
8. Previous placenta previa (4%–8%)
9. Non-White ethnicity
10. Low socioeconomic status
11. Smoking
12. Cocaine use

C. COMPLICATIONS

1. Hemorrhage, including rebleeding (planning delivery and control of hemorrhage are critical in cases of placenta previa as well as placenta accreta, increta, and percreta)
2. Higher rates of blood transfusion
3. Placental abruption

4. Preterm delivery
5. Increased incidence of postpartum endometritis
6. Mortality rate (2%–3%); in the United States, the maternal mortality rate is 0.03%, the great majority of which is related to uterine bleeding and the complication of disseminated intravascular coagulopathy (DIC; Baker, 2016)

D. HISTORY

1. Painless vaginal bleeding occurring after the 20th week of gestation
2. Backache
3. Abdominal pain
4. Decreased or absent fetal movement
5. Fatigue, dizziness, or lightheadedness

E. PHYSICAL EXAMINATION

1. Whenever a patient presents with painless vaginal bleeding in the second or third trimester, ***do not*** perform a pelvic, bimanual, or speculum exam unless there is an ultrasound report documenting the location of the placenta.
2. Vital signs: Signs of hypovolemic shock may be demonstrated
3. Skin: Pale, cold, clammy with significant blood loss
4. Abdomen
   a. Soft, nontender uterus
   b. Presenting part not engaged; fetus may be in an abnormal lie, that is, transverse, oblique, or breech
   c. Assess fetal heart tones, which are usually normal unless the patient is in shock
5. External genitalia
   a. May reveal bright red vaginal bleeding in varying amounts

F. LABORATORY/DIAGNOSTIC STUDIES

1. Ultrasound exam
2. External fetal monitoring
3. CBC with differential
4. Blood type and Rh if not already known; crossmatch for four units
5. Oxygen saturation if maternal hypoxia is suspected
6. Coagulation studies if DIC is suspected
7. Urinalysis (UA; catheter specimen)

G. DIFFERENTIAL DIAGNOSES

1. Intrauterine pregnancy at ______ weeks' gestation ruling out
   a. Placenta previa
   b. Abruptio placentae
   c. Cervical- or vaginal-wall laceration
   d. Premature rupture of membranes
   e. Cervicitis/vaginitis
   f. Preterm labor
   g. Bloody show
   h. Hypovolemic shock

H. MANAGEMENT/CONSULTATION

1. Consult with physician on any patient presenting with second- and third-trimester bleeding.
2. If the patient is actively bleeding, arrange STAT transport to labor and delivery by stretcher.

3. Provide cardiovascular support by inserting an intravenous line to begin fluid replacement.
4. If the patient is hemodynamically stable, collaborate on plan of care
   a. Supplement with iron and folate as a safety margin in the event of repeat bleeding.
   b. RhoGAM may be indicated; Kleihauer–Betke test will reveal quantity of fetal cells in maternal circulation.

Abruptio Placentae

A. DEFINITION

1. Abruptio placentae is defined as the premature separation of the placenta from the uterus. Patients with placental abruption typically present with bleeding, uterine irritability or contractions, and possible fetal distress. As the placenta separates from the uterus, hemorrhage into the decidua basalis occurs, leading to hematoma formation, which subsequently leads to uterine irritability and further separation of the placenta. Vaginal bleeding usually follows, although the presence of a concealed hemorrhage in which the blood pools behind the placenta is possible.
2. Classification of placental abruption is based on the extent of separation (i.e., partial vs. complete) and location of separation (i.e., marginal vs. central). Clinical classification is as follows:
   a. Class 0: Asymptomatic (diagnosed after delivery)
   b. Class 1: Mild (~48%)
   c. Class 2: Moderate (~27%)
   d. Class 3: Severe (~24%)
3. Placental abruption occurs in 1% of pregnancies but leads to 12% of all perinatal fetal/infant deaths. The rate is higher when there is a significant maternal smoking history. Placental abruption is responsible for 6% of maternal deaths.

B. ETIOLOGY/RISK FACTORS

1. Cause is largely unknown.
2. Risk factors include the following:
   a. Maternal hypertension (~44% of cases)
   b. Extremes of maternal age: younger than 20 years or older than 35 years
   c. Maternal trauma (e.g., motor vehicle accidents, assaults, falls) causes 1.5% to 9.4% of all cases
   d. Increased parity
   e. Previous cesarean birth
   f. Short umbilical cord
   g. Substance use: Alcohol, cocaine, and tobacco
   h. Low socioeconomic status
   i. Sudden decompression of the uterus (e.g., premature rupture of membranes, delivery of first twin, or in pregnancies complicated by polyhydramnios)
   j. Male fetal gender
   k. Previous placental abruption (risk recurrence is 4%–12%)
   l. Bleeding in the second or third trimester
   m. Prolonged rupture of membranes
   n. Chorioamnionitis
   o. Subchorionic hematoma
   p. Retroplacental fibromyoma
   q. Retroplacental bleeding from needle puncture (i.e., postamniocentesis)

C. HISTORY

1. Vaginal bleeding, the patient may be asymptomatic (does not correlate with degree of abruption)
2. Most common presentation is mild, nonacute bleeding in second or third trimester with or without contractions or back pain.
3. Uterine tenderness
4. Uterine irritability that may present as idiopathic preterm labor
5. Abdominal pain
6. Blood-stained amniotic fluid if membranes ruptured
7. Decreased or absent fetal movement
8. Fatigue, dizziness, or lightheadedness
9. History of recent trauma

D. PHYSICAL EXAMINATION

1. Whenever a patient presents with painless vaginal bleeding in the second or third trimester, ***do not*** perform a pelvic, bimanual, or speculum exam unless there is an ultrasound report documenting the location of the placenta. More than 50% of placental abruptions are missed on ultrasound, so normal findings do not rule out abruption.
2. Vital signs: May demonstrate signs of hypovolemic shock. Shock Index (SI) can be determined by dividing the heart rate by the systolic BP for an indication of hemodynamic instability and hypovolemia. The normal range for healthy, nonpregnant adults is 0.5 to 0.7, and an SI > 0.9 was associated with increased mortality. A study on pregnant individuals revealed an SI <0.9 was reassuring, but an SI ≥ 1.7 required urgent attention (Nathan et al., 2015).
3. Skin: Pale, cold, clammy with significant blood loss
4. Abdomen
   a. Tenderness (minimal to extreme): Placental abruption will cause uterine irritability and tenderness.
   b. Uterine irritability (tender to palpation; low-level contractions with electronic monitoring)
      i. Uterine resting tone may vary from soft to firm to board-like; may occur with tetanic contractions.
      ii. Assess fetal heart tones.
   c. External genitalia
5. May reveal bright red or dark red vaginal bleeding in varying amounts

E. LABORATORY/DIAGNOSTIC STUDIES

1. Ultrasound exam
2. External fetal monitoring
3. CBC with differential
4. Blood type and crossmatch at time of diagnosis
5. Oxygen saturation if maternal hypoxia is suspected
6. Coagulation studies if DIC is suspected
7. UA (catheter specimen)

F. DIFFERENTIAL DIAGNOSES

1. Intrauterine pregnancy at ________ weeks' gestation ruling out
   a. Abruptio placentae
   b. Placenta previa
   c. Urinary tract infection
   d. Appendicitis
   e. Premature rupture of membranes
   f. Cervicitis/vaginitis

g. Preterm labor
h. Onset of normal labor
i. Fibroid degeneration
j. Hypovolemic shock

G. MANAGEMENT/CONSULTATION

1. Consult with a physician on any patient presenting with second and third-trimester bleeding.
2. Arrange STAT transport to labor and delivery by stretcher as needed for true abruption.
3. Provide cardiovascular support by inserting an intravenous line to begin fluid replacement as clinically indicated.
4. Transfer care to physician.

H. PATIENT EDUCATION

1. Educate patient about reversible risk factors, such as smoking, prior to future pregnancies.
2. Assess for intimate partner violence at the postpartum visit.

Grief Following Pregnancy Loss

A. DESCRIPTION

Pregnancy loss and infant death are experienced in every culture, but expressions of grief vary by individual and among cultures. The experience is profound for most families and engenders a deep sense of sorrow. The NP needs to take time to respond to the needs of the patient and partner (if present/available) with the understanding that cultural tradition must be taken into account. First-trimester loss may be particularly challenging because of the relative lack of U.S. traditions to support couples experiencing loss during early pregnancy. What couples are particularly attuned to is the caring attitude of the NP during the experience of loss, even if the words are not remembered. However, many patients do remember phrases that were said at this emotional time decades after the experience.

B. POINTS OF CARE

1. Pregnancy loss is a profound experience for most families.
2. "Disenfranchised grief": This refers to a unique kind of mourning that lacks societal support accompanying the death of a close relative or friend. It denies the grieving person the affirmation of the pregnancy or the hoped-for child and deprives him or her of the support associated with other losses.
3. Prenatal and perinatal providers may contribute to the grief by using medical terminology such as *products of conception* instead of saying *your baby*.
4. Acknowledge the suffering. Phrases to use include the following:
   a. "I am so sorry for your loss. How can I help you?"
   b. "Is there someone I can call for you?"
   c. "Has anyone in your family had this experience? How did they handle it?"
5. The experience of miscarriage or perinatal loss is remembered forever and has great impact. Interpersonal communication skills are of critical importance in providing care.
   a. Assess the meaning and significance of the loss for the couple.
   b. Assess the couple's perception of the events of the loss.
   c. Asking whether or not the pregnancy was planned is **not** helpful.

6. The NP may accompany the patient to the ultrasound exam when fetal heart tones are not heard. If so, do reach out and hold the patient's hand for comfort. Tell the patient that you are sorry that this has happened in a calm, reassuring manner. Have a tissue ready for use.

7. Many patients conclude immediately that they must have "done something wrong" to cause the death. Reassurance at this time is very important.

8. Anxiety and depressive symptoms not only relate to the event but may be affected by the physiologic changes of hormone levels, thus affecting behavior. Attention to the mental and emotional health of the couple experiencing pregnancy loss is essential. Responses may range from overwhelming grief and depression to relief. Use of a depression screening tool may be helpful during the follow-up care visits.

9. The NP should take the lead in making sure the patient has follow-up appointments, educating the couple on what may occur with the experience of miscarriage or perinatal loss to facilitate them getting through the experience.

- **a.** Acknowledge that the loss may place a strain on the couple's relationship.
- **b.** Assess the couple's coping strategies.
- **c.** Acknowledge that family and friends may remain silent out of fear of inflicting emotional pain; discuss comments the couple is likely to hear.
- **d.** Acknowledge that holidays, the due date of the lost baby, anniversaries, or other meaningful dates may cause the feelings of grief to resurface.

10. Gender differences: It is important to recognize that men and women grieve differently as the grief experience may be a source of distress in the couple's relationship.

- **a.** *Incongruent grief* is a term used to refer to grief experienced by each parent.
- **b.** Mothers experience longer periods and higher levels of grief
  - **i.** More emotionally expressive, sharing feelings
  - ii. More likely to participate in support groups
  - iii. Bereavement: A nonlinear process often characterized by paradoxes that are not easily resolved (not a pathologic process) that persists up to 6 months or more in approximately 20% of patients; mother can be depressed and yearn for the lost baby.
- c. Fathers
  - **i.** Supportive of his partner, but dealing with his own grief
  - ii. Expectation of the male role may not be clear, so he may suppress his feelings.
  - iii. May not feel "real" unless it is a second- or third-trimester loss
  - iv. Intense feelings of isolation, loneliness, and pain
  - v. Stages: Confirming the news, working it through, getting on with life
- **d.** Naming the baby
  - **i.** Some couples may be open to naming the baby. They may choose a gender-neutral name if the gender is unknown. This action may make the experience "more real."
  - ii. Naming the baby may also be consistent with spiritual care.

11. Resources and referral

- **a.** Offer a referral to professional support for those with poor coping skills or who have expressed interest in seeing a mental health professional.
- **b.** Offer support group resources

c. Refer to appropriate online resources, for example:
   i. www.nationalshare.org
   ii. www.babylosscomfort.com/grief-resources

12. Interconception care after loss
   a. Discuss the possibility of future pregnancies.
   b. Address the future referral to a genetic counselor or high-risk obstetric care as indicated by the type of loss.
   c. Give preconception health advice that allows the couple to make an informed decision on timing the next pregnancy.

Bibliography

American College of Obstetrics and Gynecologists Practice. (2018). Early pregnancy loss. Bulletin no. 200. *Obstetrics & Gynecology, 132*(5), e197–e207. https://doi.org/10.1097/AOG.0000000000002899

Ananath, C. V., & Kinzler, W. L. (2015). *Placental abruption: Clinical features and diagnosis*. http://www.uptodate.com/contents/placental-abruption-clinical-features-and-diagnosis

Baker, R. (2016). *Placenta previa*. http://emedicine.medscape.com/article/262063-overview

Callister, L. (2006). Perinatal loss: A family perspective. *Journal of Perinatal & Neonatal Nursing, 20*(3), 227–236. https://doi.org/10.1097/00005237-200607000-00009

Casey, P. M., Long, M. E., & Marnach, M. L. (2011). Abnormal cervical appearance: What to do, when to worry? *Mayo Clinic Proceedings, 86*(2), 147–151. https://doi.org/10.4065/mcp.2010.0512

Center for Science in the Public Interest. (2021). *Caffeine chart*. https://cspinet.org/eating-healthy/ingredients-of-concern/caffeine-chart

Chang, J., Elam-Evans, L. D., Berg, C. J., Herndon, J., Flowers, L., Seed, K. A., & Syverson, C. J. (2003). Pregnancy-related mortality surveillance—United States, 1991–1999. *MMWR Surveillance Summary, 52*(2), 1–8.

Creanga, A. A., Berg, C. J., Syverson, C., Seed, K., Bruce, F. C., & Callaghan, W. M. (2015). Pregnancy-related mortality in the United States, 2006-2010. *Obstetrics & Gynecology, 125*(1), 5–12. https://doi.org/10.1097/AOG.0000000000000564

Cunningham, F. G., Leveno, K. J., Bloom, S. L., Spong, C. Y., Dashe, J. S., Hoffman, B. L., Casey, B. M., & Sheffield, J. S. (2014). *William's obstetrics* (24th ed.). McGraw-Hill.

Curtis, M., Antoniewicz, L., & Linares, S. (2014). Early pregnancy failure and ectopic pregnancy. In M. Curtis (Ed.), *Glass' office gynecology* (7th ed.). Wolters-Kluwer.

Fields, L., & Hathaway, A. (2017). Key concepts in pregnancy of unknown location: Identifying ectopic pregnancy and providing patient-centered care. *Journal of Midwifery and Women's Health, 62*, 172–179. https://doi.org/10.1111/jmwh.12526

Kilpatrick, C. C., & Verghese, G. (2014). Early pregnancy failure and ectopic pregnancy. In M. Curtis, L. Linhares, & L. Antoniewicz (Eds.), *Glass' office gynecology* (pp. 233–243). Wolters-Kluwer.

Marshall, N. E., Fu, R., & Guise, J. M. (2011). Impact of multiple cesarean deliveries on maternal morbidity: A systematic review. *American Journal of Obstetrics & Gynecology, 205*(3), 262.e1–262.e8. https://doi.org/10.1016/j.ajog.2011.06.035

Moore, T., Parrish, H., & Black, B. (2011). Interconception care for couples after perinatal loss: A comprehensive review of the literature. *Journal of Perinatal & Neonatal Nursing, 25*(1), 44–51. https://doi.org/10.1097/JPN.0b013e3182071a08

Murphy, F., & Merrell, J. (2009). Negotiating the transition: Caring for women through the experience of early miscarriage. *Journal of Clinical Nursing, 18*(11), 1583–1591. https://doi.org/10.1111/j.1365-2702.2008.02701.x

Naimi, A. I., Perkins, N. J., Sjaarda, L. A., Mumford, S. L., Platt, R. W., Silver, R. M., & Schisterman, E. F. (2021). The effect of preconception-initiated low-dose aspirin on human chorionic gonadotropin-detected pregnancy, pregnancy loss, and live birth: Per protocol analysis of a randomized trial. *Annals of Internal Medicine, 174*, 595–601. https://doi.org/10.7326/M20-0469

Nathan, H. L., El Ayadi, A., Hezelgrave, N. L., Seed, P., Butrick, E., Miller, S., Briley, A., Bewley, S., & Shennan, A. H. (2015). Shock index: An effective predictor of outcome in postpartum haemorrhage? *BJOG, 122*(2), 268–275. https://doi.org/10.1111/1471-0528.13206

Neugebauer, R., & Ritsher, J. (2005). Depression and grief following early pregnancy loss. *International Journal of Childbirth Education, 20*(3), 21–24.

Norwitz, E. R., & Park, J. S. (2020). *Overview of the etiology and evaluation of vaginal bleeding in pregnant women*. https://www.uptodate.com

Pruiksma, R. (2006). Level of HCG for considering an ectopic pregnancy. *American Family Physician, 73*(8), 1331.

Robinson, G. (2011). Dilemmas related to pregnancy loss. *Journal of Nervous & Mental Disease, 199*(8), 571–574. https://doi.org/10.1097/NMD.0b013e318225f31e

Rowlands, I., & Lee, C. (2010). 'The silence was deafening': Social and health service support after miscarriage. *Journal of Reproductive & Infant Psychology, 28*(3), 274–286. https://doi.org/10.1080/02646831003587346

Sepilian, V. P., Wood, E., & Rivlin, M. E. (2012). *Ectopic pregnancy*. http://emedicine.medscape.com/article/2041923-overview

Swanson, K., Chen, H., Graham, J., Wojnar, D., & Petras, A. (2009). Resolution of depression and grief during the first year after miscarriage: A randomized controlled clinical trial of couples-focused interventions. *Journal of Women's Health, 18*(8), 1245–1257. https://doi.org/10.1089/jwh.2008.1202

UpToDate. (2020). Patient education: Miscarriage (beyond the basics). *UpToDate*. http://www.uptodate.com/contents/miscarriage-beyond-the-basics?Source=see_link

Wasabi, H. A., Fayed, A. A., Esmaeil, S. A., & Al Zeidan, R. A. (2011). Progestogen for treating threatened miscarriage. *Cochrane Database of Systematic Reviews*, 7(12), cd005943. https://doi.org/10.1002/14651858.CD005943.pub4

Wyatt, P., Owolabi, T., Meier, C., & Huang, T. (2005). Age-specific risk of fetal loss observed in a second trimester serum screening population. *American Journal of Obstetrics & Gynecology, 192*(1), 240–246. https://doi.org/10.1016/j.ajog.2004.06.099

16. Gestational Diabetes Mellitus

MARY LEE BARRON | KELLY D. ROSENBERGER

Pregnancy is characterized by insulin resistance and hyperinsulinemia and thus may predispose some individuals to diabetes. These metabolic changes stem from the placental hormones that ensure that the fetus has an abundant and continuous supply of nutrients: growth hormone, cortisol, placental lactogen, prolactin, and progesterone. Additional factors include increased maternal adipose deposition, decreased exercise, and increased caloric intake. When pancreatic function is not sufficient to overcome insulin resistance, diabetes occurs. Gestational diabetes mellitus (GDM) is defined as carbohydrate intolerance that begins or is first recognized during pregnancy. The condition is associated with increased maternal, fetal, and neonatal risks. Diabetes complicates approximately 6% to 7% of all pregnancies in the United States, and 90% of these cases are complicated by GDM (American College of Obstetricians and Gynecologists [ACOG], 2018a). The prevalence is increased in U.S. individuals who are Latinx, African American, Native American, Asian American, and Pacific Islanders. With increases in obesity and sedentary lifestyles, the problem is on the rise globally. See Table 16.1 for the prevalence of GDM in individuals with polycystic ovarian syndrome (PCOS), as determined by the World Health Organization (WHO) criteria.

GDM is associated with increased risks for the fetus and the newborn, including macrosomia, shoulder dystocia, birth injuries, hyperbilirubinemia, hypoglycemia, respiratory distress syndrome, hypocalcemia, polycythemia, and childhood obesity. Maternal risks include preeclampsia, polyhydramnios, gestational hypertension, cesarean delivery, and diabetes occurring later in life.

In 2010, the International Association of Diabetes and Pregnancy Study Groups (IADPSG) recommended new terminology to classify diabetes occurring during pregnancy: *overt* or *gestational*. The rationale for this recommendation is that an increasing number of individuals have personal risk factors, such as being overweight or obese, for *overt* but as yet unrecognized diabetes.

About 10% of formerly diagnosed GDM pregnant individuals have circulating islet-cell antibodies, a latent form of type 1 diabetes, although the risk of developing type 1 diabetes is unknown. These individuals are a part of the overt diabetes group. This is important because diagnosing diabetes early in

TABLE 16.1 GDM INCIDENCE WITH PCOS

INCIDENCE (%)	GESTATIONAL AGE (WEEKS)
9.20	12
18.70	19
25.60	32

GDM, gestational diabetes mellitus; PCOS, polycystic ovarian syndrome.

pregnancy may decrease the associated risk of congenital anomalies and diabetes-associated maternal risk of nephropathy and retinopathy.

All pregnant individuals should be screened, but there is no universal screening approach that has been promulgated. There is both a one-step and a two-step approach for screening. The American Diabetes Association (ADA) recommends either the IADPSG screening measures or the two-step approach (see Section A). The ACOG does not endorse the IADPSG recommendations at present because the organization believes that recommendations will not lead to clinically significant improvements in maternal and neonatal outcomes and would lead to a significant increase in healthcare costs. This position was supported in 2013, by the Eunice Kennedy Shriver National Institute of Child Health and Human Development Consensus Development Conference on diagnosing GDM, which recommended the two-step approach. Notably, the adoption of IADPSG guidelines would result in GDM being diagnosed in approximately 18% of all pregnant individuals.

A. TIMING AND ADMINISTRATION OF SCREENING

1. Overt diabetes is diagnosed at the initial prenatal visit and up to 24 weeks' gestation when any of the following criteria is met:

a. Fasting plasma glucose ≥126 mg/dL (7.0 mmol/L)

b. A1c ≥6.5%

c. Random plasma glucose ≥200 mg/dL (11.1 mmol/L), which is subsequently confirmed by elevated fasting plasma glucose or A1c, as noted earlier

2. GDM, defined as carbohydrate intolerance that begins or is first recognized during pregnancy:

a. IADPSG: One-step criteria (82% sensitivity and 94% specificity compared to two-step strategy

i. Fasting glucose ≥92 mg/dL (5.1 mmol/L) but <126 mg/dL (7.0 mmol/L) at the first prenatal visit or

ii. Two-hour 75-g oral glucose tolerance test (OGTT) at 24 to 28 weeks' gestation with at least one abnormal result

iii. Fasting: ≥92 mg/dL (5.1 mmol/L), 1 hour: ≥180 mg/dL (10.0 mmol/L), 2 hours: ≥153 mg/dL (8.5 mmol/L)

b. ACOG: Two-step approach

i. Glucose challenge test (GCT)

ii. Give 50 g oral glucose load (without regard to time of day). If unable to tolerate 50 g glucola and alternative is 10 Twizzlers.

Screening thresholds have varied from 130, 135, to 140 mg/dL with varying sensitivities and reported sensitivities. Existing data do not support the use of one over the other. The current 1-hour glucose (plasma or serum) screening level is equal to or greater than 140 mg/dL. If elevated, do the 3-hour glucose tolerance test: A positive diagnosis requires that two or more thresholds be met or exceeded. ADA recommends a cutoff value for the GCT of either 140 mg/dL (7.8 mmol/L), which is said to identify 80% of women with GDM, or 130 mg/dL (7.2 mmol/L), which should identify 90%. Problems have also been reported for the GCT: There are many false positives, and sensitivity is only 86% at best (Menato et al., 2008).

iii. Nonfasting random plasma glucose greater than 200 mg/dL on screening plus confirmation of fasting greater than 126 mg/dL is indicative of diabetes mellitus, and no OGTT is necessary for diagnosis.

3. Screening has traditionally been performed at 24 to 28 weeks. It can and should be conducted earlier if there is a high degree of suspicion that a patient has undiagnosed type 2 diabetes (glycosuria, obesity [body mass index (BMI) >30], excessive weight gain during the first 18–24 weeks of gestation, personal history of GDM or PCOS, history of birth of an infant equal or greater than 9 pounds [4,000 g], or a strong family history of diabetes). The U.S. Preventive Services Task Force (USPSTF) currently recommends GDM screening at or after 24 weeks in asymptomatic individuals to reduce the risk for primary cesarean deliveries, preterm deliveries, preeclampsia, macrosomia, large-for-gestational-age (LGA), birth injuries, and neonatal intensive care unit admissions (USPSTF, 2021).

4. The 3-hour OGTT
   a. The test is administered after a fast of at least 8 hours, but with the patient consuming her usual unrestricted daily diet in the days preceding the test. On the day of the test, only water may be consumed, and cigarette smoking should be avoided.
   b. Two abnormal values are necessary for diagnosis. If only one level is elevated, repeat testing at a later gestation may be ordered or dietary restriction recommended. Approximately 15% to 20% of those with GDM will develop overt diabetes mellitus (Table 16.2). In 2017, ACOG stated while two or more abnormal values is typically utilized for GDM diagnosis, some clinicians may opt to make the diagnosis based on one elevated value.

B. RISK FACTORS

1. Age older than 25
2. First-degree relative or personal health history of diabetes or GDM*
3. Previous delivery of an infant weighing less than 6 lb or greater than 9 lb (4,000 g)*
4. A1c ≥5.7%, or impaired glucose tolerance
5. BMI ≥30 kg/m² **or** a BMI ≥25 kg/m² **PLUS** one or more of the risk factors (BMI ≥23 kg/m² in Asian Americans)
6. Non-White race (African American, Latinx, Native American, Asian Americans, Pacific Islander)
7. Previous unexplained perinatal loss or birth of a child with congenital anomalies
8. PCOS
9. Glycosuria on more than one visit in current pregnancy
10. Essential hypertension or pregnancy-related hypertension
11. Current use of glucocorticoids
12. History of cardiovascular disease

TABLE 16.2 TWO-STEP APPROACH FOR DIAGNOSING GDM

TIMING	CARPENTER AND COUSTAN CRITERIA (ACOG; mg/dl)	NATIONAL DIABETES GROUP CRITERIA (mg/dl)
Fasting	95	105
1 hour	180	190
2 hours	155	165
3 hours	40	145

ACOG, American College of Obstetricians and Gynecologists; GDM, gestational diabetes mellitus.

*See the Risk Factors section. High risk (one or more required) and initial screening should occur at the first prenatal visit and be repeated between 24 and 28 weeks if gestational diabetes mellitus is not diagnosed earlier.

13. High-density lipoprotein cholesterol level <35 mg/dL and/or triglycerides level >250 mg/dL
14. Physical inactivity
15. Acanthosis nigricans

C. DIFFERENTIAL DIAGNOSES

1. Overt diabetes
2. Gestational diabetes
3. Other causes of hyperglycemia:
   a. Corticosteroids
   b. Antiretrovirals
   c. Calcium channel blockers
   d. Stress related (infection, hepatic or renal insufficiency)
   e. Endocrine disorders such as Cushing's syndrome, hyperthyroidism
   f. Pancreatic insufficiency
   g. Amylophagia (consumption of purified starch)

D. MANAGEMENT

Initial treatment includes moderate physical activity, dietary changes, support from diabetes educators and nutritionists, and glucose monitoring. If the patient's glucose is not controlled after these initial interventions, the patient may be prescribed medication (either insulin or oral hypoglycemic agents), and have increased surveillance in prenatal care or changes in delivery management (USPSTF, 2021). Insulin is the preferred treatment if pharmacologic therapy is indicated. For individuals declining insulin or unable to afford or safely administer insulin, metformin is an alternative (ACOG, 2018a). Glyburide is no longer a first choice as studies demonstrate it does not have outcomes equivalent to insulin (ACOG, 2018a).

1. Schedule more frequent visits (every 2 weeks) from diagnosis to 36 weeks' gestation, and weekly visits from 36 weeks until delivery.
2. Perform routine prenatal evaluation at each visit and add careful review of glucose records.
3. Provide nutritional counseling for patients with a diagnosis of GDM and patients with one abnormal value on OGTT.
   a. Goals
      i. Achieve normoglycemia
      ii. Prevent ketosis
      iii. Provide adequate weight gain
      iv. Contribute to fetal well-being
   b. Nutritional requirements
      i. Calories
      ii. Pregnant individuals often require 1,800 to 2,500 kcal/d to achieve weight gain, blood glucose goals, and adequate nutrient intake
      iii. Calculate ideal body weight
         a) Start with 100 lb + 5 lb per inch over 5 feet.
         b) Add 30 lb for pregnancy.
         c) Convert to kilograms: number of pounds divided by 2.2.
      iv. Calculate required calories
         a) Option 1: calories/d = ideal weight (in kilograms) × 35 kcal/kg
         b) Option 2: (if BMI greater than 30 kg/m^2, calories/d = actual weight [in kilograms] × 25 kcal/kg)
      v. Underweight patients may require caloric needs up to 35 to 40 kcal/kg/d.

vi. Normal-weight patients require 30 kcal/kg/d.
vii. Overweight patients may require 22 to 25 kcal/kg/d.
viii. Morbidly obese patients may require 12 to 14 kcal/kg/d depending on present pregnant weight.
ix. Carbohydrate intake (40% of calories) needs to be distributed across meals and snacks to blunt postprandial hyperglycemia. Emphasize the use of complex high-fiber carbohydrates with the exclusion of concentrated sweets and sugar-sweetened beverages (soft drinks, fruit drinks) and drink water instead.
x. Protein intake (20% of calories) must be distributed throughout the day and included in all meals to promote satiety. A bedtime snack may be needed to prevent accelerated ketosis overnight.
xi. Fat (40% of calories; saturated fats <7% of total calories)

c. Individual assessment with close follow-up is needed to assess and modify specific nutrition recommendations. Weight gain should be monitored for excessive gains (above Institute of Medicine [IOM] guidelines), which are associated with LGA infants, preterm birth (PTB), and cesarean delivery. Suboptimal weight gain, which decreases the need for medical therapy, increases the risk of small-for-gestational-age (SGA) infants.

d. Weight loss in pregnancy is *not* recommended.

4. Blood glucose monitoring
   a. Although there is a lack of evidence for the optimal frequency of daily monitoring, ACOG (2018a) recommends measuring the glucose level at least four times daily (fasting and 1 or 2 hours after the first bite of a meal). For some well-controlled patients, the frequency of monitoring may be reduced to fasting and one postprandial measurement daily.
   b. Record results in a glucose log, along with dietary information.
      i. Dietary information along with glucose results helps to interpret trends and recognition of glycemic patterns.
      ii. Postprandial monitoring is associated with:
         a) Better glycemic control
         b) Lower incidence of LGA
         c) Lower rate of cesarean delivery
   c. ACOG and ADA blood glucose concentration target goals:
      i. Fasting level: <95 mg/dL (5.3 mmol/L)
      ii. One-hour postprandial: <140 mg/dL (7.8 mmol/L)
      iii. Two-hour postprandial: <120 mg/dL (6.7 mmol/L)
5. Hemoglobin A1c (HbA1c) levels
   a. HbA1c levels are not affected by blood glucose levels alone. They are also altered in hemolytic anemias, hemoglobinopathies, acute and chronic blood loss, and pregnancy. Vitamin B12, folate, and iron-deficiency anemias have also been shown to affect HbA1c levels.
   b. A1c values tend to be lower in pregnancy because average blood glucose concentration is about 20% lower because of a rise in red cell mass and a slight decrease in red blood cell (RBC) life span.
   c. A1c levels tend to be higher in African American, Latinx, and Asian individuals.
   d. In patients diagnosed early in pregnancy (before 20 weeks), it may be helpful to determine whether diabetes is overt.
   e. Not clear whether HbA1c is useful later in pregnancy.
6. Urine ketone measurement for self-monitoring; may be recommended for GDM patients with severe hyperglycemia or weight loss, but there is no evidence that such monitoring improves fetal outcomes.

7. Exercise
   a. Cardiovascular conditioning improves glycemic control from increased tissue sensitivity to insulin.
   b. Circuit resistance training improves glycemic control.
   c. In some pregnant individuals, the need for insulin may be eliminated because both fasting and postprandial blood glucose concentrations improve.
   d. Moderate exercise is recommended for pregnant individuals with no medical or obstetrical complications: Encourage exercise daily for 30 minutes (for all capable pregnant individuals). Brisk walking is ideal. Exercise may make the need for insulin less likely.
8. Pharmacologic therapy
   a. Initiated if nutritional therapy is not adequately effective.
   b. Antihyperglycemic agents: Insulin is the preferred treatment, and metformin is an alternative medication for GDM (ACOG, 2018a; ADA, 2020b).
      i. Insulin
         a) Recommended for pregnant individuals who do not achieve adequate glycemic control with nutritional therapy and exercise alone. Research suggests antibodies against insulin may cross the placenta, causing inappropriate fetal weight gain. The use of human insulin decreases the development of these antibodies.
         b) Protocol: Calculate daily insulin dosing.
      ii. Insulin types: No evidence for the superiority of a specific insulin or insulin regimen (see Table 16.3)
         a) Rapid and short acting: Regular or lispro
         b) Intermediate and long acting: NPH or ultralente
         c) Note that Lantus and Levemir are not recommended because of a lack of data in pregnant individuals.

TABLE 16.3 MAIN TYPES OF INSULIN

TYPE	ONSET	PEAK	DURATION	COMMENTS
Rapid Acting: Humalog, Lispro NovoLog, Aspart Apidra, Glulisine	<15 min <15 min <15 min	60–90 min 60–120 min 60–90 min	3–5 hr 3–5 hr 1–2.5 hr	Can inject at start of meal or 10–15 minutes before meal. Used with longer-acting insulin
Short Acting: Regular, Novolin, Actrapid, or Humulin Velosulin	30–60 min 30–60 min	2–5 hr 2–3 hr	6–8 hr 2–3 hr	Inject at least 20–30 min before meals
Intermediate: NPH Lente	1–2 hr 1–2.5 hr	4–12 hr 3–10 hr	18–24 hr 18–24 hr	Used to control levels between meals. May be combined with rapid or short-acting insulin
Long Acting: Ultralente Lantus, Glargine Levemir, Detemir	30 min – 3 hr 1–1.5 hr 1–2 hr	10–20 hr No peak 6–8 hr	20–36 hr 20–24 hr Up to 24 hr	Usually once a day and covers insulin needs for 24 hr. May be combined with rapid or short-acting insulin

iii. For elevated fasting glucose levels:

a) Begin with single dose of bedtime NPH (usual starting dose = 0.2 units/kg body weight).

b) Use injections of short-acting insulin to cover postprandial hyperglycemia.

c) Insulin per day (based on prepregnancy weight):

i) Some providers use starting dose of 0.7 u/kg/d

ii) First half of pregnancy: 0.6 u/kg/d

iii) Second half of pregnancy: 0.9 u/kg/d

d) Divide insulin dosing over the course of a day: Morning: two thirds of insulin

e) NPH insulin: two thirds

f) Regular insulin: one third

g) Evening: one third of insulin

i) NPH insulin: one half

ii) Regular insulin: one half

c. Oral antihyperglycemic agents

i. Metformin and glyburide have been increasingly used in pregnant individuals with GDM, although not approved by the Food and Drug Administration (FDA). The benefit is that they work in controlling blood glucose levels and do not increase the risk for fetal anomaly or adverse perinatal outcomes. However, 20% to 40% of pregnant individuals require both insulin and oral agents.

ii. In 2018, ACOG advised glyburide should not be used as a first choice. If used, glyburide dose: 2.5 to 5 mg/d by mouth in divided doses or 1.25 mg by mouth if at risk for hypoglycemia, given with first meal. Up to 30 mg may be necessary to achieve control in some pregnant individuals. More complications of preeclampsia, hyperbilirubinemia, and stillbirth when glyburide was compared with insulin.

iii. Metformin: Primarily used in individuals with PCOS and/or pregestational diabetes. In individuals with PCOS, metformin is continued until the end of the first trimester as there is evidence it reduces first-trimester loss. There is some evidence for reducing other adverse perinatal outcomes, such as macrosomia and cesarean delivery rates, as well (Table 16.4). Risks include no long-term

TABLE 16.4 METFORMIN DOSING

Immediate release:	
	Initial dose: 500-mg orally twice a day or 850 mg orally once a day
	Dose titration: Increase in 500-mg weekly increments or 850 mg every 2 weeks as tolerated
	Maintenance dose: 2,000 mg daily
	Maximum dose: 2,550 mg daily
Extended release:	
	Initial dose: 500–1,000 mg orally once a day
	Dose titration: Increase in 500-mg weekly increments
	Maintenance dose: 2,000 mg daily
	Maximum dose: 2,550 mg daily

studies, crosses the placenta, and may be associated with PTB. Check creatinine at baseline and advise to take with meals.

iv. Early comparisons of metformin and glyburide showed the failure rate of metformin to be twice that of glyburide in achieving glycemic control in GDM. Although the mean birth weights in the metformin group were lower, other neonatal outcomes, including macrosomia, did not differ between the two groups. A 2017 large systematic review comparing insulin and oral hypoglycemic agents also demonstrated no substantial difference between the two approaches in safety, effectiveness, and maternal and neonatal outcomes, but several other outcomes were not evaluated. However, a recent 2020 meta-analysis revealed Metformin did have benefits when compared to glyburide with lower mean birth weights, less macrosomia, and less gestational weight gain.

9. Evaluate fetal well-being: Antenatal surveillance is indicated starting at 32 weeks (see Chapter 6) and third-trimester ultrasound growth scan.

E. COMPLICATIONS

1. Macrosomia
2. Neonatal hypoglycemia
3. Higher incidence of preeclampsia
4. Increased risk of cesarean delivery
5. Although GDM usually resolves after delivery, up to 33% of affected individuals have diabetes or impaired glucose metabolism at their postpartum screening. An estimated 15% to 50% will develop diabetes in the decades following the affected pregnancy.

F. REFERRAL/CONSULTATION

1. Comanage with physician or consider referral to physician if the patient requires insulin.
2. Refer to a nutritionist.
3. Refer the patient to a certified diabetic educator if available.

G. PATIENT EDUCATION

1. Discuss GDM and its short- and long-term implications regarding maternal and neonatal outcomes and future risk of diabetes.
2. Stress the importance of following dietary recommendations, exercise recommendations, self-monitoring of blood glucose, and keeping frequent appointments.
3. Explain the procedure of blood glucose monitoring.
4. See Chapter 6 and Appendix A regarding kick counts (initiated at 28 weeks) and other testing.
5. Encourage postpartum follow-up.
6. Address other issues of routine prenatal and postpartum care such as breastfeeding, parenting, family planning, and so on.

H. FOLLOW-UP

1. Glucose intolerance is very frequent in the early postpartum period in individuals with GDM based on the 2013 WHO criteria (Benhalima et al., 2016). Order a 6- to 12-week postpartum follow-up; screen with fasting plasma glucose or a 75-g 2-hour OGTT. Screening for type 2 diabetes mellitus should then be performed every 1 to 3 years (ADA, 2020b). Touching base with the patient is very important as follow-up rates on postpartum testing are highly variable, with up to 75% of patients failing to follow through.

2. Between 35% and 60% of individuals develop type 2 diabetes within 10 years of having GDM. Risk factors include the following:
   a. Obesity
   b. Diagnosis before 24 weeks' gestation
   c. Insulin use during pregnancy
   d. Encourage intensive lifestyle interventions directed to decreasing weight (if overweight or obese) and cardiovascular risk. These interventions and metformin are effective in preventing or delaying diabetes in individuals with GDM history for at least 10 years. Preeclampsia is independently associated with a twofold increase in future diabetes (Wu et al., 2016).

Bibliography

American College of Obstetricians and Gynecologists. (2018a). Gestational diabetes mellitus (Practice Bulletin no. 190). *Obstetrics & Gynecology, 131*(2), 406–408. https://doi.org/10.1097/AOG.0000000000002498

American College of Obstetricians and Gynecologists. (2018b). Pregestational diabetes mellitus (Practice Bulletin no. 201). *Obstetrics & Gynecology, 132*(6), e228–e248. https://doi.org/10.1097/AOG.0000000000002960

American Diabetes Association. (2020a). Management of diabetes in pregnancy: Standards of medical care in diabetes—2020. *Diabetes Care, 43*(Suppl. 1), S183–192. https://doi.org/10.2337/dc20-S014

American Diabetes Association. (2020b). Standards of medical care in diabetes—2020. *Diabetes Care, 43*(Suppl. 1), S1–151. https://doi.org/10.2337/dc20-Sint

Baptiste-Roberts, K., Barone, B., Gary, T., Golden, S., Wilson, L., Bass, E., & Nicholson, W. (2009). Risk factors for type 2 diabetes among women with gestational diabetes: A systematic review. *American Journal of Medicine, 122*(3), 207.e4–214.e4. https://doi.org/10.1016/j.amjmed.2008.09.034

Benhalima, K., Jegers, K., Devlinger, R., Verhaeghe, J., & Mathieu, C. (2016). Glucose intolerance after a recent history of gestational diabetes based on the 2013 WHO criteria. *PLOS ONE, 11*(6). https://doi.org/10.1371/journal.pone.0157272

Dietz, P. M., Vesco, K. K., Callaghan, W. M., Bachman, D. J., Bruce, F. C., Berg, C. J., England, L. J., & Hornbrook, M. C. (2008). Postpartum screening for diabetes after a gestational diabetes mellitus-affected pregnancy. *Obstetrics & Gynecology, 112*(4), 868–874. https://doi.org/10.1097/AOG.0b013e318184db63

Durnwald, C. (2020a). *Diabetes mellitus in pregnancy: Screening and diagnosis.* http://www.uptodate.com

Durnwald, C. (2020b). *Gestational diabetes mellitus: Glycemic control and maternal prognosis.* http://www.uptodate.com

Eggleston, E. M., LeCates, R. F., Zhang, F., Wharam, J. F., Ross-Degnan, D., & Oken, E. (2016). Variation in postpartum glycemic screening in women with a history of gestational diabetes mellitus. *Obstetrics & Gynecology, 128*(1), 159–167. https://doi.org/10.1097/AOG.0000000000001467

Family Practice Notebook. (n.d). *Gestational diabetes insulin management.* http://www.fpnotebook.com/endo/OB/GstnlDbtsInslnMngmnt.htm

Hunt, K. J., & Conway, D. L. (2008). Who returns for postpartum glucose screening following gestational diabetes mellitus? *American Journal of Obstetrics & Gynecology, 198*(4), 404.e1–404.e6. https://doi.org/10.1016/j.ajog.2007.09.015

International Association of Diabetes and Pregnancy Study Groups Consensus Panel, ., Metzger, B. E., Gabbe, S. G., Persson, B., Buchanan, T. A., Catalano, P. A., Damm, P., Dyer, A. R., Leiva, A., Hod, M., Kitzmiller, J. L., Lowe, L. P., McIntyre, H. D., Oats, J. J. N., Omori, Y., & Schmidt, M. I. (2010). International Association of Diabetes and Pregnancy Study Groups recommendations on the diagnosis and classification of hyperglycemia in pregnancy. *Diabetes Care, 33*(3), 676–682. https://doi.org/10.2337/dc09-1848

Kim, C., Bullard, K. M., Herman, W. H., & Beckles, G. L. (2010). Association between iron deficiency and A1C levels among adults without diabetes in the National Health and Nutrition Examination Survey, 1999–2006. *Diabetes Care, 33*(4), 780–785. doi:10.2337/dc09–0836

Landon, M. B., Spong, C. Y., Thom, E., Carpenter, M. W., Ramin, S. M., Casey, B., Wapner, R. J., Varner, M. W., Rouse, D. J., Thorp, J. M. Jr., Sciscione, A., Catalano, P., Harper, M., Saade, G., Lain, K. Y., Sorokin, Y., Peaceman, A. M., Tolosa, J. E., Anderson, G. B., & . . . Eunice Kennedy Shriver National Institute of Child Health and Human Development Maternal-Fetal Medicine Units Network. (2009). A multicenter, randomized trial of treatment for mild gestational diabetes. *New England Journal of Medicine, 361*, 1339–1348. https://doi.org/10.1056/NEJMoa0902430

Maxson, P. J., Edwards, S. E., Ingram, A., & Miranda, M. L. (2012). Psychosocial differences between smokers and non-smokers during pregnancy. *Addictive Behaviors, 37*(2), 153–159. https://doi.org/10.1016/j.addbeh.2011.08.011

Menato, G., Bo, S., Signorile, A., Gallo, M. L., Cotrino, I., Poala, C. B., & Massobrio, M. (2008). Current management of gestational diabetes mellitus. *Expert Review of Obstetrics & Gynecology, 3*, 73–91. https://doi.org/10.1586/17474108.3.1.73

Moore, L. E., Clokey, D., Rappaport, V. J., & Curet, L. B. (2010). Metformin compared with glyburide in gestational diabetes: A randomized controlled trial. *Obstetrics & Gynecology, 115*(1), 55–59. https://doi.org/10.1097/AOG.0b013e3181c52132

Nicholson, W., Bolen, S., Witkop, C. T., Neale, D., Wilson, L., & Bass, E. (2009). Benefits and risks of oral diabetes agents compared with insulin in women with gestational diabetes: A systematic review. *Obstetrics & Gynecology, 113*(1), 193–205. doi:10.1097/AOG.0b013e318190a459

Rowan, J. A., Hague, W. M., Gao, W., Battin, M. R., Moore, M., & MiG Trial Investigators. (2008). Metformin versus insulin for the treatment of gestational diabetes. *New England Journal of Medicine, 358*(19), 2003–2015. https://doi.org/10.1056/NEJMoa0707193

Singh, S. R., Ahmad, F., Lah, A., Yu, C., Bai, Z., & Bennett, H. (2009). Efficacy and safety of insulin analogues for the management of diabetes mellitus: A meta-analysis. *Canadian Medical Association Journal, 180*(4), 385–397. https://doi.org/10.1503/cmaj.081041

Sinha, N., Mishra, T. K., Singh, T. S., & Gupta, N. (2012). Effect of iron deficiency anemia on Hemoglobin A1C levels. *Annals of Laboratory Medicine, 32*(1), 17–22. https://doi.org/10.3343/alm.2012.32.1.17

Standards of Medical Care in Diabetes. III. Detection and Diagnosis of Gestational Diabetes Mellitus. (2012). *National guideline clearinghouse.* http://guideline.gov/content.aspx?id=35246&search=gestational+diabetes

U.S. Preventive Services Task Force. (2021). *Screening for gestational diabetes mellitus: U.S. Preventive Services Task Force recommendation statement.* https://www.uspreventiveservicestaskforce.org/uspstf/recommendation/gestational-diabetes-mellitus-screening

Washington University School of Medicine. Department of Obstetrics and Gynecology. (2015). *Resident handbook 2011–2012. OB guide 2014–2015.* Washington University.

Wu, P., Kwok, C. S., Haththotuwa, R., Kotronias, R. A., Babu, A., Fryer, A. A., Myint, P. K., Chew-Graham, C. A., & Mamas, M. A. (2016). Pre-eclampsia is associated with a twofold increase in diabetes: A systematic review and meta-analysis. *Diabetologia, 59*(12), 2518–2526. https://doi.org/10.1007/s00125-016-4098-x

17. Obesity and Pregnancy

MARY LEE BARRON | KELLY D. ROSENBERGER

The prevalence of obesity as a worldwide epidemic has increased dramatically over the past two decades. In the United States, the prevalence of obesity is increasing at an alarming rate. Obesity is reported as 31.8%, increasing to 58.5% when combining overweight and obese categories. From 1999 to 2018, the rate of obesity has increased from 28.4% to 39.7% in women aged 20 to 39 years and is higher in non-Hispanic African American and Mexican American women (National Center for Health Statistics, 2016, 2020). Almost two-thirds of women and three-fourths of men are overweight or obese, as are nearly 50% of women of reproductive age and 17% of their children ages 2 to 19 years (American Society for Reproductive Medicine [ASRM], 2015).

Obesity before and during pregnancy is associated with fertility problems and numerous maternal and perinatal risks such as pregnancy loss, preeclampsia, gestational diabetes mellitus (GDM), urinary tract infections, dysfunctional labor, preterm premature rupture of membranes, preterm delivery, and postterm birth. In addition, obstructive sleep apnea may be exacerbated during pregnancy and may increase the risk of preeclampsia and GDM. The risks increase with greater degrees of obesity. Postpartum issues include longer hospital stays, infection (wound, episiotomy, and endometritis), and venous thromboembolism. Some obese individuals have more difficulty initiating and maintaining lactation, partly because of the complications and their effect on a good start to breastfeeding. Specifically, overweight/obese individuals have a lower prolactin response to suckling in the first week postpartum, which may contribute to early lactation failure.

However, it is not clear whether obesity is a direct cause of adverse pregnancy outcome. An alternate theory questions whether the association between obesity and adverse pregnancy outcomes is the result of shared characteristics of both mother and baby genotypes, such as high maternal body mass index (BMI) associated with higher birthweight in the infant, fetal macrosomia, and shoulder dystocia (Tyrrell et al., 2016). Excess adipose tissue is an active endocrine organ and may have effects on the metabolic, vascular, and inflammatory pathways during pregnancy affecting outcomes (Ramsay et al., 2002). Adverse outcomes due to insulin resistance and pathway changes are associated with maternal diabetes and altered placental growth and function. Nondiabetic obese patients and patients with GDM are also at greater risk for adverse outcomes such as preeclampsia. The cause is complex and, at minimum, is neither well understood nor straightforward. Furthermore, it is difficult to study because of the complexity of the relationships among the maternal metabolic milieu, the developing fetus, and factors such as lifestyle and environment.

A. DEFINITION

1. Obesity is defined as pregnancy BMI ≥30 kg/m^2 (Table 17.1).

TABLE 17.1 WORLD HEALTH ORGANIZATION CLASSIFICATION BY BMI CATEGORIES

BMI	CLASSIFICATION
<18.5	Underweight
18.5–24.9	Normal weight
25.0–29.9	Overweight
30.0–34.9	Class I obesity
35.0–39.9	Class II obesity
40.0–49.9	Class III obesity

BMI, body mass index.

2. Associated complications with obesity and pregnancy
   - **a.** Maternal complications during pregnancy: Increased risk of gestational diabetes, gestational hypertension, preeclampsia, and cesarean delivery
   - **b.** Fetal and neonatal complications: Increased risk of adverse fetal and neonatal outcomes. Obese individuals have a higher rate of prematurity resulting from maternal conditions such as preeclampsia. The risk for neural tube defects in fetuses of obese individuals is roughly twice that of those with normal weight prior to pregnancy. Obese, and especially morbidly obese, pregnant individuals have a higher likelihood of having a fetus with congenital anomalies and increased risks of late stillbirths. However, the diagnosis of these disorders and fetal weight may be hampered by the poor ultrasound (US) resolution obtained in obese and morbidly obese pregnant patients.
   - **c.** Intrapartum complications: Many obese and morbidly obese individuals may experience an indicated preterm delivery because of complications such as preeclampsia. Others are induced because of post dates gestation. However, many who spontaneously start labor experience slower labors than those with a normal BMI and may require labor augmentation. There is also the challenge of electronic maternal and fetal monitoring in morbidly obese patient. Because of fetal macrosomia, the risk for shoulder dystocia, and therefore birth trauma, is increased.
   - **d.** Anesthesia complications: Consultation with the anesthesia staff is important. Many obese patients have poor Mallampati scores (used to predict the ease of intubation). Because of difficulty in locating landmarks, spinal anesthesia may be difficult to place. Epidural anesthesia is encouraged in these patients because of the associated decreased oxygen consumption in labor and increased cardiac output.
   - **e.** Cesarean delivery: Obese pregnant patients have an increased risk for both emergent and elective cesarean deliveries. Emergent cesarean deliveries are difficult due to anesthesia challenges if an epidural is not already placed or is not functioning well; presence of the pannus; adiposity that must be gone through even with elevation of the pannus; and difficulty of locating the fundus for assistance of fetal delivery. In obese pregnant individuals, deliveries by cesarean section result in higher estimated blood losses, longer operative times, and increased rates of wound infection (Flick& Artal, 2013). Rho(D) immune globulin should be administered intravenously to prevent failures. It may be necessary to give a higher dose of antibiotics to reach adequate therapeutic levels.
   - **f.** Postpartum complications include postpartum hemorrhage, increased risk of venous thromboembolism, endometritis, decreased

breastfeeding initiation with early discontinuation, and postpartum depression.

B. HISTORY

1. Assess for demographic, lifestyle, obstetric, and medical/biologic risk factors
   a. Bariatric surgery: Infants of mothers with a previous bariatric operation had a greater likelihood of perinatal complications compared with infants of nonoperative mothers. Operation-to-birth intervals of less than 2 years were associated with higher risks for prematurity, neonatal intensive care unit (NICU) admission, and small-for-gestational-age (SGA) status compared with longer intervals.
2. Assess for gestational age if unknown (see Chapter 3).
3. Assess a 3-day diet history that includes:
   a. The person who prepares the meals in the home
   b. Frequency of eating at restaurants and consumption of ready-to-eat processed foods
4. Assess past dietary practices, dieting practices, and attitudes toward pregnancy weight gain.
5. Assess for obstructive sleep apnea during pregnancy which increases the risk for preeclampsia and GDM.
   a. Screening questions:
      i. Do you snore?
      ii. Do you wake up tired after a full night of sleep?
      iii. Do you fall asleep during the day?
      iv. Have you been told you stop breathing at night while you are asleep?
      v. Do you have a history of hypertension?

   If the answer is "yes" to two or more questions, refer to a sleep specialist.

C. PHYSICAL EXAMINATION

1. As indicated by guidelines (see Chapter 3) and gestational age
2. Calculate BMI.
3. Screen for known complications of overweight/obesity, such as gestational diabetes, hypertension, and preeclampsia, as identified in relevant topic chapters.

D. LABORATORY AND DIAGNOSTIC STUDIES

1. Routine prenatal laboratory testing as indicated by gestational age
   a. GDM screening should be conducted earlier if there is a high degree of suspicion that a patient has undiagnosed type 2 diabetes (glycosuria, obesity [BMI ≥30], personal history of GDM, or a strong family history of diabetes). Screening can be performed with a 50-g, 1-hour glucose challenge test. In some centers, the hemoglobin A1c is also used as this has been found to correlate well.
2. Ultrasound screening
   a. Overweight and obese individuals have higher rates of menstrual irregularities and infertility. Because the patient may not realize she is pregnant, there may be a delay in prenatal care initiation. Therefore, early US should be performed to verify dating for accurate gestational age, exclude multiple gestations, and diagnoses abnormal pregnancies early: ectopic, missed abortion, or congenital anomalies.
   b. Consider additional US screening for fetal growth and/or presentation based on clinical judgment. Because of additional adipose tissue,

usual measurements for following fetal growth (McDonald's or fundal height measurement) may not be accurate. Depending on the size of the patient and consistency of the fundal height with gestational age, this may mean US screening every 4 to 6 weeks or an extra screening at 32 weeks. As detecting fetal presentation and position may be difficult, consider US at 36 weeks to verify.

c. Biophysical profiles: Fetal heart rate testing can be difficult to perform because of the patient's adiposity. For some patients, US for biophysical profiles are the only option to monitor fetal health.

E. MANAGEMENT

1. Counseling

a. Nutritional needs in pregnancy (see Chapter 3): Consider that the obese patient is "malnourished." Obesity does not equate with eating too much of a healthy diet. Rather, there may be overconsumption and the consumption of so-called "empty calories." The importance of good nutrition during pregnancy cannot be underestimated. Maternal undernutrition and malnutrition are major problems, especially in patients with low socioeconomic status, leading to low birth weight and fetal growth restriction. From animal models, maternal malnutrition creates a pro-inflammatory environment that leads to inhibition of placental tissue growth (Claycombe et al., 2013).

b. Recommendation for appropriate weight gain at the initial visit and periodically throughout the pregnancy

i. The 2009 Institute of Medicine (IOM) guidelines recommend a total of 15 to 25 lb. weight gain (6.8–11.3 kg) for overweight individuals and 11 to 20 lb. (5.0–9.1 kg) for all obese individuals (BMI $\geq$ 30; see Chapter 3) during pregnancy. Most American women gain weight below or above the IOM ranges. In a recent Centers for Disease Control and Prevention (CDC) report, gestational weight gain was within the recommended range for only 32% of patients giving birth to full-term, singleton infants in 2015, with 48% gaining more weight and 21% less weight than recommended. Approximately 44% of individuals who were underweight before pregnancy gained *within* the recommendations, compared with 39% of individuals who were normal weight, 26% of individuals who were overweight, and 24% of individuals with obesity before pregnancy. Weight gain *above* the recommendations was highest among individuals who were overweight (61%) or had obesity (55%) before pregnancy. However, there are individuals who gain less than what is recommended in the IOM guidelines. The American College of Obstetricians and Gynecologists (ACOG) considers that in an obese pregnant individual who is gaining less weight than recommended, but has an appropriately growing fetus, there is no existing evidence that encouraging increased weight gain to conform with the updated IOM guidelines will improve maternal or fetal outcomes (ACOG, 2013a).

ii. Changes are required in the patient's behavior and in care management. High-quality evidence indicates that diet, exercise, or both lower the risk of cesarean delivery, macrosomia, and neonatal respiratory morbidity. Maternal hypertension is also reduced. Respecting the patient's autonomy and dignity is paramount, especially in light of the societal stigma regarding obesity. At the initial visit, counseling should include overall health before and after pregnancy. Nutritional counseling should be the focus that is integrated into the first and repeat prenatal visits, that is, focus on healthy eating rather than the "numbers."

There is "no such BMI level at which an individual crosses from being healthy to unhealthy" (ACOG, 2013b).

iii. Motivational interviewing (MI) involves assessing a patient's motives for change and acting as a supportive partner who empowers the patient in the process. This counseling technique is a goal-oriented, client-centered approach that elicits behavior change by helping clients to explore and resolve ambivalence. Pregnant individuals are often open to change as they are concerned about having a healthy baby. However, with MI, there is recognition that people who need to make changes are at different levels of readiness to do so. There are four general processes used:

a) Engaging: This process involves the client by talking about issues, concerns, and hopes, and establishes a trusting relationship with a counselor.

b) Focusing: This process is used to narrow the conversation to habits or patterns that clients want to change.

c) Evoking: This process elicits client motivation for change by increasing clients' sense of the importance of change, their confidence about change, and their readiness to change.

d) Planning: This process is used to develop the practical steps clients want to use to implement the changes they desire.

More information on the MI technique is available (www.motivationalinterviewing.org)

2. With the increasing prevalence of obesity in the United States and worldwide, there is the need for the prevention of hypertensive disorders of pregnancy in this population. Obese pregnant individuals with additional risk factors for preeclampsia may benefit from treatment with low-dose aspirin (81 mg). When initiated after 12 weeks (optimally before 16 weeks) of gestation, aspirin is effective in preventing hypertensive disorders of pregnancy in high-risk obese patients, but questions regarding appropriate dosing in the obese population remain unanswered (ACOG, 2018).

F. PATIENT EDUCATION

Obesity education (apart from routine prenatal education) should occur within the context of the medical, cultural, and social issues of the patient and should be incorporated into the appropriate prenatal visit as clinically relevant. For example, discussing maternal complications may be appropriate during the first trimester, and discussing cesarean delivery may be best done in the third trimester.

TABLE 17.2 RECOMMENDATIONS FOR TOTAL AND RATE OF WEIGHT GAIN DURING PREGNANCY

PREPREGNANCY BMI	TOTAL WEIGHT GAIN IN POUNDS	RATE OF GAIN IN SECOND AND THIRD TRIMESTERS IN POUNDS/WEEK
Underweight (<18.5 kg/m^2)	28–40	1 (1–3)
Normal weight (18.5–24.9 kg/m^2)	25–35	1 (0.8–1)
Overweight (25–29.9 kg/m^2)	15–25	0.6 (0.5–0.7)
Obese (≥30 kg/m^2)	11–20	0.5 (0.4–0.6)

G. CONSULTATION/REFERRAL

1. Consult with a physician and refer for care if the patient is morbidly obese (Class II or III). It is likely that the patient is best served with interdisciplinary team care. The patient may be designated as high risk from the beginning of prenatal care.

2. Refer to the dietician for nutritional counseling if available. The optimal diet should be worked with a registered dietician and tailored for pregnant individuals of different classes of obesity by recommending a nutrient-dense caloric intake in the range of 2,000 to 2,500 cal/d to provide adequate calories and nutrients to support fetal growth. This caloric intake results in a gestational weight gain of 11 lb or less and, in some, a net negative weight gain. Limited weight gain in obese pregnant individuals has the potential for setting the foundation for a healthier lifestyle over the lifespan, including during interconceptional periods and during subsequent pregnancies. Pregnant individuals should be encouraged to continue most prepregnancy exercise programs or begin an exercise program avoiding vigorous activities. Table 17.2 provides recommendations for both the total and rate of weight gain in singleton pregnancies based on prepregnancy BMI. Note that in pregnancies with multiple gestations the weight gain recommendations are higher.

Bibliography

American College of Obstetricians and Gynecologists. (2013a). ACOG Committee opinion no. 548 (Reaffirmed 2020): Weight gain during pregnancy. *Obstetrics & Gynecology, 121*, 210–212. https://doi.org/10.1097/01.AOG.0000425668.87506.4c

American College of Obstetricians and Gynecologists. (2013b). Practice Bulletin no. 549: Obesity in pregnancy. *Obstetrics & Gynecology, 126*(6), e112–e126. https://doi.org/10.1097/AOG.0000000000001211

American College of Obstetricians and Gynecologists. (2015). Practice Bulletin no. 156 summary: Obesity in pregnancy (Reaffirmed 2020). *Obstetrics & Gynecology, 126*(6), e112–e126. https://doi.org/10.1097/AOG.0000000000001211

American College of Obstetricians and Gynecologists. (2018). ACOG Committee opinion no. 743: Low dose aspirin use during pregnancy. *Obstetrics & Gynecology, 132*, e44–212. https://doi.org/10.1097/AOG.0000000000002708

American Society for Reproductive Medicine. (2015). Obesity and reproduction: A committee opinion. *Fertility & Sterility, 104*(5), 1116–1126. https://doi.org/10.1016/j.fertnstert.2015.08.018

Blomberg, M. I., & Källén, B. (2010). Maternal obesity and morbid obesity: The risk for birth defects in the offspring. *Birth Defects Research Part A: Clinical and Molecular Teratology, 88*, 35–40. https://doi.org/10.1002/bdra.20620

Campbell, E. E., Dworatzek, P. N., Penava, D., de Vrijer, B., Gilliland, J., Matthews, J. I., & Seabrook, J. A. (2016). Factors that influence excessive gestational weight gain: Moving beyond assessment and counselling. *Journal of Maternal-Fetal & Neonatal Medicine, 29*(21), 3527–3531. https://doi.org/10.3109/14767058.2015.1137894

Claycombe, K. J., Uthus, E. O., Roemmich, J. N., Johnson, L. K., & Johnson, W. T. (2013). Prenatal low-protein and postnatal high-fat diets induce rapid adipose tissue growth by inducing Igf2 expression in Sprague Dawley rat offspring. *Journal of Nutrition, 143*, 1533–1539. https://doi.org/10.3945/jn.113.178038

Denison, F. C., Price, J., Graham, C., Wild, S., & Liston, W. A. (2008). Maternal obesity, length of gestation, risk of postdates pregnancy and spontaneous onset of labour at term. *British Journal of Obstetrics and Gynecology, 115*, 720–725. https://doi.org/10.1111/j.1471-0528.2008.01694.x

Flick, A., & Artal, M. (2013). Obesity and weight gain in pregnancy: The fact is that pregnancy is an ideal time for obese patients to make lifestyle changes. *Contemporary OB/GYN. 58*(7), 26–36. http://images2.advanstar.com/pixelmags/obgyn/pdf/2013-07.pdf

Heery, E., Wall, P. G., Kelleher, C. C., & McAuliffe, F. M. (2016). Effects of dietary restraint and weight gain attitudes on gestational weight gain. *Appetite, 107*, 510. https://doi.org/10.1016/j.appet.2016.08.103

Lindberg, S., DeBoth, A., & Anderson, C. (2016). Effect of a best practice alert on gestational weight gain, health services, and pregnancy outcomes. *Maternal & Child Health Journal, 20*(10), 2169–2178. https://doi.org/10.1007/s10995-016-2052-7

Maggard, M. A., Yermilov, I., Li, Z., Maglione, M., Newberry, S., Suttop, M., Hilton, L., Santry, H. P., Morton, J. M., Livingston, E. H., & Shekelle, P. G. (2008). Pregnancy and fertility following bariatric surgery: A systematic review. *Journal of the American Medical Association, 300*, 2286–2296. https://doi.org/10.1001/jama.2008.641

Muktabhant, B., Lawrie, T. A., Lumbiganon, P., & Laopaiboon, M. (2015). Diet or exercise, or both, for preventing excessive weight gain in pregnancy. *Cochrane Database of Systematic Reviews, 2015*(6), CD007145. https://doi.org/10.1002/14651858.CD007145.pub3

National Center for Health Statistics. (2016). QuickStats: Gestational weight gain among women with full-term, singleton births, compared with recommendations—48 states and the District of Columbia, 2015. *Morbidity and Mortality Weekly Report, 65*, 1121. https://doi.org/10.15585/mmwr.mm6540a10

National Center for Health Statistics. (2020). *Prevalence of obesity and severe obesity among adults: United States, 2017 – 2018 (NCHS Data Brief no. 360)*. https://www.cdc.gov/nchs/products/databriefs/db360.htm

Parent, B., Martopullo, I., Weiss, N. S., Khandelwal, S., Fay, E. E., & Rowhani-Rahbar, A. (2017). Bariatric surgery in women of childbearing age, timing between operation and birth, and associated perinatal complications. *JAMA Surgery, 152*(2), 1–8. https://doi.org/10.1001/jamasurg.2016.3621

Practice Committee of the American Society for Reproductive Medicine. (2015). Obesity and reproduction: A committee opinion. *Fertility & Sterility, 104*(5), 1116–1126. https://doi.org/10.1016/j.fertnstert.2015.08.018

Ramsay, J. E., Ferrell, W. R., Crawford, L., Wallace, A. M., Greer, I. A., & Sattar, N. (2002). Maternal obesity is associated with dysregulation of metabolic, vascular and inflammatory pathways. *The Journal of Clinical Endocrinology and Metabolism, 87*(9), 4231–4237. https://doi.org/10.1210/jc.2002-020311

Tooher, R., Gates, S., Dowswell, T., & Davis, L. J. (2010). Prophylaxis for venous thromboembolic disease in pregnancy and the early postnatal period. *Cochrane Database Systematic Reviews, 2010*(5), CD001689. https://doi.org/10.1002/14651858.CD001689.pub2

Tyrrell, J., Richmond, R. C., Palmer, T. M., Feenstra, B., Rangarajan, J., Metrustry, S., Cavadino, A., Paternoster, L., Armstrong, L. L., De Silva, N. M. G., Wood, A. R., Horikoshi, M., Geller, F., Myhre, R., Bradfield, J. P., Kreiner-Møller, E. K., . . . Freathy, R. M. (2016). Genetic evidence for causal relationships between maternal obesity-related traits and birth weight. *Journal of the American Medical Association, 315*, 1129–1140. https://doi.org/10.1001/jama.2016.1975

Vallejo, M. C. (2007). Anesthetic management of the morbidly obese parturient. *Current Opinion in Anaesthesiology, 20*, 175–180. https://doi.org/10.1097/ACO.0b013e328014646b

18. Hypertensive Disorders of Pregnancy

NANCY J. CIBULKA | KELLY D. ROSENBERGER

There are four categories of major hypertensive disorders of pregnancy: preeclampsia (PEC), chronic/preexisting hypertension, chronic hypertension with superimposed PEC, and gestational hypertension (American College of Obstetricians and Gynecologists [ACOG], 2013). Affected pregnancies are at increased risk for maternal and fetal complications and poor outcomes. Hypertensive disorders complicate up to 10% of pregnancies worldwide and are one of the leading causes of maternal morbidity and mortality. In developed nations, PEC is associated with a doubling of the rate of adverse neonatal events (sepsis, seizures, and death) and accounts for 16% of maternal deaths (Bicocca et al., 2020). The U.S. Preventative Services Task Force (USPSTF) reported PEC is the second most common cause of maternal morbidity and mortality in the world. PEC occurs in 4% of U.S. pregnancies, accounts for 6% of preterm births, and 19% of medically indicated preterm deliveries in the United States (USPSTF, 2021).

The pathophysiology of PEC is not fully understood but is thought to involve maternal, paternal, fetal, and placental factors that contribute to abnormal development of placental vasculature in early pregnancy. Placental ischemia/hypoxia appears to be a key element of the disease. The factors currently considered to be most important are (a) maternal immunologic issues; (b) abnormal placental implantation; (c) genetic, nutritional, and environmental factors; and (d) cardiovascular and inflammatory changes (Lim, 2016). A cascade of physiologic events results in widespread maternal systemic endothelial dysfunction and vasospasm, which occurs after 20 weeks gestation and as late as 4 to 6 weeks postpartum. About 10% of maternal deaths are caused by a hypertensive disorder of pregnancy in the postpartum period. PEC is a known risk factor for future cardiovascular and renal disease.

A. DEFINITION

1. PEC: A multisystem disorder unique to pregnancy characterized by new-onset hypertension and either proteinuria or end-organ dysfunction, most often occurring after 20 weeks gestation. Diagnosis is not always straightforward.

a. Mild PEC, now known as *preeclampsia without severe features*: Blood pressure (BP) ≥140/90 mmHg on two measurements at least 6 hours apart and proteinuria of ≥0.3 g in a 24-hour specimen or 1+ or more on a dipstick (Table 18.1) in a patient who was previously normotensive.

b. PEC with severe features: BP ≥160/110 mmHg on two measurements at least 6 hours apart and evidence of end-organ damage as listed in Table 18.1.

TABLE 18.1 MILD PEC VERSUS PEC WITH SEVERE FEATURES

SIGNS/SYMPTOMS	MILD PEC	SEVERE PEC
BP	≥140/90 × 2, 4–6 hr apart	≥160/110 × 2, 4–6 hr apart
Proteinuria	≥0.3 g in 24 hr ≥1+ on dipstick	≥5 g in 24 hr ≥3 + dipstick × 2
Reflexes	May be normal	Hyperreflexia ≥3+, possible ankle clonus
Urine output	Matching intake, or ≥30 mL/hr	Oliguria, ≥20 mL/hr or <500 mL in 24 hr
Headache	Absent or transient	Persistent, severe
Visual disturbances	Absent	Blurred, scotomata, sparkles, photophobia
Changes in mentation	Absent or transient	Altered mental status
RUQ of abdomen or epigastric pain	Absent	May be present
Pulmonary edema/cyanosis	Absent	May be present
Placental perfusion	Somewhat reduced	Decreased with possible IUGR, abnormal FHR
Thrombocytopenia	Absent	<100,000/mm^3
Serum creatinine Protein/creatinine ratio	Normal 0.3 mg/dL	Elevated, >1.1 mg/dL >0.3 mg/dL
AST and ALT Uric acid	Normal May be normal	Doubled or greater >5.5 mg/dL

ALT, alanine transaminase; AST, aspartate transaminase; FHR, fetal heart rate; IUGR, intrauterine growth restriction; PEC, preeclampsia; RUQ, right upper quadrant.

c. *Eclampsia* refers to the progression of this condition to the development of new-onset grand mal seizures without another cause.

d. Hemolysis, elevated liver enzymes, and low platelets (HELLP) syndrome: Unknown whether this syndrome is a severe form of PEC or an independent disorder (15%–20% of patients do not have hypertension or proteinuria).

2. Chronic/preexisting hypertension: Systolic pressure ≥140 mmHg and/or diastolic pressure ≥90 mmHg that predates the pregnancy or is found before 20 weeks gestation on at least two occasions or persists longer than 12 weeks postpartum. Chronic hypertension during pregnancy is associated with increased risk for premature birth, superimposed PEC, intrauterine growth restriction (IUGR), oligohydramnios, fetal demise, and placental abruption.

3. Chronic hypertension with superimposed PEC: Diagnosed by a sudden increase in BP that was previously well controlled or new-onset or sudden increase in proteinuria after 20 weeks gestation in a patient with preexisting hypertension; may also be characterized by the development of other signs/symptoms of severe PEC noted in Table 18.1.

4. Gestational hypertension: Hypertension without proteinuria or other signs/symptoms of PEC that first appears after 20 weeks gestation or within 48 to 72 hours after delivery and resolves by 12 weeks postpartum. This is a temporary diagnosis for individuals who do not meet the criteria for either PEC or chronic hypertension. In time, some patients will develop proteinuria or the end-organ dysfunction that characterizes PEC, whereas others may be diagnosed with chronic hypertension if BP elevations persist beyond 12 weeks postpartum. It is unknown whether this condition is a mild stage of PEC or an independent disorder.

B. RISK FACTORS

1. PEC or gestational hypertension in a previous pregnancy increases the risk sevenfold in a subsequent pregnancy.
2. First pregnancy (nulliparity)
3. Family history of PEC in a first-degree relative (mother or sister)
4. Paternal history of PEC in mother or previous partner
5. Maternal age older than 35 years or younger than 18 years
6. Preexisting medical conditions: chronic hypertension, renal disease, pregestational diabetes mellitus, antiphospholipid antibody syndrome or inherited thrombophilia, vascular or connective tissue disease
7. African American ethnicity
8. Body mass index >26
9. Hyperglycemia, insulin resistance, and dyslipidemia (metabolic syndrome)
10. Twin or multifetal pregnancy
11. Hydatidiform mole
12. Hydrops fetalis
13. Unexplained IUGR
14. Mother herself had growth restriction in utero
15. IUGR, placental abruption, or fetal demise in a previous pregnancy
16. In vitro fertilization

C. HISTORY

1. Assess for demographic, familial, paternal, obstetric, and medical/biologic risk factors (see Section B).
2. With mild PEC, the patient may be asymptomatic. Differences between mild and severe PEC are listed in Table 18.1.
3. Signs/symptoms of PEC most often occur after 34 weeks gestation, including during labor, known as *late-onset PEC*. Early-onset PEC develops before 34 weeks gestation (10% of cases), and postpartum PEC (5% of cases) usually occurs within 48 hours of delivery but can present as late as 4 to 6 weeks postpartum.
4. Signs and symptoms are highly variable and may include the following:
   a. Edema in the face and hands
   b. Persistent and/or severe headache unrelieved by acetaminophen
   c. Visual disturbances such as spots or sparkles, photophobia, blurred vision, or scotomata
   d. Nausea, vomiting, and/or upper abdominal or epigastric pain
   e. Oliguria (<500 mL in 24 hours)
   f. Shortness of breath and chest pain
   g. Fatigue, malaise, and mental confusion
   h. Abdominal pain
   i. Clonus (may indicate impending convulsions)
   j. Decreased fetal movement

D. PHYSICAL EXAMINATION

1. General appearance: Observe for anxiety and evidence of distress.
2. Check vital signs for BP elevation, tachycardia, and tachypnea
   a. To reduce inaccurate readings, be sure to use appropriate cuff size.
   b. Take BP in an upright position after a minimum of a 10-minute rest.
   c. Patient should not use tobacco or caffeine in preceding 30 minutes.

3. Check maternal weight: Gain of 5 lb or more in 1 week is significant.

4. Auscultate fetal heart rate for tachycardia or bradycardia.

5. Check fundal height for suspicion of IUGR.

6. Auscultate lungs and heart.

7. Neurologic examination: Assess for normal/abnormal mentation, check deep tendon reflexes for evidence of hyperreflexia and presence of ankle clonus.

8. Abdominal examination: Check for right upper quadrant (RUQ) tenderness (liver capsule distention).

9. Skin: Inspect and palpate for generalized nondependent edema of hands and face and check lower extremities (2+ to 4+ edema); observe for cyanosis, petechiae, ecchymosis, and jaundice.

E. LABORATORY AND DIAGNOSTIC STUDIES

1. Complete blood count (CBC): Hemolysis or hemoconcentration or both may occur; thrombocytopenia is <100,000/mm^3.

2. Elevated serum creatinine (>1.1 mg/dL)

3. Liver function tests (LFTs): elevated alanine transaminase (ALT)/aspartate transaminase (AST) levels

4. Uric acid elevation (>5.5)

5. Lactate dehydrogenase (LDH) is markedly elevated in HELLP syndrome.

6. Urine dipstick, urine protein/creatinine ratio, or 24-hour urine for protein (>1+ on dipstick or 0.3 g/24 hr)

7. Coagulation studies and peripheral smear, if indicated

8. Antenatal surveillance: Nonstress test (NST) or biophysical profile (BPP), ultrasound for growth and amniotic fluid volume (AFV), Doppler studies if indicated

F. DIFFERENTIAL DIAGNOSES

1. PEC (mild or severe) or eclampsia

2. Chronic/preexisting hypertension with or without superimposed PEC

3. Gestational hypertension

4. HELLP syndrome

5. Renal disease

6. Liver disease (e.g., hepatitis)

7. Autoimmune disorders

8. Idiopathic thrombocytopenia purpura (ITP)

G. MANAGEMENT OF PEC AND GESTATIONAL HYPERTENSION

1. The only cure for PEC/eclampsia is delivery. Management decisions must balance maternal and fetal risks, especially if early preterm. Administration of betamethasone for preterm gestations and antihypertensive therapy for severe BP ranges are important considerations.

2. Expectant management in the ambulatory care setting may be appropriate if less than 37 weeks and diagnosis is PEC without severe features (mild) or gestational hypertension.

- **a.** Weekly or twice weekly prenatal visits needed to evaluate for PEC worsening from mild to severe; repeat laboratory tests weekly.
- **b.** Assess fetal well-being: Daily movement counts (kick counts); twice weekly NSTs and/or BPPs; ultrasound to assess growth and AFV every 3 weeks; Doppler studies if IUGR.
- **c.** Frequent rest periods at home in side-lying position; daily BP monitoring; weight, and urine dipstick for protein can be initiated; explain parameters and give clear instructions if exceeded.

3. If pregnancy is complicated by mild PEC after 37 weeks gestation, then the infant should be delivered. Induction of labor may be an option.

4. Management of PEC with severe features and/or HELLP syndrome is best accomplished in the hospital with an experienced obstetrician–gynecologist or maternal–fetal medicine subspecialist. Seizure prophylaxis with magnesium sulfate, antihypertensive therapy, and intensive monitoring are usual for intrapartum management. Prompt delivery may be necessary, even if distant from the due date.

5. Acute-onset severe hypertension (systolic ≥160 mmHg or diastolic ≥110 mmHg) persisting 15 minutes or more is considered a hypertensive emergency and should be treated with intravenous labetalol or hydralazine or oral nifedipine in a hospital setting.

6. For patients requiring antihypertensive therapy, the following are often used. Generally, antihypertensive therapy is not initiated for mild hypertension defined as BP <150/100 mmHg. Severe hypertension (systolic ≥160 and/or diastolic ≥110 mmHg) should be treated to prevent maternal complications such as stroke or heart failure. Goal range is systolic 120 to 160 and diastolic 80 to 110 mmHg. A lower threshold of ≥150/100 mmHg is advised by ACOG for patients with end-organ cardiac or renal disease.

- **a.** Nifedipine XL 30 mg orally daily, maximum dose 120 mg
- **b.** Labetalol 200 mg orally, every 8 to 12 hours, maximum daily dose 2,400 mg
- **c.** Methyldopa 250 mg orally, every 8 to 12 hours, maximum daily dose 3000 mg. Note that methyldopa has been used but has a slow onset of action, is only a mild antihypertensive agent, and has been associated with postpartum depression and psychosis with sedation as a common side effect.
- **d.** May add if needed, hydralazine 10 to 25 mg orally, every 6 to 12 hours, maximum daily dose of 200 mg combined with nifedipine, labetalol, or methyldopa. Due to reflex tachycardia, monotherapy with hydralazine is no longer recommended.
- **e.** Avoid angiotensin-converting enzyme (ACE) inhibitors, angiotensin-2 receptor blockers, and direct renin inhibitors.
- **f.** No absolute contraindications to breastfeeding with these medications, but transfer to human milk is variable. The patient will need follow-up within 1 week after birth for BP check.

H. MANAGEMENT OF CHRONIC HYPERTENSION DURING PREGNANCY

1. If the patient has previously undiagnosed or known chronic hypertension, assess for end-organ damage before 20 weeks of pregnancy.

- **a.** EKG
- **b.** Urine protein/creatinine ratio or 24-hour urine for protein and creatinine and creatinine clearance
- **c.** Baseline labs: CBC, creatinine, LFTs
- **d.** Retinal examination

2. If antihypertensives are not needed for BP control during pregnancy, advise twice daily kick counts starting at 28 weeks (see Appendix A), and obtain third-trimester ultrasound to assess growth.

3. If antihypertensives are required during pregnancy, the patient should be managed by a physician or comanaged. Obtain third-trimester serial ultrasounds for growth and antenatal surveillance starting at 32 weeks or sooner if evidence of IUGR (see Chapter 6). Suggested medications are:

- **a.** Nifedipine XL 30 mg orally daily, maximum dose 120 mg

b. Labetalol 200 mg orally every 12 hours, maximum daily dose 2,400 mg

c. Avoid ACE inhibitors and atenolol (possible risk of teratogenicity in first trimester and fetal/neonatal harm, including IUGR, oligohydramnios, and decreased placental perfusion). Avoid starting hydrochlorothiazide (HCTZ) because of the possible risk of decreased placental perfusion and adverse neonatal effects, but these side effects have not been observed if the patient was using HCTZ before conception.

I. STRATEGIES TO REDUCE COMPLICATIONS

1. Patient education and counseling after 20 weeks gestation: Report concerning symptoms such as severe headache, visual changes, upper extremity and/or facial edema, epigastric or RUQ pain, nausea/vomiting, decreased urine output, vaginal bleeding, signs of ruptured membranes or preterm labor, and decreased fetal movement.

2. Online patient education resources on PEC are listed in Appendix A.

3. Inform patient that delayed postpartum PEC/eclampsia usually occurs by 48 hours but may occur as late as 4 to 6 weeks postpartum.

4. Prevention: Pregnant individuals at high risk for PEC should take a low-dose 81-mg aspirin at bedtime starting at 12 weeks gestation (ACOG, 2016; Henderson et al., 2014; LeFevre, 2014, USPSTF, 2021). Consider low-dose aspirin for the following patients:

a. History of PEC in a prior pregnancy, especially if early onset at less than 34 0/7 weeks

b. Multifetal gestation

c. Chronic hypertension

d. Type 1 or 2 diabetes

e. Renal disease

f. Autoimmune disease (i.e., systematic lupus erythematosus, antiphospholipid syndrome)

g. Patients with more than one of the moderate risk factors (first pregnancy, maternal age 35 years or more, BMI ≥30, family history of PEC, sociodemographic characteristics, and personal history factors).

5. Randomized controlled trials investigating calcium supplementation, vitamin C, and vitamin E have not shown beneficial results. Calcium may be useful in populations with low calcium intake.

6. There is no evidence that bed rest or salt restriction reduces the risk of PEC.

7. ACOG advises the following timing of delivery recommendations for patients with chronic hypertension:

≥38 0/7ths to 39 6/7ths weeks gestation for patients not requiring medication

≥37 0/7ths to 39 6/7ths weeks gestation for patients with hypertension controlled with medication

34 0/7ths to 36 6/7ths for patients with severe hypertension that is not well controlled.

These ranges are on a case-by-case basis with clinician judgment and consideration of all other maternal and fetal factors.

J. COMPLICATIONS

1. Placental abruption

2. Liver and renal failure

3. Subcapsular hepatic hematoma

4. Preterm delivery

5. IUGR
6. Oligohydramnios
7. Intracranial hemorrhage related to eclampsia
8. Disseminated intravascular coagulopathy (DIC)
9. Acute-onset severe hypertension
10. Maternal cerebral hemorrhage or infarction (stroke)
11. Maternal and/or fetal death

K. CONSULTATION/REFERRAL

1. Consult with a physician if gestational hypertension, evidence of PEC, or pregnancy complicated by chronic preexisting hypertension. Refer or comanage with the physician if a pregnant individual has chronic/preexisting hypertension requiring antihypertensives; refer if there is severe or unstable hypertension or any evidence of IUGR, oligohydramnios, or risk of life-threatening complications.
2. Refer, preferably to a tertiary care center, for PEC with severe features, HELLP syndrome, eclampsia, and acute-onset severe hypertension with PEC or eclampsia.

L. FOLLOW-UP

1. Postpartum follow-up within 1 week for BP monitoring and assessment for signs/symptoms of postpartum PEC.
2. Consider the risk of recurrence in subsequent pregnancies and give recommendations for future prenatal care and birth control.
3. PEC is associated with an increased future risk of developing hypertension, ischemic heart disease, venous thromboembolism, kidney disease, and stroke. Therefore, screen patients with a history of hypertensive disorder during pregnancy for cardiac risk factors. Educate and manage as indicated.
4. At 6 weeks postpartum, refer to a primary care provider for evaluation and treatment of chronic hypertension if BP remains elevated.
5. Patients with chronic/preexisting hypertension should continue with their previous medication regimen and regular care with a primary care provider.

Bibliography

American College of Obstetricians and Gynecologists. (2013). Executive summary: Hypertension in pregnancy. *Obstetrics & Gynecology, 122,* 1122–1131. https://doi.org/10.1097/01.AOG.0000437382.03963.88

American College of Obstetricians and Gynecologists. (2016). *Practice advisory on low-dose aspirin and prevention of preeclampsia: Updated recommendations.* http://www.acog.org

American College of Obstetricians and Gynecologists. (2020). Practice bulletin summary, number 222: Gestational hypertension and preeclampsia. *Obstetrics & Gynecology, 135*(6), 1492–1495. https://doi.org/10.1097/AOG.0000000000003892

American College of Obstetricians and Gynecologists. Committee on Obstetric Practice. (2015). ACOG Committee Opinion #638: First-trimester risk assessment for early-onset preeclampsia. *Obstetrics & Gynecology, 126,* e25–e27. https://doi.org/10.1097/01.AOG.0000471176.72443.88

American College of Obstetricians and Gynecologists. Committee on Obstetric Practice. (2019). Emergent therapy for acute-onset, severe hypertension during pregnancy and the postpartum period (ACOG Committee Opinion #767 replaced #623). *Obstetrics & Gynecology, 133*(2), 409–412.

August, P. (2016a). Management of hypertension in pregnant and postpartum women. *UpToDate.* http://www.uptodate.com

August, P. (2016b). Preeclampsia: Prevention. http://www.uptodate.com

August, P., & Sibai, B. (2016). *Preeclampsia: Clinical features and diagnosis.* http://www.uptodate.com

August, P., & Sibai, B. (2020). *Hypertensive disorders in pregnancy: Approach to differential diagnosis.* http://www.acog.org

Bicocca, M. J., Mendez-Figueroa, H., Chauhan, S. P., & Sibai, B. M. (2020). Maternal obesity and the risk of early-onset and late-onset hypertensive disorders of pregnancy. *Obstetrics & Gynecology, 136*(1), 118–127. https://doi.org/10.1097/AOG.0000000000003901

Henderson, J. T., Whitlock, E. P., O'Connor, E., Senger, C. A., Thompson, J. H., & Rowland, M. G. (2014). Low-dose aspirin for prevention of morbidity and mortality from preeclampsia: A systematic evidence review for the U.S. Preventive Services Task Force. *Annals of Internal Medicine, 160*, 695–703. https://doi.org/10.7326/M13-2844

Jeyabalan, A., & Larkin, J. (2020). *Chronic hypertension in pregnancy: Management and outcome.* http://www.acog.org

LeFevre, M. (2014). Low-dose aspirin use for the prevention of morbidity and mortality from preeclampsia: U.S. Preventive Services Task Force recommendation statement. U.S. Preventive Services Task Force. *Annals of Internal Medicine, 161*, 819–826. https://doi.org/10.7326/M14-1884

Lim, K. (2016). *Preeclampsia.* http://emedicine.medscape.com/article/1476919-overview#a3

Magloire, L., & Funai, E. F. (2016). Gestational hypertension. *UpToDate.* http://www.uptodate.com

Norwitz, E. R., & Repke, J. T. (2016). Preeclampsia: Management and prognosis. *UpToDate.* http://www.uptodate.com

Sibai, B. (2016). HELLP syndrome. *UpToDate.* http://www.uptodate.com

U.S. Preventive Services Task Force. (2021). Aspirin use to prevent morbidity and mortality from preeclampsia: Preventive medicine. *USPSTF recommendation statement.* https://www.uspreventiveservicestaskforce.org/uspstf/draft-recommendation/aspirin-use-to-prevent-preeclampsia-and-related-morbidity-and-mortality-preventive-medication1

19. Preterm Labor

KELLY D. ROSENBERGER | NANCY J. CIBULKA

Preterm birth (PTB), defined as birth before 37 completed weeks of pregnancy, occurs in one in ten pregnancies and is a leading cause of neonatal and infant morbidity and mortality in the United States (March of Dimes, 2020a). There were 383,061 preterm births in the United States, representing 10.2% of all live births in 2019. In the United States from 2016 to 2018, preterm birth rates were highest for African American infants (13.8%), followed by American Indian/Alaskan Natives (11.6%), Hispanics (9.8%), Caucasians (9.1%), and Asian/Pacific Islanders (8.7%) (March of Dimes, 2020a). According to a report from the March of Dimes and leading health organizations including the World Health Organization, the 10 countries with the highest preterm birth numbers include Brazil, the United States, India, and Nigeria, demonstrating that preterm birth is truly a global problem. (March of Dimes, the Partnership for Maternal, Newborn & Child Health, Save the Children, & World Health Organization, 2012). Although neonatal nursing and intensive care have improved the survival rate for premature infants, those surviving may face lifelong health problems. When compared to infants born at term, preterm infants are at greater risk for neonatal and infant mortality; respiratory distress, neurological, and gastrointestinal neonatal problems; visual and hearing impairments; and lifelong motor and cognitive deficits. According to the March of Dimes (2020b), PTBs cost the United States at least $26.2 billion annually.

Although the mechanism for preterm labor (PTL) and delivery is not fully understood, significant progress has been made toward identifying individuals who are at risk of preterm delivery and initiating effective prevention strategies. PTL is defined as contractions causing progressive effacement and cervical dilation between 20 and 37 completed weeks of pregnancy. PTL, preterm and premature spontaneous rupture of membranes (PPROM), and cervical incompetence are all significant contributors to PTB. This chapter considers risk factors, prevention, assessment, and management for the prevention of PTL and PTB. Treatment of PTL is not addressed in full detail because the management of this high-risk pregnancy complication typically occurs in an inpatient hospital setting. However, an algorithm is provided as an overview for informational purposes and to answer patient questions regarding PTL triage and management that often begins in the office setting and may result in hospital admission.

A. RISK FACTORS

1. Ideally, risk factors should be identified before conception or early in pregnancy so that preventive measures can be initiated. However, PTL and PTB often occur in individuals with no risk factors.

2. Prior PTB: This is the strongest risk factor for PTL or PTB; recurrences often happen at the same gestational age. The risk is highest when there is a history of more than one PTB and when the PTB was the most recent birth (Robinson & Norwitz, 2021).

3. Twins, triplets, or other multiples
4. Uterine or cervical abnormalities or a history of uterine or cervical surgery (e.g., bicornuate uterus, large fibroids, loop electrosurgical excision procedure, cone biopsy, other excisional procedure on the cervix, multiple dilation and evacuation procedures)
5. Short cervical length measured by transvaginal ultrasonography (less than 25 mm in midtrimester)
6. Other obstetric risks
   a. Polyhydramnios
   b. Vaginal bleeding
   c. Placenta previa or abruption
   d. Certain birth defects in the fetus
   e. PPROM
   f. Conceiving through in vitro fertilization
   g. Multiple miscarriages
   h. Preeclampsia
7. Short interval between pregnancies (less than 6 months)
8. Anxiety, depression, and extremely stressful life events (e.g., divorce and death)
9. History of an infant who died from sudden infant death syndrome (SIDS)
10. Medical/biologic factors
    a. Genital and urinary tract infections, for example, sexually transmitted infections (STIs)
    b. Medical problems such as pyelonephritis, diabetes, hypertension, anemia, clotting disorders, renal disease, moderate to severe asthma, and pneumonia
    c. Nutritional disorders such as being underweight or obese before pregnancy
    d. Possible periodontitis
    e. Abdominal surgery during pregnancy
11. Demographic risks
    a. African American
    b. Low socioeconomic status
    c. Younger than 17 years and older than 35 years
    d. Not married
    e. Did not graduate from high school
12. Lifestyle risks
    a. Late or no prenatal care
    b. Unplanned pregnancy
    c. Multiple abortions
    d. Poor nutrition or poor weight gain; low maternal prepregnancy weight
    e. Smoking
    f. Drinking alcohol
    g. Illicit drug use
    h. Domestic violence
    i. Physical trauma
    j. Excessive stress
    k. Lack of social support
13. Occupational issues
    a. Increased risk of PTL or PTB has been associated with working more than 42 hours per week
    b. A high degree of heavy physical work with exertion
    c. Prolonged standing, more than 6 hours per day

d. Mental or environmental stress
e. Low job satisfaction

14. No paternal risk factors have been identified. PTL/PTB risk is not affected by the father's history of preterm children with other partners.

15. No valid risk scoring systems or biomarkers for prediction of PTB are currently available for asymptomatic nulliparous pregnant individuals. However, cervicovaginal fetal fibronectin (fFN) mat be a useful biomarker for predicting PTB within 7 to 14 days in individuals with contractions and mild cervical dilation and effacement, especially when combined with ultrasound assessment of cervical length measurements. fFN may also be useful for predicting risk of PTB in asymptomatic high-risk individuals with a history of previous PTB.

B. HISTORY

1. Assess for demographic, lifestyle, obstetric, and medical/biologic risk factors
2. Assess for gestational age, if unknown (see Chapter 3)
3. Assess for any prior spontaneous PTB or PPROM
4. Assess for signs of PTL at every visit after 20 weeks' gestation
5. Patient may complain of signs of PTL including:
   a. Mild contractions or "balling up" every 10 to 15 minutes or more often
   b. Cramps that feel like a menstrual period
   c. Change in vaginal discharge (increase, bloody show, and mucus plug)
   d. Leaking fluid or a sudden gush of fluid from the vagina
   e. Pelvic pressure
   f. Constant, low, dull backache
   g. Abdominal cramps with or without diarrhea
   h. General, vague feeling that "something is not right"
6. Assess for symptoms of genital and urinary tract infection (e.g., abnormal discharge, symptoms of urinary tract infection, and uterine tenderness, see Chapters 12 and 13).

C. PHYSICAL EXAMINATION

1. Check all vital signs for normalcy (maternal fever and tachycardia may indicate chorioamnionitis).
2. Auscultate fetal heart rate (fetal tachycardia >160 beats per minute may indicate infection).
3. Sterile speculum examination for evidence of infection or PPROM with a wet nonlubricated speculum (lubricants interfere with fFN test). Collect a cervicovaginal fluid specimen in case the fFN test is desired after transabdominal ultrasound by rotating the swab in the posterior fornix for 10 seconds. Collect other specimens as indicated. See Section D.6.
4. Palpate uterus for contractions, noting frequency, length, and intensity.
5. Palpate uterus for tenderness and fetal size.
6. Assess fetal position and presenting part by Leopold maneuvers.
7. Perform an additional physical examination as indicated by the patient's complaints.

D. LABORATORY AND DIAGNOSTIC STUDIES

1. Screen for urinary tract infection with urinalysis or urine culture.
2. Screen for group B Streptococcus (GBS) colonization, STIs if indicated, and perform a wet mount to screen for vaginitis.

3. Perform a complete blood count (CBC) and other laboratories (e.g., urine drug screen) as indicated.

4. Shortened cervical length, with or without funneling, as measured with transvaginal ultrasonography in the second trimester has been associated with an increased risk of PTL or PTB. Currently, the American College of Obstetricians and Gynecologists (ACOG) considers transvaginal ultrasound measurement of cervical length useful for supporting or excluding the diagnosis of PTL.

   a. A cervix is considered short when ≤20 mm and borderline short at 21 to 25 mm before 24 weeks' gestation.

   b. Short cervical length at 24 weeks' gestation in singleton pregnancies has been found to correlate with a risk of PTB before 35 weeks.

5. Routine ultrasound if needed to confirm or establish due date and presence of any fetal, placental, or maternal abnormalities; confirmation of fetal presentation; assessment of amniotic fluid volume and estimated fetal weight.

6. While performing a sterile speculum examination, test for rupture of membranes using the AmniSure Rupture of Membranes (ROM) test or, if not available, use the following procedures:

   a. Observe for amniotic fluid coming from the cervical canal and pooling in the vagina.

   b. Using a sterile cotton swab, obtain a fluid sample and apply to nitrazine paper—a dark-blue color, indicating pH 7.0 to 7.5, is a positive test; however, false-positive readings can occur, especially with the use of lubricants or a history of recent intercourse, resulting in semen in the vaginal secretions.

   c. Place a sample of fluid on a glass slide and air-dry for 5 to 7 minutes under low-power microscopy, look for a ferning pattern.

   d. Observe the color and odor of the fluid.

   e. Avoid digital examination unless necessary to check for imminent birth. Only after ruling out PPROM and placenta previa, and collecting all necessary specimens may a digital examine be performed to assess for cervical effacement and dilation. Baseline cervical characteristics should be documented at an initial prenatal visit or previous examination (position, consistency, length in centimeters, and whether any dilation). If patient has complaints consistent with PTL, the following assessments are significant: cervical changes from baseline, 3 cm or more dilation and a cervix less than 25 mm in length.

7. Use electronic fetal monitoring (EFM) with tocodynamometry to assess for the presence of regular contractions.

8. Routine testing for fFN or bacterial vaginosis and home uterine monitoring is not recommended in asymptomatic pregnant individuals because there is no evidence that these interventions improve perinatal outcomes (ACOG, 2012, 2016a).

9. Researchers are currently working on new tests to measure cell-free messenger RNA from pregnant individuals' plasma. Unlike DNA, which can only measure static aspects of pregnancy like chromosomal abnormalities, RNA changes over time and thus reflects how the fetus is developing. The tests are being conducted worldwide looking at molecular prediction methods for both PTL and preeclampsia. If this new approach using molecular genetics is accurate, pregnancies that are at risk of preeclampsia and PTB will be able to be identified up to 2 months before delivery. The RNA tests have the potential to redefine prenatal care, prevent serious complications, and save lives (Nurse-Midwives Smart Brief, 2021).

10. The diagnosis of PTL is based on clinical criteria of regular painful contractions with cervical changes. The following criteria may be used for the diagnosis of PTL: Uterine contractions ≥4 every 20 minutes or ≥8 in 60 minutes **and**

- Cervical dilation ≥3 cm, **or**
- Cervical length <20 mm on transvaginal ultrasound, **or**
- Cervical length 20 to 30 mm on transvaginal ultrasound and a positive fFN test.

E. DIFFERENTIAL DIAGNOSES

1. PTL
2. Dehydration
3. Gastrointestinal disorder causing cramps
4. PPROM
5. Chorioamnionitis
6. Ruling out vaginitis, STIs, urinary tract infection, and pyelonephritis
7. Fetal anomaly complicating maternal medical or obstetric condition

F. MANAGEMENT

1. Treat any genitourinary infection as indicated (see Chapters 12 and 13).

2. Advise and assist with smoking cessation and avoiding alcohol and illicit drug use (especially cocaine).

3. Advise individuals at risk of PTL or PTB to reduce occupational stress and fatigue.

4. Encourage a healthy diet and appropriate weight gain.

5. Educate all patients between 20 and 37 weeks' gestation about the signs of PTL (Table 19.1) and triage actions to be taken (see Figure 19.1). Advise patients to call their provider right away or go to the hospital if they notice any symptoms of PTL, vaginal bleeding, or leaking fluid.

6. If there is a history of midtrimester loss due to loss of cervical integrity, cervical cerclage may be indicated and is usually placed at 13 to 17 weeks (Berghella, Rafael, Szychowski, Rust, & Owen et al., 2011). Cerclage may also

TABLE 19.1 PRETERM LABOR

SIGNS AND SYMPTOMS	REDUCING RISK FOR PRETERM BIRTH
■ Regular or frequent contractions or uterine tightening, often painless ■ Increases or change in vaginal discharge (watery, mucus, or bloody) ■ Feels like baby is "balling up" ■ Pressure or pain in the lower abdomen or thighs ■ Pelvic pressure—may feel like baby might "fall out" ■ Constant or irregular, low, dull backache ■ Cramps with or without diarrhea ■ Menstrual-like cramps ■ Clear, pink, or brownish fluid (water) leaking from vagina	■ Start getting regular prenatal checkups; go to every appointment ■ Tell your health-care provider if you have ever had a pregnancy that ended early or labor that started before the 37th week of pregnancy ■ Do not use tobacco or drink alcohol; avoid secondhand smoke ■ Do not use illegal drugs and tell your healthcare provider about any prescription or over-the-counter medicines you are taking ■ Eat a healthy diet and take any supplements recommended by your healthcare provider ■ Call your healthcare provider if you feel any burning or pain when you go to the bathroom; you may have an infection that needs to be treated ■ Avoid stress as much as possible

be beneficial in pregnant individuals with singleton pregnancy, prior spontaneous PTB at less than 34 weeks' gestation, and short cervical length (less than 25 mm) before 24 weeks' gestation (ACOG 2012). Refer to an obstetrician or maternal–fetal medicine specialist.

7. Studies support use of progesterone to reduce the risk of PTD if there is a prior history of PTL or PPROM and PTB (Meis et al., 2003; Norwitz, 2016).

8. In February 2011, the Food and Drug Administration (FDA) approved the use of 17-alpha-hydroxyprogesterone caproate injections (17P; Makena, KV Pharmaceutical Co, St. Louis, MO) to reduce the risk of PTB in pregnant individuals with a singleton pregnancy and a history of prior PTB. In 2020, the FDA proposed Makena and generic equivalents be withdrawn from the market after a postmarket study failed to confirm clinical benefits. As of the initial writing on this chapter, ACOG recommendations remain the same as outlined in 2019 supporting the use of progesterone supplementation in pregnant individuals with prior spontaneous PTB. Currently, Makena and the generic equivalents are still on the market with ACOG and the FDA continuing additional analysis and providing clinical updates as necessary. In March 2021, the FDA issued this statement: "The U.S. Food and Drug Administration's Center for Drug Evaluation and Research (CDER) is aware of the recently published EPPPIC meta-analysis reporting the efficacy of various progestogens, with various routes of administration (vaginal progesterone, oral progesterone, intramuscular hydroxyprogesterone caproate [HPC]) to reduce the risk of pre-term birth (PTB) in at-risk women with singleton or multifetal pregnancies. CDER's recent proposal to withdraw the accelerated approval of Makena (HPC) was based upon a large randomized trial that failed to confirm the benefit of this drug to newborns or reduce the risk of PTB. In making the decision to propose Makena's withdrawal, CDER also reviewed results from prior studies of progestins (HPC and other similar drugs) for PTB, including studies relevant to Makena that are included in the EPPPIC meta-analysis. Therefore, the publication of the EPPPIC meta-analysis does not change CDER's proposal to withdraw the approval of Makena." As of November 2021, both ACOG and Up to Date have not changed their recommendations and continue to support progesterone supplementation for pregnant individuals who had a prior PTB or those with a short cervix on ultrasound examination.

- **a.** There is no known risk of teratogenicity, but there is a possible risk of masculinization, and hypospadias of female fetuses has been reported (based on limited human data).
- **b.** The main maternal adverse effect reported is a possible increased risk of developing gestational diabetes. Other common reactions reported include thromboembolism, hypersensitivity, pain and redness at the njection site, pruritis or urticaria, hypertension, depression, jaundice, PTL, and fluid retention.
- **c.** Contraindications to 17P are as follows: Current or history of thrombosis or thromboembolic disorder, known or suspected history or breast cancer or any hormone-sensitive cancer, cholestatic disease of pregnancy, liver tumors or active liver disease, and uncontrolled hypertension.

9. Pregnant individuals who have had a previous spontaneous PTB may receive weekly injections of 17P (250 mg) in the hip, starting at 16 to 24 weeks' gestation and continuing through 36 weeks' gestation.

10. Pregnant individuals with midtrimester cervical shortening (≤20 mm) and no prior PTB may benefit from vaginal progesterone each evening, from 16 through 36 weeks' gestation (Cahill et al., 2010; Hassan et al., 2011; Romero et al., 2012).

a. Vaginal suppository 100 or 200 mg
b. 8% vaginal gel containing 90 mg micronized progesterone per dose
c. Micronized progesterone tablet of 100 or 200 mg placed in the vagina

11. Natural progesterone administered vaginally has high uterine bioavailability by avoiding the first pass through the liver and has few systemic side effects; however, vaginal irritation can occur.
12. Carefully counsel patients that studies are not conclusive and that clinical trials are ongoing to determine best practices.
13. Current evidence does not support progesterone supplementation in pregnant individuals with a cerclage or those with multiple gestations (ACOG, 2012; Berghella et al., 2010).
14. A cervical pessary may reduce the risk of PTB in some pregnant individuals with a short cervix (Goya et al., 2012).
15. There is no evidence that more frequent prenatal visits, bed rest, hydration, prophylactic antibiotics, omega-3 fatty acids, vitamins C and E, supplemental calcium, social support, or abstinence improve outcomes.
16. Antenatal corticosteroids have been shown to reduce the complications of prematurity and have not been associated with increased risks to the mother or neonate. A single course of corticosteroids is recommended for pregnant individuals between 24 and 34 weeks' gestation who are at risk of preterm delivery within 7 days. A single course of corticosteroids may be considered at 23 weeks' gestation for pregnant individuals at risk of preterm delivery within 7 days, regardless of membrane status. Antenatal corticosteroids have been shown to be beneficial when given to patients between 34 and 36 completed weeks who are at risk of preterm delivery within 7 days and have not previously received corticosteroids.
17. A single, repeat course of antenatal corticosteroids should be considered in pregnant individuals who are less than 34 weeks' gestation who are at risk of preterm delivery within the next 7 days when the prior course was administered more than 14 days previously (ACOG, 2016a, 2017).
18. If a patient is in PTL and a delay in delivery will benefit the newborn, tocolytic therapy with beta-adrenergic receptor agonists (such as terbutaline), calcium channel blockers, or nonsteroidal anti-inflammatory drugs may be indicated for short-term use (up to 48 hours) to allow for the administration of antenatal corticosteroids. In addition, evidence suggests that magnesium sulfate reduces the severity and risk of cerebral palsy if administered when the birth is expected before 32 weeks' gestation (ACOG, 2016a, 2016b).
19. Continuing therapy with tocolytics is not indicated after 48 hours and is not indicated for pregnant individuals with preterm contractions without cervical change. There is no evidence to support the use of ongoing tocolytic therapy because serious maternal or fetal side effects may occur.
20. March of Dimes offers their Preterm Labor Assessment Toolkit free to healthcare providers (www.marchofdimes.org/professionals/preterm-labor-assessment-toolkit.aspx).
21. Online patient resources about PTB prevention are provided in Appendix A.

G. CONSULTATION/REFERRAL

Consult with a physician if the patient is at high risk for PTL/PTB based on history, physical examination, or diagnostic testing. Refer the patient to the hospital or pregnancy assessment unit for evaluation if the patient is experiencing signs or symptoms suggestive of PTL or PPROM (see Figure 19.1). Refer the patient with a prior PTB and a history suggestive of cervical incompetency or

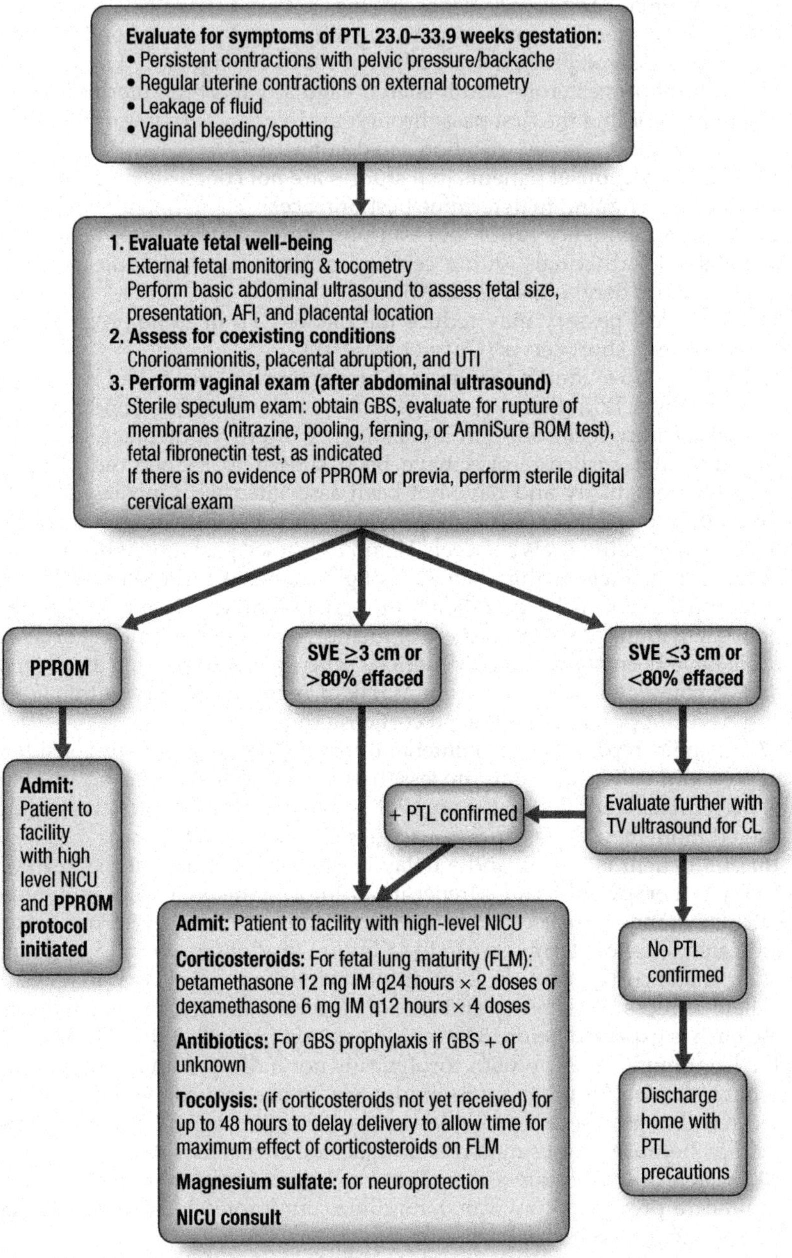

FIGURE 19.1 Preterm labor algorithm.

with short cervical length before 24 weeks' gestation. Consult with a physician if the patient meets the criteria for progesterone supplementation. Refer the patient for the management of twins or multiples or if any evidence chorioamnionitis.

H. FOLLOW-UP

1. Once the episode of threatened PTL has resolved, the patient may be discharged home.

2. Increase frequency of visits and/or telephone contact and reinforce signs of PTL and action to be taken.

3. If STI was treated, repeat culture in 3 to 4 weeks to test for cure.

4. After delivery, recommend future preconception counseling.

Bibliography

American College of Nurse-Midwives. (2018). Position statement: Prevention of labor and preterm birth. *ACNM*. https://www.midwife.org/

American College of Obstetricians & Gynecologists. (2012). Prediction and prevention of preterm birth (Practice Bulletin No. 130, reaffirmed 2019). *Obstetrics & Gynecology, 120*, 964–973. https://doi.org/10.1097/AOG.0b013e3182723b1b

American College of Obstetricians and Gynecologists. (2016a). Management of preterm labor (Practice Bulletin No. 171 interim update). *Obstetrics & Gynecology, 128*, e155–e164. https://doi.org/10.1097/AOG.0000000000001711

American College of Obstetricians and Gynecologists. (2016b). Magnesium sulfate use in obstetrics (Committee Opinion No. 652). *Obstetrics & Gynecology, 127*, e52–e53. https://doi.org/10.1097/AOG.0000000000001267

American College of Obstetricians and Gynecologists. (2016c). Premature rupture of membranes (Practice Bulletin No. 172 interim update). *Obstetrics & Gynecology, 128*, e165–e177. https://doi.org/10.1097/AOG.0000000000001712

American College of Obstetricians and Gynecologists. (2017). Antenatal corticosteroid therapy for fetal maturation. (Committee Opinion No. 713, reaffirmed 2020). *Obstetrics & Gynecology, 130*(2), e102–e109. https://www-acog-org.proxy.cc.uic.edu/clinical/clinical-guidance/committee-opinion/articles/2017/08/antenatal-corticosteroid-therapy-for-fetal-maturation

American College of Obstetricians and Gynecologists. (2021). Prediction and prevention of spontaneous preterm birth (Practice Bulletin No. 234). *Obstetrics & Gynecology, 138*(2), E65–e90. https://www.acog.org/clinical/clinical-guidance/practice-bulletin/articles/2021/08/prediction-and-prevention-of-spontaneous-preterm-birth

Berghella, V. (2016). Second-trimester evaluation of cervical length for prediction of spontaneous preterm birth in singleton gestations. *UpToDate*. http://www.uptodate.com

Berghella, V., Figueroa, D., Szychowski, J. M., Owen, J., Hankins, G. D., Iams, J. D., Shffield, J. S., Perez-Delboy, A., Wing, D. A., Guzman, E. R., & Vaginal Ultrasound Trial Consortium. (2010). 17-alpha-hydroxyprogesterone caproate for the prevention of preterm birth in women with prior preterm birth and a short cervical length. *American Journal of Obstetrics & Gynecology, 202*, 351.e1–351.e6. https://doi.org/10.1016/j.ajog.2010.02.019

Berghella, V., Rafael, T. J., Szychowski, J. M., Rust, O. A., & Owen, J. (2011). Cerclage for short cervix on ultrasonography in women with singleton gestations and previous preterm birth: A meta-analysis. *American College of Obstetricians & Gynecologists, 117*, 663–671. https://doi.org/10.1097/AOG.0b013e31820ca847

Cahill, A. G., Odibo, A. O., Caughey, A. B., Stamilio, D. M., Hassan, S. S., Macones, G. A., & Romero, R. (2010). Universal cervical length screening and treatment with vaginal progesterone to prevent preterm birth: A decision and economic analysis. *American Journal of Obstetrics & Gynecology, 202*, 548.e1–548.e8. https://doi.org/10.1016/j.ajog.2009.12.005

EPPPIC Group. (2021). Evaluating progestogens for preventing preterm birth international collaborative (EPPPIC): Meta-analysis of individual participant data from randomised controlled trials. *Lancet, 397*(10280), 1183–1194. https://www-sciencedirect-com.proxy.cc.uic.edu/science/article/pii/S0140673621002178?via%3Dihub

Goya, M., Pratcorona, L., Merced, C., Rodo, C., Valle, L., Romero, A., Juan, M., Rodríguez, A., Muñoz, B., Santacruz, B., Bello-Muñoz, J. C., Llurba, E., Higueras, T., Cabero, L., Carreras, E., & Pesario Cervical para Evitar Prematuridad (PECEP Trial Group). (2012). Cervical pessary in pregnant women with a short cervix (PECEP): An open-label randomized controlled trial. *Lancet, 379*, 1800–1806. https://doi.org/10.1016/S0140-6736(12)60030-0

Hassan, S. S., Romero, R., Vidyadhari, D., Fusey, S., Baxter, J. K., Khandelwal, M., Vijayaraghavan, J., Trivedi, Y., Soma-Pillay, P., Sambarey, P., Dayal, A., Potapov, V., O'Brien, J., Astakhov, V., Yuzko, O., Kinzler, W., Dattel, B., Sehdev, H., Mazheika, L., . . . PREGNANT Trial. (2011). Vaginal progesterone reduces the rate of preterm birth in women with a sonographic short cervix: A multicenter, randomized, double-blind, placebo-controlled trial. *Ultrasound in Obstetrics & Gynecology, 38*, 18–31. https://doi.org/10.1002/uog.9017

Lockwood, C. J. (2021). Preterm labor: Clinical findings, diagnostic evaluation, and initial treatment. *UpToDate*. http://www.uptodate.com

March of Dimes. (2020a). *2020 March of Dimes Report Card: United States*. https://www.marchofdimes.org/materials/US_REPORTCARD_FINAL_2020.pdf

March of Dimes. (2020b). *The impact of premature birth on society*. https://www.marchofdimes.org/mission/the-economic-and-societal-costs.aspx

Meis, P. J., Klebanoff, M., Thom, E., Dombrowski, M. P., Sibai, B., Moawad, A. H., & Gabbe, S. (2003). Prevention of recurrent preterm delivery by 17 alpha-hydroxyprogesterone caproate. *New England Journal of Medicine, 348*, 2379–2385. https://doi.org/10.1056/NEJMoa035140

Norwitz, E. R. (2021). Progesterone supplementation to reduce the risk of spontaneous preterm labor and birth. *UpToDate*. http://www.uptodate.com

Nurse-Midwives Smart Brief. (2021). *Maternal Health: Test predicts preeclampsia, preterm delivery*. https://www.insider.com/stanford-student-invents-test-to-detect-premature-birth-preeclampsia-2021-5

Robinson, J. N., & Norwitz, E. R. (2021). Preterm birth: Risk factors, interventions for risk reduction, and maternal prognosis. *UpToDate*. http://www.uptodate.com

Romero, R., Nicolaides, K., Conde-Agudela, A., Tabor, A., O'Brien, J. M., Cetingoz, E., Da Fonseca, E., Creasy, G. W., Klein, K., Rode, L., Soma-Pillay, P., Fusey, S., Cam, C., Alfirevic, Z., & Hassan, S. S. (2012). Vaginal progesterone in women with an asymptomatic sonographic short cervix in the midtrimester decreases preterm delivery and neonatal morbidity: A systematic review and metaanalysis of individual patient data. *American Journal of Obstetrics & Gynecology, 206*, 124.e1–124.e19. https://doi.org/10.1016/j.ajog.2011.12.003

Ross, M. G. (2018). *Preterm labor*. https://emedicine.medscape.com/article/260998-overview

U.S. Food and Drug Administration. (2021). *Makena (hydroxyprogesterone caproate injection) Information. CDER Statement*. https://www.fda.gov/drugs/postmarket-drug-safety-information-patients-and-providers/makena-hydroxyprogesterone-caproate-injection-information.

20. HIV-1 and Pregnancy: Screening, Diagnosis, and Management

NANCY J. CIBULKA | KAREN COTLER | KELLY D. ROSENBERGER

According to the Centers for Disease Control and Prevention (CDC) HIV surveillance report, adult and adolescent females comprised close to 22.4% of new HIV infections in 2020 in the United States (CDC, 2020). Most HIV-infected women are of reproductive age, and a disproportionate number are African American or Hispanic American. In 2018, an estimated 10.5% of females with HIV in the United States had undiagnosed HIV. Women comprise more than half of the people with HIV worldwide. In the United States, among females newly diagnosed with HIV, African Americans account for 57%, and 18% were Hispanic/Latinx (CDC, 2020). However, from 2014 to 2018, the number of new HIV cases diagnosed in women in the United States decreased by approximately 7%. Contributing to this successful decline includes efforts of universal testing of all pregnant individuals for HIV, use of cesarean delivery (when appropriate), and avoidance of breastfeeding. With the availability and effectiveness of highly active antiretroviral therapy (HAART), HIV has become a chronic illness in the United States and other developed countries.

HIV-positive women are infected through heterosexual contact, and many are unaware that they are infected. Since 2013, the number of perinatal HIV infections in the United States has been less than 150 cases per year among the approximately 5,000 women with HIV who give birth annually. Thus, the CDC and several professional organizations advise that all pregnant individuals should be screened for HIV infection at their first prenatal visit. Early identification and treatment of pregnant patients with HAART is the most effective way to prevent mother-to-child transmission (MTCT) of HIV. This chapter discusses the risk factors of HIV, screening for HIV during pregnancy, and management of patients who screen positive. However, it is important to keep in mind that the widespread use of HAART in developed countries has delayed illness progression and enhanced quality of life. As a result, individuals who know they are HIV infected may be contemplating motherhood. In the event that newly diagnosed or already diagnosed HIV-infected patients are comanaged for prenatal care, this chapter provides important information and current guidelines for use in ambulatory obstetric settings to prevent MTCT.

A. DEFINITIONS AND BACKGROUND

1. HIV is a retrovirus that infects helper T (CD4) cells and thereby compromises the body's immune system. Individuals with untreated HIV eventually develop a severely compromised immune system, known as AIDS. Once HIV infection progresses to AIDS, opportunistic infections and certain cancers can progress quickly. AIDS is a leading cause of death among young women worldwide.

2. HIV infection occurs primarily through sexual contact; contaminated blood or blood products, including exposure to contaminated needles and syringes; and perinatally (MTCT). The most common method of HIV transmission to women is through high-risk heterosexual contact (the cause of infection in more than 77% of females, followed by 21% with injection drug use (CDC, 2020).

3. HIV is transmitted perinatally in utero, during vaginal delivery, and through breast milk of an HIV-infected mother. Great progress has been made toward preventing MTCT of HIV in the United States, where fewer than 100 infected infants are now born annually.

4. Early identification and treatment of pregnant individuals with HAART is the most effective way to prevent MTCT and protect both mother and infant health.

5. Without any intervention, it is estimated that MTCT of HIV occurs in 15% to 45% of live births (WHO, 2016). With appropriate care, including HAART, the risk for infant infection can be 2%.

B. RISK FACTORS

1. Unprotected sex (vaginal, anal, and oral)

2. Injection drug use and other substance abuse

3. Partner who engages in risky behaviors (either known or unknown to the patient)

4. Presence of sexually transmitted diseases

5. Individuals who have experienced sexual abuse and/or a significant number of adverse childhood experiences (see Chapter 7, Section I.A.17) may be more likely to engage in risky behavior.

6. Socioeconomic conditions are associated with factors that increase the risk for HIV infection, including poor access to healthcare and exchange of sex for drugs, money, or for other reasons.

7. Occupational exposure to blood and blood products (healthcare workers, first responders, military in combat, etc.)

8. Travel to high-incidence countries or partners of unknown HIV status from such countries

9. A comprehensive self-assessment tool for HIV risk is available on the CDC website (https://hivrisk.cdc.gov/)

C. SCREENING

1. The CDC, American College of Obstetricians and Gynecologists (ACOG), and the Association of Women's Health, Obstetric and Neonatal Nurses (AWHONN) recommend that all pregnant individuals should be offered an HIV screening test.

2. After the patient is notified of the testing, unless the patient declines (opt-out screening), HIV testing is recommended along with the routine panel of prenatal labs for all pregnant individuals.

3. Reasons for declining HIV testing should be explored and documented. In addition, patients should receive education about HIV, consequences of the infection for mother and infant, the transmission of HIV, and treatment. Online patient education resources for HIV prevention and pregnancy are available in Appendix A.

4. The CDC advocates that separate written consent for HIV testing should not be required.

5. Repeat HIV antibody testing in the third trimester is recommended for pregnant individuals who are known to engage in risky behavior, are receiving care in facilities that have an HIV incidence in pregnant individuals of at least 1 per 1,000 per year, are incarcerated, or reside in communities with elevated rates of HIV infection.

6. Rapid HIV testing is an option in intrapartum settings for patients who were not tested during pregnancy and for those at high risk for HIV.

7. Guidelines providing a practical means to HIV testing in pregnancy are provided in Appendix C.

8. Positive HIV tests must be reported to the local health department by the laboratory performing the test. Healthcare providers are then contacted and asked to complete a report for newly diagnosed cases of HIV and AIDS. The health department handles partner notification.

D. HISTORY

1. Assess for risk factors as listed in the previous section.

2. Gynecologic history (including sexually transmitted infections [STIs], abnormal Pap smears, and recurrent candidiasis)

3. Sexual history (sexual orientation, high-risk partners, high-risk practices, multiple partners, and use of condoms); assess whether the partner is known to have HIV infection

4. Psychosocial history for substance abuse and high-risk partner characteristics

5. Symptoms of early symptomatic infection (experienced by an estimated 40% to 90% of infected individuals) 2 to 4 weeks post exposure: fever, night sweats, malaise, lymphadenopathy, pharyngitis, rash, myalgias/arthralgias, oral lesions such as thrush or hairy leukoplakia, anorexia, nausea, vomiting, and headache; acute infection in pregnant and breastfeeding patients is associated with a high risk of perinatal HIV transmission.

6. Other symptoms: Enlarged liver and/or spleen; weight loss; diarrhea; cough and dyspnea; blood abnormalities such as anemia, neutropenia, and thrombocytopenia; neurological disorders such as aseptic meningitis and varicella zoster

7. Advanced AIDS: Signs of opportunistic infections such as cytomegalovirus (CMV) disease, *Toxoplasma gondii, Pneumocystis jiroveci* pneumonia, disseminated *Mycobacterium avium* complex, tuberculosis, HIV wasting syndrome, cardiomyopathy, Kaposi's sarcoma, and/or HIV encephalopathy/dementia

8. If the patient has previously been diagnosed with HIV, assess for the course of illness, whether partner is HIV infected, prior care and date of the last visit, HIV viral load and CD4 count if known, and history of antiretroviral therapy (ART).

E. PHYSICAL EXAMINATION

1. Vital signs and general observation

2. Complete examination with attention to symptoms noted under Section D

3. Appropriate to the stage of pregnancy and to any presenting complaint

4. Pelvic examination (with Pap smear and STI testing as indicated)

F. LABORATORY SCREENING AND FURTHER TESTING

1. HIV antibody screening: The third-generation test is an enzyme-linked immunoabsorbent assay (ELISA) or enzyme immune assay (EIA) followed by confirmatory Western blot if ELISA or EIA is reactive.

2. Western blot results are reported as positive, negative, or indeterminate. A positive test must show a reaction with two of these three bands: P24, glycoprotein 41 (gp41), and gp120/160.

3. It takes 3 to 8 weeks (25 days on average) for a newly infected person to produce detectable antibodies. This is known as the "window period" when an individual is in the acute phase of illness and highly infectious to others, but the HIV-antibody test is negative.

4. The newer, fourth-generation HIV test looks for both antibodies and the p24 antigen. The fourth-generation tests are accurate 3 to 4 weeks after exposure because that is when the p24 antigen is high enough to measure. A polymerase chain reaction test (PCR) is completed as confirmatory testing.

5. The PCR can identify early HIV infection before antibodies are apparent by detecting the RNA of the HIV. When acute HIV infection is suspected during pregnancy or breastfeeding, an HIV RNA test should be obtained along with an HIV antibody test and, if negative, repeat both tests in 2 weeks.

6. Repeat HIV testing in the third trimester is recommended for patients known to be at increased risk (see Section B).

7. HIV preexposureprophylaxis (PrEP) to reduce the risk of acquiring HIV during Preconception, Antepartum and Postpartum periods recommended for patients at risk (IV drug user, sex worker, serodiscordinant partner,) (HIV.gov, 2020)

8. Maternal HIV testing and identification of perinatal HIV exposure for pregnant individuals with STI or with signs and symptoms of acute HIV and that expedited HIV testing during labor is recommended for those who are at risk of HIV infection and not retested in the third trimester. (HIV.gov, 2020)

9. The United States Food and Drug Administration (FDA) has approved several rapid tests for point-of-care or laboratory testing. OraQuick Advance® Rapid HIV-1/2 Antibody Test (OraSure Technologies, Inc., Bethlehem, PA) is approved for oral fluid, fingerstick, or venipuncture whole-blood samples and is acceptable for testing patients in hospital-based labor and delivery units. Results can be read within 20 to 30 minutes. Reveal™ Rapid HIV-1 Antibody Test (MedMira Laboratories, Inc., Halifax, Nova Scotia) is approved for use with serum or plasma testing in clinical laboratories. Other rapid HIV tests are available. Positive tests need to be confirmed with a third- or fourth-generation antibody as soon as possible, and ART should be started while awaiting results.

10. Laboratory testing needed after confirmation of HIV infection: HIV RNA viral load; CD4 count and percentage; HIV resistance testing to guide initial ART choice; complete blood count (CBC) with differential; serum chemistry; serologies for hepatitis A, B, and C, syphilis, toxoplasmosis, and CMV; screening for gonorrhea and chlamydia; Pap smear; tuberculosis screening; genotypic tests for resistance to ART medications. Additional labs may be considered, for example, G6PD, HLA-B 5701, and others.

G. DIFFERENTIAL DIAGNOSES

1. HIV infection during pregnancy, confirmed by diagnostic testing
2. Immune deficiency disorder
3. Cancer
4. Viral syndrome and/or mononucleosis
5. Chronic infection
6. Others based on presenting symptoms

H. MANAGEMENT OF HIV-INFECTED PREGNANT INDIVIDUALS

1. Refer pregnant patients to an HIV/AIDS infectious disease (ID) specialist and to a pregnancy center that manages HIV-infected patients. Maintain strict confidentiality regarding test results and maternal records.

2. If the patient is newly diagnosed with HIV, ensure that she has education and counseling about the diagnosis. Immediate counseling should address transmission of HIV, confidentiality, and disclosure issues.

3. Address any emergent mental health issues, including suicidal or homicidal ideation, severe depression, anxiety, and/or panic. It is important to be aware of the increase in psychosocial effects of COVID-19 during pregnancy, including intimate partner violence, substance abuse, and depression.

4. Discuss the need for partner testing and the risk of transmission to an uninfected partner. Advise 100% condom use during sexual relations.

5. Educate the patient about the importance of early management of HIV infection during pregnancy and that the risk of MTCT will be greatly reduced with appropriate care.

6. Three-drug combination HAART treatment, designated by an ID specialist, is recommended for HIV-infected pregnant individuals to reduce the risk of MTCT. Treatment may be delayed until 12 weeks gestation unless the immune system is severely compromised; however, data support safe early initiation of therapy for all pregnant individuals to most effectively reduce in utero transmission of the virus. Emphasize the importance of 100% adherence to HAART therapy. Patients already on HAART should continue (if not contraindicated).

7. Guidelines for care to prevent MTCT

- **a.** Antepartum: Maternal HAART therapy during pregnancy with the goal of reducing the maternal HIV RNA viral load to undetectable
- **b.** Intrapartum: Continue HAART. Intravenous zidovudine (also known as ZDV or AZT) at least 1 hour before a vaginal birth and 3 hours before cesarean section if HIV RNA is ≥400 copies/mL or unknown. Intravenous ZDV is no longer required if HIV RNA is <400 copies/mL but may be given at the discretion of the provider. Vaginal birth is an option if the HIV viral load is less than 1,000 copies/mL; if higher, a cesarean section is recommended
- **c.** Postpartum: Continue HAART for mother until further assessment of immune status and preferences. Infant receives ZDV orally starting 2 hours after birth, dosage determined by body weight and gestational age, given every 12 hours for the first 6 weeks of life. Other ART may be used in addition to ZDV, determined by neonatal ID specialist. Breastfeeding is contraindicated.

8. If the patient is comanaged, ensure that repeat laboratory testing, including HIV RNA viral load, CD4, CBC, and liver function tests (LFTs), is accomplished approximately every 6 weeks to assess response to therapy.

9. The primary goals of HAART are to improve and/or protect immune system function and to reduce HIV-associated morbidity and mortality.

10. Address other salient issues that increase the risk of MTCT, such as substance abuse, mental health issues, domestic violence, high-risk behaviors, need for economic assistance, and other factors that might impair the ability to adhere to treatment and/or promote HIV transmission. Coordination of multiple services may be needed.

11. Choice of HAART regimens should be based on similar principles used for nonpregnant individuals and account for resistance profile of the virus, safety, and efficacy of the medications for the mother and fetus, convenience and adherence of the regimen, potential for drug interactions, and pharmacokinetic data in pregnancy. Current guidelines support the initiation of HAART therapy sooner rather than later. The latest adult and adolescent treatment guidelines are available (www.aidsinfo.nih.gov/guidelines).

- **a.** Most HAART drugs are safe in pregnancy.
- **b.** Bictegravir and tenofovir alafenamide should not be used in pregnancy due to limited clinical experience and lack of pharmacokinetic data.

12. The National Perinatal HIV Hotline (1-888-448-8765) provides free consultation to providers caring for HIV-infected patients and infants.

13. Recommendations for HIV management during pregnancy evolve rapidly. The most recent information can be found on the HIVinfo website (hiv-info.nih.gov/).

14. Provide educational resources at the appropriate time (see Appendix A).

I. MANAGEMENT OF INDIVIDUALS AT HIGH RISK OF INFECTION

1. Patients who are not infected with HIV but are partnered with someone who is known to be infected with HIV (serodifferent or serodiscordinant couples) may be candidates for preexposure prophylaxis (PrEP).

2. PrEP is a single pill, tenofovir 300 mg and emtricitabine 200 mg (Truvada), that is taken once daily. Before providing PrEP and for ongoing care, consider the following:

- **a.** Document negative HIV status prior to starting PrEP.
- **b.** Screen for hepatitis B and C infections; screen and treat for STIs.

3. Follow up visit after 1 month of starting PrEP. Check for adherence and side effects.

4. Check creatinine at baseline, 3 months after the initial check, then every 6 months.

5. Check urinalysis at baseline.

6. Repeat HIV-antibody test and STI screening every 3 months.

7. Assess for high-risk behaviors and counsel patient for risk reduction, stressing the importance of avoiding infection during pregnancy and breastfeeding.

8. Evaluate medication adherence at each follow-up visit.

J. COMPLICATIONS

1. Maternal disease progression

2. Opportunistic infection

3. Perinatal infection of infant

4. Increased risk of preterm labor (associated with certain ART drugs)

5. Medication toxicity or untoward side effects for mother and/or infant or long-term health effects to ART medications (information is mostly unknown)

K. CONSULTATION/REFERRAL

1. Refer to HIV/AIDS specialist and to maternal-fetal medicine specialist with experience caring for pregnant women with HIV infection; always consult about treatment options.

2. Refer for psychological and/or spiritual support.

3. Refer to pediatric HIV/AIDS specialist before delivery.

4. Refer to HIV/AIDS local support group.

L. FOLLOW-UP

1. Contact patient within 48 hours of new diagnosis to assess the psychological status and assist with care coordination.

2. Discuss confidentiality and disclosure issues with the patient.

3. Maintain contact and supportive relationship with the patient to facilitate future return for well-woman care and family planning.

4. Following delivery, all contraceptive choices are available to patients infected with HIV. However, drug interactions may occur between hormonal contraceptives and ART medications. For more information, refer to the section on antiretroviral drug interactions (www.cdc.gov/mmwr/preview/mmwrhtml/rr5904a14.htm).

5. Continue to emphasize 100% use of barrier protection during sexual activity.

Bibliography

American College of Obstetricians and Gynecologists Committee on Ethics. (2007). Human immunodeficiency virus (Committee Opinion No. 389, reaffirmed 2015). *Obstetrics & Gynecology, 110*, 1473–1478. https://doi.org/10.1097/01.AOG.0000291572.09193.7f

American College of Obstetricians and Gynecologists Committee on Gynecologic Practice. (2014a). Preexposure prophylaxis for the prevention of human immunodeficiency virus (Committee Opinion No. 595, reaffirmed 2016). *Obstetrics & Gynecology, 123*, 1133–1136. https://doi.org/10.1097/01.AOG.0000446855.78026.21

American College of Obstetricians and Gynecologists Committee on Gynecologic Practice. (2014b). Routine human immunodeficiency virus screening (Committee Opinion No. 596, reaffirmed 2016). *Obstetrics & Gynecology, 123*, 1137–1139. https://doi.org/10.1097/01.AOG.0000446828.64137.50

American College of Obstetricians and Gynecologists Committee on Health Care for Underserved Women. (2012). Human immunodeficiency virus and acquired immunodeficiency syndrome and women of color (Committee Opinion No. 536). *Obstetrics & Gynecology, 120*, 735–739. https://doi.org/10.1097/00006250-201209000-00042

American College of Obstetricians and Gynecologists Committee on Obstetric Practice. (2000). Scheduled cesarean delivery and the prevention of vertical transmission of HIV infection (Committee Opinion No. 234, reaffirmed 2016). *International Journal of Gynecology & Obstetrics, 73*, 279–281. https://doi.org/10.1016/S0020-7292(01)00412-X

American College of Obstetricians and Gynecologists Committee on Obstetric Practice and HIV Expert Work Group. (2015). Prenatal and perinatal human immunodeficiency virus testing: Expanded recommendations (Committee Opinion No. 635, reaffirmed 2016). *Obstetrics & Gynecology, 125*, 1544–1547. https://doi.org/10.1097/01.AOG.0000466370.86393.d2

Carpenter, R. J. (2015). *Early symptomatic HIV infection*. http://emedicine.medscape.com/article/211873-overview

Centers for Disease Control and Prevention. (2012). Update to CDC's U.S. medical eligibility criteria for contraceptive use, 2010: Revised recommendations for the use of hormonal contraception among women at high risk for HIV infection or infected with HIV. *Morbidity and Mortality Weekly Report, 61*, 449–452. http://www.cdc.gov/mmwr/preview/mmwrhtml/mm6124a4.htm?s_cid=mm6124a4_e%0D%0A

Centers for Disease Control and Prevention. (2016). *HIV among pregnancy women, infants, and children*. http://www.cdc.gov/hiv/group/gender/pregnantwomen/index.html

Centers for Disease Control and Prevention. (2019). *HIV surveillance report: Diagnoses of HIV infection in the United States and dependent areas 2019*. https://www.cdc.gov/hiv/library/reports/hiv-surveillance/vol-32/index.html

Center for Disease Control and Prevention. (2020). Estimated HIV Incidence and Prevalence in the United States, 2014-2018. *HIV Surveillance Supplemental Report, 25*(1), 1–77.

Cibulka, N. J. (2006). Mother-to-child transmission of HIV in the United States. *American Journal of Nursing, 106*(7), 56–63. https://doi.org/10.1097/00000446-200607000-00029

Clark, R. A., Maupin, R. T., & Hammer, J. H. (2004). *A woman's guide to living with HIV infection*. Johns Hopkins University Press.

Fantasia, H. C., Harris, A. L., & Fontenot, H. B. (2020). *Guidelines for nurse practitioners in gynecologic settings* (12th ed.). Springer Publishing.

Greenwald, J. L., Burstein, G. R., Pincus, J., & Branson, B. (2006). A rapid review of rapid HIV antibody tests. *Current Infectious Disease Reports, 8*, 125–131. https://doi.org/10.1007/s11908-006-0008-6

Hughes, B., & Cu-Uvin, S. (2020). *Antiretroviral selection and management in pregnant women with HIV in resource-rich settings*. https://www.uptodate.com/contents/antiretroviral-selection-and-management-in-pregnant-women-with-hiv-in-resource-rich-settings

Panel on Treatment of Pregnant Women with HIV and Prevention of Perinatal Transmission (2020). *Use of antiretroviral drugs in the transmission in the United States*. https://clinicalinfo.hiv.gov/en/guidelines

Panel on Opportunistic Infections in Adults and Adolescents with HIV. (2021). *Guidelines for the prevention and treatment of opportunistic infections in adults and adolescents with HIV: Recommendations from the Centers for Disease Control and Prevention, the National Institutes of Health, and the HIV*

Medicine Association of the Infectious Diseases Society of America. https://clinicalinfo.hiv.gov/sites/default/files/guidelines/documents/Adult_OI.pdf

Panel on Treatment of Pregnant Women with HIV Infection and Prevention of Perinatal Transmission (2021). *Recommendations for the use of antiretroviral drugs in pregnant women with HIV infection and interventions to reduce perinatal HIV transmission in the United States*. https://clinicalinfo.hiv.gov/en/guidelines/perinatal/overview-2?view=full

Sheth, S., & Coleman, J. (2015). HIV in pregnancy. In C. T. Johnson, J. L. Hallock, J. L. Bienstock, H. E. Fox, & E. E. Wallach (Eds.), *Johns Hopkins manual of gynecology and obstetrics* (5th ed., pp. 265–281). Wolters Kluwer.

World Health Organization. (2016). *Mother-to-child transmission of HIV*. http://www.who.int/hiv/topics/mtct/en

21. Zika Virus and Pregnancy

NANCY J. CIBULKA | KELLY D. ROSENBERGER

The Zika virus (ZIKV) and other viruses and/or vector-borne diseases are emerging infectious global health threats. Because of an increasingly mobile worldwide population, nurse practitioners need to be knowledgeable about many diseases that might originate in other parts of the world.

The purpose of this chapter is to review current knowledge of Zika infection, including risk of exposure, presentation, and potential maternal and fetal effects. Guidelines for preventing and managing this infection during pregnancy will be provided based on data that are known at this time. Although this chapter focuses on Zika infection, healthcare providers need to stay informed about all new emerging infectious agents that may pose a threat to their patients. Those who care for women and infants are encouraged to stay informed by frequently reviewing websites and guidelines provided by the Centers for Disease Control and Prevention (CDC), the American Academy of Nurse Practitioners (AANP), Nurse Practitioners in Women's Health (NPWH), the American College of Obstetricians and Gynecologists (ACOG), the Society for Maternal–Fetal Medicine (SMFM), the American Academy of Pediatrics (AAP), the Infectious Disease Society of America (ISDA), and any other relevant organizations.

A. BACKGROUND

1. ZIKV is a flavivirus that is closely related to other flaviviruses, such as West Nile, Japanese encephalitis, yellow fever, and dengue, which it most resembles.
2. ZIKV is spread to people through the bite of an infected mosquito of the *Aedes* genus (*Aedes aegypti* and *Aedes albopictus*). When the female mosquito bites, virus particles are deposited into the victim's epidermis and dermis. Mosquitoes that spread ZIKV bite both during the dawn and daytime as well as in the evening; they are aggressive (ACOG, 2016; McNeill et al., 2016).
3. Prior to 2015, ZIKV outbreaks occurred in parts of Africa, Southeast Asia, and the Pacific Islands. In May 2015, a health alert for ZIKV was issued for Brazil. Current outbreaks are occurring in many countries. Alerts are posted for travel destinations in the Caribbean, Central and South America, Southeast Asia, the Pacific Islands, and North America. The mosquitoes that carry ZIKV are not found at elevations above 6,500 feet (see current travel notices at wwwnc.cdc.gov/travel/page/zika-information).
4. In addition to the bite of an infected mosquito, ZIKV is transmitted to humans through maternal–fetal transmission, which results in a congenital infection; intrapartum transmission from a viremic mother to the newborn; sexual transmission from an infected partner; blood products or organ/tissue transplantation with infected materials; and possibly through saliva, sweat, or tears.

5. Clinical illness is generally mild; the most common symptoms include acute onset of fever, maculopapular rash (sometimes pruritic), arthralgia, and conjunctivitis. Not everyone has symptoms. ZIKV is confirmed by laboratory testing (CDC, 2016a, 2016b).

6. ZIKV that occurs during pregnancy can cause adverse outcomes in all trimesters, including fetal loss, microcephaly and other serious brain abnormalities, fetal growth restriction, and ocular anomalies (ACOG, 2016; CDC, 2016a).

7. In the United States, confirmed cases of ZIKV escalated during 2016. Most cases were associated with travel (99%) or residence in areas with ongoing ZIKV or exposure through unprotected sex with someone who had traveled to these areas. Half of all cases were reported from four states: New York, Florida, California, and Texas; the median age was 39 years (CDC, 2016a). No new cases of ZIKV were reported in the continental United States in 2018, 2019, and 2020 from local mosquito-borne transmission, but cases were reported in travelers returning from affected areas (CDC, 2020).

8. Of the 1% of ZIKV cases that were not associated with travel, more than 90% were reported from Florida, where *Ae. Aegypti* mosquitoes were identified in the Miami, Florida, area (CDC, 2016a).

9. ZIKV cases are unpredictable, and outbreaks are likely to occur again in the United States and in other countries. Congenital ZIKV is associated with severe congenital anomalies, with greatest risk if infection occurs during the first trimester. Clinical features of congenital ZIKV syndrome include microcephaly, facial disproportion, hypertonia/spasticity, hyperreflexia, seizures, irritability, arthrogryposis, ocular abnormalities, sensorineural hearing loss, and neuroradiologic abnormalities.

B. HISTORY

1. Assess the patient for symptoms. Clinical manifestations of ZIKV in a pregnant individual are the same as those in nonpregnant adults. Symptoms are usually mild and may last for several days to a week.

- **a.** Fever
- **b.** Maculopapular rash (sometimes pruritic)
- **c.** Arthralgia
- **d.** Conjunctivitis

2. Assess patient for recent travel or history of residing in an area with local transmission of ZIKV within the past 6 months.

3. Ask whether patient has had contact (including sex) with a confirmed or suspected case or with someone who traveled to an area with local transmission of ZIKV within the past 6 months.

4. Assess patient for nausea, vomiting, diarrhea, and jaundice—these symptoms are not characteristic of ZIKV infection.

5. If patient is pregnant, assess for number of weeks gestation and any prior problems with current pregnancy.

C. COMPLICATIONS

1. In all trimesters, infection from ZIKV has been associated with fetal abnormalities, most notably microcephaly.

2. Fetal loss, stillbirth, intrauterine growth restriction, hydrops fetalis (Lockwood, Ros, & Nielson-Saines, 2020)

3. Fetal ocular abnormalities and temporary hearing loss

4. Other malformations of the fetal brain and central nervous system have been linked to ZIKV infection; investigation is ongoing.

5. Guillain–Barré syndrome in adults (rare)

D. DIFFERENTIAL DIAGNOSES

1. ZIKV
2. Dengue or other flavivirus
3. Any viral illness

E. LABORATORY AND DIAGNOSTIC STUDIES

1. Because of the risks and complications of ZIKV in pregnancy, all pregnant individuals should be assessed for possible ZIKV exposure at each prenatal visit (CDC, 2016a).
2. All pregnant individuals who reside in or have traveled to areas with ZIKV or whose partners have been in these areas in the past 6 months should be tested, even if asymptomatic (ACOG, 2016; CDC, 2016a).
3. Pregnant individuals with no epidemiological exposure to ZIKV do not need testing.
4. ZIKV is a reportable illness. Testing is performed at the CDC Arbovirus Diagnostic Laboratory, most state health departments, and some commercial laboratories. Contact your local or state health department for instructions for specimen handling and testing.
5. Follow the CDC testing algorithm for testing during pregnancy (www.cdc.gov/zika/pdfs/testing_algorithm.pdf).
6. The incubation period for ZIKV is 3 to 14 days. Viremia in ZIKV occurs several days before onset of symptoms and lasts approximately 10 days. Symptomatic pregnant individuals who are evaluated less than 2 weeks after symptom onset should have serum and urine ZIKV real-time reverse transcription-polymerase chain reaction (rRT-PCR) testing. Symptomatic patients evaluated 2 to 12 weeks after symptom onset and asymptomatic patients should have a Zika immunoglobulin (IgM) antibody test; if the test is positive or inconclusive, serum and urine rRT-PCR testing should be done (CDC, 2016b).
7. A positive test is diagnostic for infection, but a negative or inconclusive test does not completely exclude the possibility of ZIKV infection. An inconclusive test should be considered positive until confirmatory testing is completed (ACOG, 2016).
8. Laboratory evaluation of test results can be complex because of cross-reactivity with related flaviviruses. Cross-reactivity can occur in patients with previous infection to Zika or current infection to dengue fever, West Nile, or yellow fever virus. Confirmatory testing with the plaque reduction neutralization test (PRNT) can differentiate between true- and false-positive test results (CDC, 2016b).
9. Asymptomatic pregnant individuals with nonrecurring exposure to ZIKV should have IgM testing 2 to 12 weeks after exposure and, if results are anything other than negative, offer PRNT titers. If ZIKV exposure is ongoing, testing is indicated when prenatal care is initiated. If the test is negative, repeat at 18 to 20 weeks and in the event of fetal abnormalities noted on ultrasound.
10. ZIKV is a reportable infectious disease. Healthcare providers should report all suspected cases of ZIKV to state health departments.

F. TREATMENT

1. Treat ZIKV infections in pregnant individuals with symptomatic measures. The CDC recommends the following (www.cdc.gov/zika/symptoms/treatment.html):
    a. Treat the symptoms
    b. Get plenty of rest

c. Drink plenty of fluids to prevent dehydration
d. Take acetaminophen for fever and pain
e. To reduce risk of bleeding, do not take aspirin or nonsteroidal anti-inflammatory drugs until dengue fever can be ruled out

2. If you are pregnant or take other medication, contact your healthcare provider right away

G. FETAL AND NEWBORN SCREENING

1. A baseline fetal ultrasound at 18 to 20 weeks is advised for symptomatic and asymptomatic individuals with ZIKV exposure.
2. If the baseline ultrasound examination is normal in patients with ZIKV exposure, even without positive or inconclusive laboratory testing for ZIKV, consider serial ultrasounds every 3 to 4 weeks. Decisions regarding amniocentesis should be made on a case-by-case basis (ACOG, 2016). However, the World Health Organization advises serial ultrasounds every 4 weeks for pregnant individuals living in areas where ZIKV is endemic only for symptomatic patients with positive or inconclusive testing for the virus, but not if testing is negative.
3. If microcephaly or intracranial calcifications are detected on ultrasound in a pregnant individual who tested negative for ZIKV, retest and consider amniocentesis for ZIKV testing.
4. Newborns born to mothers with positive or inconclusive laboratory test results for ZIKV should have testing within 24 hours of birth, as should infants with microcephaly or intracranial calcifications born to mothers with possible ZIKV infection.

H. CONSULTATION/REFERRAL

1. Refer to a maternal–fetal specialist or comanage if serum or amniotic fluid is positive or inconclusive for ZIKV.

I. PREVENTION AND PATIENT EDUCATION

1. There is no specific treatment for ZIKV infection, and currently there is no vaccine. Therefore, discuss plans for conception and desired timing with all patients of childbearing age. Advise the patient and her partner to avoid travel to all areas where ZIKV transmission is known to occur. Educate on safer alternative travel destinations (ACOG, 2016; CDC, 2016c). Advise patients the CDC posts up-to-date travel health information at wwwnc.cdc.gov/travel/page/zika-information.
2. If the patient is pregnant, couples should use barrier methods consistently or abstain from sex for the remainder of the pregnancy.
3. If a patient previously diagnosed with ZIKV infection desires conception, advise to wait at least 8 weeks after symptom onset before conceiving. If a male partner was diagnosed with ZIKV, the couple should wait at least 3 months and should use condoms or abstinence during that time (ACOG, 2019).
4. Men who may have been exposed to the ZIKV but did not develop symptoms of ZIKV disease: Wait at least 3 months to try to conceive.
5. Advise travelers of precautions to prevent mosquito bites (CDC, 2016c):
   a. Wear lightweight clothing that covers arms and legs completely. Use permethrin to treat clothing as mosquitoes can bite through clothing.
   b. Use Environmental Protection Agency–registered insect repellents containing DEET (*N,N*-diethyl-*m*-toluamide). DEET is safe to use during pregnancy (avoid insect repellent on infants younger than 2 months of age). Follow the instructions on the label for application.

c. Use mosquito netting over beds, cribs, and strollers and make sure that all windows and doors have intact screens on them.

d. Inspect home and yard for standing water that can serve as a breeding ground for mosquitoes. Eliminate old tires and any container that might collect water.

6. Postpartum patients with ZIKV exposure may breastfeed as at this time there is no evidence ZIKV is transmitted through breast milk, although the virus has been detected in breast milk.

7. These recommendations could change as more information becomes available. Patients and healthcare providers can stay current on recommendations and care for ZIKV by going to the CDC and ACOG websites at: www.cdc.gov/zika/index.html, www.cdc.gov/zika/pregnancy/index.html, and www.acog.org/womens-health/resources-for-you#q=zika%20virus

8. Patient handouts on ZIKV, mosquito bite prevention, and other protective measures are available at: www.cdc.gov/zika/symptoms/treatment.html

9. Additional patient education resources are provided in Appendix A and through the March of Dimes at: www.marchofdimes.org/complications/zika-virus-and-pregnancy.aspx

J. FOLLOW-UP

1. ZIKV infection in an individual who is not pregnant would not pose a risk for birth defects in future pregnancies after the virus has cleared from the blood. Based on what is known about other similar infections, once a person has been infected with ZIKV, they are likely to be protected from a future Zika infection.

2. ZIKA testing is recommended for infants as noted in Section G.4. In addition, infants should have a complete and thorough physical exam, including ophthalmologic and hearing evaluation.

3. CDC guidelines for measuring head circumference in infants can be found at the CDC website: www.cdc.gov/zika/pdfs/microcephaly_measuring.pdf

Bibliography

American College of Obstetricians and Gynecologists. (2016). *Zika Virus: Protect yourself. Protect your pregnancy.* https://www.acog.org/womens-health/infographics/zika-virus-and-pregnancy

American College of Obstetricians and Gynecologists. (2019). Management of patients in the context of zika virus: ACOG Committee Opinion, number 784. *Obstetrics & Gynecology, 134*(3), e64–e70. https://doi.org/10.1097/AOG.0000000000003399

American College of Obstetricians and Gynecologists and the Society for Maternal–Fetal Medicine. (2016). *Practice advisory on ZIKA virus.* https://www.smfm.org/publications/220-acog-smfm-joint-practice-advisory-interim-guidance-for-care-of-obstetric-patients-during-a-zika-virus-outbreak

Brooks, J. T., Friedman, A., Kachur, R. E., LaFlam, M., Peters, P. J., & Jamieson, D. J. (2016). Update: Interim guidance for prevention of sexual transmission of Zika virus—U.S. July 2016. *Morbidity and Mortality Weekly Report, 65*(29), 745–747. https://doi.org/10.15585/mmwr.mm6529e2

Centers for Disease Control and Prevention. (2016a). Zika virus -cases-50 states and the district of Columbia, January 1–July 31, 2016. *Morbidity and Mortality Weekly Report, 65*(36), 983–986. https://doi.org/10.15585/mmwr.mm6536e5

Centers for Disease Control and Prevention. (2016b). *Diagnostic testing.* https://www.cdc.gov/zika/laboratories/types-of-tests.html

Centers for Disease Control and Prevention. (2016c). *Zika virus: Prevention.* https://www.cdc.gov/zika/prevention/index.html

Centers for Disease Control and Prevention. (2020). *Zika Virus: Case counts in the U.S. 2018–2020.* https://www.cdc.gov/zika/reporting/2021-case-counts.html

LaBeaud, A. D. (2016). *Zika virus infection: An overview.* https://www.uptodate.com/contents/zika-virus-infection-an-overview

Lockwood, C. J., Ros, S. T., & Nielson-Saines, K. (2020). *Zika virus infection: Evaluation and management of pregnant women*. https://www.uptodate.com/contents/zika-virus-infection-evaluation-and-management-of-pregnant-women?search=Lockwood,%20Ros%20zika%20virus&source=search_result&selectedTitle=3~150&usage_type=default&display_rank=3

McNeill, C., Shreve, M. D., Jarrett, A., & Perry, C. (2016). Zika: What providers need to know. *Journal for Nurse Practitioners, 12*, 359–367. https://doi.org/10.1016/j.nurpra.2016.04.009

World Health Organization. (2016). *Zika virus disease*. http://www.who.int/csr/disease/zika/case-definition/en

See the following for more information for healthcare providers:

American College of Obstetricians and Gynecologists at http://www.acog.org Click on Zika information link, updated frequently

Centers for Disease Control and Prevention. (2019). *Zika virus: For pregnant women*. https://www.cdc.gov/zika/pregnancy/index.html

Centers for Disease Control and Prevention. (2021). *Zika travel notices*. https://wwwnc.cdc.gov/travel/page/zika-information

Medscape. (2016). *Zika virus resource center*. http://www.medscape.com/resource/zika-virus

22. Disaster Planning for Pregnancy and Postpartum

NANCY J. CIBULKA | ANNA J. FISCHER COLBY | KELLY D. ROSENBERGER

Assessment for Disaster Planning

This chapter discusses disaster planning for pregnant and postpartum individuals and their infants and provides guidelines for care whether evacuating or sheltering in place. Because injuries are common during disasters, guidelines for assessment and management of minor trauma are also provided.

More attention has been given to the need for disaster preparedness as a result of terrorist attacks and natural calamities, such as devastating hurricanes, tornadoes, wildfires, tsunamis, and earthquakes, in various parts of the world. Despite these incidents, the public is still not adequately prepared to respond to a major disaster. In particular, emergency plans that address the needs of women and infants are not well developed in the United States (American College of Obstetricians and Gynecologists, Committee on Health Care for Underserved Women, 2010). A recently updated Association of Women's Health, Obstetric and Neonatal Nursing (AWHONN) position statement encourages nurses to participate in all phases of disaster planning (2020). Obstetric, neonatal, and women's healthcare providers can serve a vital role in addressing the many health needs of pregnant individuals, new mothers, and infants and reduce risk and morbidities.

Pregnant individuals, those who have recently given birth, and infants are vulnerable populations that are disproportionately harmed in a mass casualty event. Although each disaster is unique and must be handled according to the local situation, this chapter offers some general suggestions for the care of childbearing individuals and their infants. Obstetric considerations for the assessment and management of minor trauma are included. Although many nurses and healthcare providers want to assist in mass casualty events, most are not educated in the best ways to respond, communicate with disaster management teams, triage patients, or provide care to victims and their families. Online courses for healthcare providers seeking to improve competencies in disaster preparedness are included in Appendix A, along with a list of resources for healthcare providers and patients.

A. POTENTIAL RISKS TO PREGNANT INDIVIDUALS AND INFANTS

1. Larger number of women will receive late or no prenatal care.
2. Loss of continuity of care resulting from missing prenatal records
3. Increased rate of intrauterine growth restriction, low birth weight, and small head circumference
4. Increased rate of preterm births and fetal demise
5. Increased risk of placental abruption or uterine rupture related to trauma

6. Separation of mother and infant when a critically ill infant is transported to a different facility
7. Difficulty in feeding infant because of contaminated water supply
8. Increased incidence of posttraumatic stress disorder (PTSD), anxiety, depression, and grief
9. Increased risk of sexual assault when safety breakdowns occur
10. Increased risk of future unplanned pregnancy and short interval between pregnancies when contraception is not available

B. EVACUATION PLANNING AND ANTICIPATORY GUIDANCE

1. All individuals need an emergency plan for disasters.
2. Pregnant individuals and those with infants need to develop an evacuation plan for disasters and should evacuate if possible. The Centers for Disease Control and Prevention (CDC) and the American Red Cross offer helpful information for pregnant individuals and families online. A web page for various natural disasters and weather emergencies is available (www.cdc.gov/disasters/index.html). Ready.gov at www.ready.gov/ provides detailed information for making a disaster plan. NPs may download the Federal Emergency Management Agency (FEMA) app to receive real-time alerts and access to resources such as local emergency shelters and recovery centers (www.fema.gov/mobile-app).
3. Healthcare providers should give patients copies of their prenatal records because existing written records may not be available and interruption of electricity may prevent accessing electronic records. In addition, discuss key prenatal issues of importance with the patient so that she can verbally communicate information that may affect care.
4. Remind patients to take all medications with them when they evacuate.
5. Be aware of the local community action plan and assist pregnant patients in locating designated facilities for obstetric care. It is the responsibility of local public health officials to designate care facilities in a disaster area.
6. Families should store at least 3 days of supplies, including food, water, medications, ready-to-feed formula, and personal care items. See Box 22.1 for a list of suggested items.
7. Educate all patients about signs of preterm labor, preeclampsia, risk of placental abruption resulting from trauma, and other obstetric emergencies.
8. Childbirth education classes often cover emergency birth procedures and are an excellent venue for addressing safety issues as well as identifying local resources for care.
9. Encourage patients to put together an emergency birth kit; for a list of suggested items, see Exhibit 22.1.
10. Provide parents with a copy of emergency birth instructions, available from the American College of Nurse-Midwives: www.midwife.org/ACNM/files/ccLibraryFiles/Filename/000000000731/Emergency%20Preparedness%20for%20Childbirth.pdf
11. Encourage patients to have a backup plan for getting to the hospital.
12. Encourage all parents to take a class on infant and child life support through the American Red Cross or the American Heart Association.
13. Encourage breastfeeding as there may not be access to clean water for cleaning bottles or mixing formula. In addition, breastfeeding will promote more rapid recovery from childbirth. Learn more about breastfeeding during emergencies, including relactation within 6 months after birth, on the La Leche League website: (www.llli.org/emergency.html).
14. Ready-to-feed formula is advised in the event that the mother's milk supply is inadequate or she is unable to breastfeed.

BOX 22.1 FAMILY EMERGENCY SUPPLIES NEEDED IN CASE OF DISASTER*

- Water—each person needs 1 gallon per day
- Food—nonperishable, canned, dried, or boxed foods that can be easily prepared
- Nonelectric can opener
- Personal care items—soap, toothbrush and toothpaste, feminine hygiene products, hand sanitizers, and so forth.
- Clothing and sturdy shoes, weather appropriate
- Infant care items—diapers, wipes, bottles, ready-to-feed formula (however, breastfeeding is strongly recommended)
- Prescription and nonprescription medications, prenatal vitamins, contraceptives (if not pregnant), and other medical supplies
- Extra eyeglasses, contact lenses, contact lens solution
- First-aid kit
- Flashlight and extra batteries
- Battery-powered or crank radio or National Oceanic and Atmospheric Administration weather radio
- Bedding or sleeping bags and towels
- Cell phone and chargers
- Copies of important records and personal documents such as passports; Social Security cards; birth certificates; insurance cards and policies; medical records, including prenatal and immunization records; medication lists, and so forth. Keep all in waterproof bags with seals.
- If evacuating, bring cash and other financial necessities such as credit and debit cards and bank account information.
- Extra house keys and car keys
- Contact information for family, relatives, neighbors, and resources
- Pet food and pet supplies (e.g., collar, leash, and carrier), if needed
- A few trash bags

*This list is not intended to be all inclusive and will vary depending on the circumstances.

EXHIBIT 22.1 INSTRUCTIONS AND CONTENTS FOR AN EMERGENCY BIRTH KIT

Keep a contact list of anyone who may be able to help, including the phone numbers for your provider and hospital. If labor begins, call your provider and/or hospital. Have a full tank of gas and a drivable car if approaching your due date. If unable to travel to the hospital when labor begins, call a friend or neighbor to help. Have the following items ready in a waterproof bag in a safe and accessible place.

ITEMS FOR BIRTH AND INFECTION CONTROL

- Antiseptic handwash such as chlorhexidine topical (Hibiclens, Hexicleans, Betasept, Hibistat, Dyna-Hex, etc.) or hand sanitizer
- Approximately 10 large absorbent blue underpads (Chux)
- Small bottle of isopropyl alcohol
- One package of cotton balls or a small box of alcohol prep pads
- One box of disposable gloves
- Six packs of sterile lubricant
- Sterile gauze pads
- Flashlight that doesn't require batteries or extra batteries
- Sharp, sterilized scissors (to cut the cord)
- Two plastic cord clamps or white shoelaces to tie umbilical cord (sterilize by placing in a pan of boiling water for 15 minutes)

(continued)

EXHIBIT 22.1 INSTRUCTIONS AND CONTENTS FOR AN EMERGENCY BIRTH KIT (*CONTINUED*)

- Several clean towels
- Large bowl and a medium-sized plastic trash bag for placenta
- Two or three large trash bags for dirty laundry and supplies
- Written instructions on emergency birth (see Section B.10)

ITEMS FOR THE INFANT

- One bulb syringe (for infant nasal/oral suction)
- Receiving blanket and extra baby blankets
- Newborn cap
- Infant clothing
- One package of disposable infant diapers (need 10 per day)
- Twelve cans of ready-to-feed formula to be used if the mother is unable to breastfeed
- Hot-water bottle filled with warm water
- A digital thermometer and non-aspirin liquid infant pain reliever (the American Academy of Pediatrics advises rectal thermometers are most accurate for infants.) American Red Cross Quick Read Digital Rectal Thermometer: www.whattoexpect.com/baby-products/baby-care/best-baby-thermometers#best-travel-baby-thermometer

ITEMS FOR THE MOTHER

- Fluids such as juices, clean or bottled water, or sports drinks
- One plastic Peri-Bottle (must have clean water supply) or small box obstetrical towelettes
- Twelve large sanitary pads
- Change of clothing
- Nursing bra and pads
- Acetaminophen or ibuprofen

**This list is not intended to be all inclusive and will vary depending on the circumstances.*

C. SELF-CARE WHILE SHELTERING

1. Close all windows and doors, turn off air conditioning, move to a designated "safe" place.

2. Patients should inform staff that they are pregnant or have recently given birth, advise of any medications taken, any special needs, or have concerns about any emerging complications.

3. Advise patients to continue prenatal care, if possible, even if with a different provider.

4. Advise the following self-care actions for mother and infant:

a. Be attentive to food and water safety and drink plenty of water if a clean water supply is available.

b. Rest often.

c. Use good hand-hygiene practices because pregnant individuals and infants are more susceptible to infections.

d. Breastfeed infant.

e. Keep a newly born infant warm using skin-to-skin contact, blankets, and a newborn cap.

D. RECOVERY AFTER DISASTER

1. Connect patients with mental health services to help them deal with anxiety, stress, depression, and grief. Patients are at risk of developing PTSD after a disaster (Bonanno et al., 2007).

2. Agencies that may offer counseling include FEMA; the Red Cross; March of Dimes; and local organizations, including churches, schools, and community centers.

3. Contact the Organization of Teratology Information Specialists (OTIS) if the information is needed about the effects of any exposures at mothertobaby.org/ or 1-866-626-6847.

4. The CDC offers information and resources for coping with a disaster or traumatic event (www.cdc.gov/mentalhealth/).

5. Healthcare professionals can assist individuals with regaining normalcy by helping them connect with community resources for housing, transportation, food, and other essential needs.

Assessment and Management of Minor Trauma: Obstetric Considerations

A. BACKGROUND

1. Trauma to the gravid maternal abdomen may not be obvious and increases the risk of placental abruption or uterine rupture as a result of blasts, falls, or flying debris.

2. Emergency triage is essential; life-threatening injuries must be identified and addressed immediately.

3. Most injuries to pregnant individuals are minor in nature and can be managed without significant risk to the mother or fetus.

B. HISTORY

1. Take a complete history pertinent to the chief complaint of trauma, including the type of trauma and time of occurrence

2. Ask the patient if she had noted any vaginal bleeding, abdominal pain, leaking fluid, or uterine contractions

3. Assess perception of fetal movement

4. Emergency findings include abdominal pain, the uterus is tender and firm to touch, increased vaginal bleeding, chest pain resulting from irritation of blood below the diaphragm, and hypovolemic shock.

C. PHYSICAL EXAMINATION

1. Vital signs

2. Complete physical examination, thoroughly assessing any maternal injury

3. Abdominal assessment for tenderness to palpation, board-like abdomen, and uterine contractions

4. Assess fetal heart rate and pattern if the equipment is available to do so.

5. Perform sterile speculum examination for evidence of bleeding or rupture of membranes.

6. Digital cervical examination (unless contraindicated) to check for cervical dilation

7. Assess for signs of shock.

D. LABORATORY AND DIAGNOSTIC STUDIES

1. Complete blood count, blood type, and Rh

2. Additional laboratories if concern for hemorrhage or serious injury; however, prothrombin time, partial thromboplastin time, and fibrinogen are not necessary after minor trauma

3. Rh-negative women may need Kleihauer–Betke test to guide administration of RhoGAM®, especially after massive fetomaternal hemorrhage when additional dose may be needed.

4. External fetal monitoring with Doppler to assess infant and tocometer to assess uterine activity

5. Ultrasound and MRI are the imaging techniques of choice during pregnancy, but radiography, CT scan, or nuclear medicine imaging techniques can generally be done at safe exposure levels if needed in addition to ultrasound or MRI (American College of Obstetricians and Gynecologists Committee on Obstetric Practice, 2016).

E. DIFFERENTIAL DIAGNOSES

1. Preterm labor
2. Premature rupture of membranes
3. Placental abruption
4. Uterine rupture
5. Fetal distress
6. Maternal minor injury (specify)
7. Confirmation of absence of serious maternal injury

F. MANAGEMENT

1. Before 24 weeks gestation, confirm the presence of fetal cardiac activity using Doppler.
2. At or beyond 24 weeks, continuous fetal monitoring is recommended for 2 to 6 hours following possible or confirmed abdominal trauma.
3. Use ultrasound, if available, to assess the placenta, fetus, amniotic fluid volume, and presence of intra-abdominal fluid and estimated fetal weight/size if gestational age is uncertain.
4. If a pregnancy complication is found (e.g., preterm labor, preterm premature rupture of membranes, placental abnormality, or fetal distress), transport the patient to the hospital for emergency management.
5. Rh-negative pregnant patients should be given anti-D immune globulin 300 mcg within 72 hours of trauma that results in any fetomaternal bleeding.
6. Tetanus and diphtheria and tetanus, diphtheria, and pertussis vaccines can be given during pregnancy, if indicated. Refer to the CDC website for additional information if vaccinations are needed in pregnant and breastfeeding individuals:
   www.cdc.gov/vaccines/pregnancy/hcp-toolkit/guidelines.html?CDC_AA_refVal=https%3A%2F%2Fwww.cdc.gov%2Fvaccines%2Fpregnancy%2Fhcp%2Fguidelines.html
7. If antibiotics are needed, use clindamycin, Augmentin, or amoxicillin. Avoid doxycycline because of the risk of staining teeth and defective enamel development.
8. Neonatal survival is possible when a cesarean section is performed within 5 minutes of unsuccessful maternal cardiac resuscitation.

G. CONSULTATION/REFERRAL

1. Transfer to a tertiary care emergency facility with a NICU if serious maternal or neonatal injuries are suspected or detected.
2. Consult with a physician or refer to a hospital if any obstetric complications are found or if fetal well-being is not confirmed.

H. FOLLOW-UP

1. If there are no complications, continue the usual schedule of prenatal care visits.
2. Consider telephone follow-up 48 hours after trauma if possible.

Bibliography

American College of Obstetricians and Gynecologists, Committee on Health Care for Underserved Women. (2010). Preparing for disasters: Perspectives on women (Committee Opinion No. 457, reaffirmed 2016). *Obstetrics & Gynecology, 115*, 1339–1342. https://doi.org/10.1097/AOG.0b013e3181e45a6f

American College of Obstetricians and Gynecologists Committee on Obstetric Practice. (2016). Guidelines for diagnostic imaging during pregnancy and lactation (Committee Opinion No. 656). *Obstetrics & Gynecology, 127*, e75–e80. https://doi.org/10.1097/00006250-201602000-00055

Association of Women's Health, Obstetric, and Neonatal Nurses. (2012). The role of the nurse in emergency preparedness. AWHONN position statement. *Journal of Obstetric, Gynecologic, & Neonatal Nursing, 41*, 322–324. https://doi.org/10.1111/j.1552-6909.2011.01338.x

Association of Women's Health, Obstetric, and Neonatal Nurses. (2020). *Emergency care for patients during pregnancy and the postpartum period: Emergency nurses association and association of women's health, obstetric and neonatal nurses consensus statement*. https://www.awhonn.org/wp-content/uploads/2020/11/ENA-AWHONN-Consensus-Statement-Final-11.18.2020.pdf

Badakhsh, R., Harville, E., & Banerjee, B. (2010). The childbearing experience during a natural disaster. *Journal of Obstetric, Gynecologic, and Neonatal Nursing, 39*, 489–497. https://doi.org/10.1111/j.1552-6909.2010.01160.x

Bonanno, G., Galea, S., Bucciarelli, A., & Vlahov, D. (2007). What predicts psychological resilience after disaster? The role of demographics, resources, and life stress. *Journal of Consulting and Clinical Psychology, 75*, 671–682. https://doi.org/10.1037/0022-006X.75.5.671

Centers for Disease Control and Prevention. (2021a). *Safety messages for pregnant, postpartum, and breastfeeding women during natural disasters and severe weather*. https://www.cdc.gov/reproductivehealth/emergency/safety-messages.htm?CDC_AA_refVal=https%3A%2F%2Fwww.cdc.gov%2Freproductivehealth%2Femergency%2Fwildfires.htm

Centers for Disease Control and Prevention. (2021b). *Toolkit for pregnant people and new parents*. https://www.cdc.gov/coronavirus/2019-ncov/communication/toolkits/pregnant-people-and-new-parents.html

Giarratano, G., Sterling, Y. M., Orlando, S., Mathews, P., Deeves, G., Bernard, M. L., & Danna, D. (2010). Targeting prenatal emergency preparedness through childbirth education. *Journal of Obstetric, Gynecologic, and Neonatal Nursing, 39*, 480–488. https://doi.org/10.1111/j.1552-6909.2010.01159.x

Jorgensen, A. M., Mendoza, G. J., & Henderson, J. L. (2010). Emergency preparedness and disaster response core competency set for perinatal and neonatal nurses. *Journal of Obstetric, Gynecologic, and Neonatal Nursing, 39*, 450–467. https://doi.org/10.1111/j.1552-6909.2010.01157.x

Joseph, N. T., Curtis, B. H., & Goodman, A. (2020). *Disaster settings: Care of pregnant patients*. http://www.uptodate.com/contents/disaster-settings-care-of-pregnant-patients?search=Disaster%20settings%20pregnant&source=search_result&selectedTitle=1~150&usage_type=default&display_rank=1

Langan, J. C., & James, D. C. (2005). *Preparing nurses for disaster management*. Pearson Prentice Hall.

Stokowski, L. A. (2015). *Ready, willing, and able: Preparing nurses to respond to disasters*. http://www.medscape.com/viewarticle/579888_10

U.S. Department of Health and Human Services Office on Women's Health. (2021). *Emergency preparedness*. http://www.womenshealth.gov/emergency-preparedness/

Williams, D. (2004). Giving birth "in place": A guide to emergency preparedness for childbirth. *Journal of Midwifery & Women's Health, 49*(4 Suppl. 1), 48–52. https://doi.org/10.1016/j.jmwh.2004.04.030

23. Thyroid Disorders in Pregnancy and Postpartum

KELLY D. ROSENBERGER | MICHAEL P. ROSENBERGER

Thyroid disorders are second to diabetes mellitus as the most common endocrine disorders occurring in reproductive-age women. Common pregnancy symptoms often mirror symptoms of thyroid dysfunction, creating challenges for identification. During pregnancy, poorly managed thyroid disorders are associated with adverse outcomes. Untreated thyroid disease during pregnancy has been associated with an increased risk of miscarriage, hypertensive disorders, fetal growth restriction, and placental abruption, as well as several others noted in this chapter (Stagnaro-Green, 2011). Thus, diagnosis and treatment are essential components of prenatal care to safeguard maternal and fetal well-being.

The impact of pregnancy on maternal thyroid physiology is significant to meet the increased metabolic demands during a normal pregnancy. The major changes in thyroid function during pregnancy include a slight enlargement of the thyroid gland due to hyperplasia and increased vascularity, but not enough for true goiter or significant thyromegaly. Changes in thyroid function test results occur during uncomplicated pregnancy as well as in individuals with thyroid dysfunction, and the changes vary by trimester. During normal pregnancy, the thyroid hormones total serum thyroxine (TT_4) and triiodothyronine (TT_3) concentrations increase, while the thyroid-stimulating hormone (TSH) slightly decreases within normal range due to the cross-reactivity of the alpha subunit of human chorionic gonadotropin with the TSH receptor, and the free thyroxine (FT_4) levels remain unchanged (Alexander et al., 2017). See Table 23.1 to review physiologic changes with normal and abnormal thyroid function during pregnancy.

A. DEFINITIONS/INCIDENCE/RISKS

The most common thyroid disorders in pregnancy are hypothyroidism, hyperthyroidism, postpartum thyroiditis, and goiter.

TABLE 23.1 CHANGES IN THYROID HORMONES DURING NORMAL PREGNANCY AND WITH THYROID DISEASE

MATERNAL CONDITION	TSH	FT_4	TT_3	TT_4
Normal Pregnancy	Decrease	No Change	Increase	Increase
Hypothyroidism	Increase	Decrease	Decrease or No Change	Decrease
Hyperthyroidism	Decrease	Increase	Increase or No Change	Increase

1. Hypothyroidism

During pregnancy, the incidence of overt hypothyroidism is 0.3% to 0.5%, defined as low FT_4 and elevated TSH levels. The incidence of subclinical hypothyroidism during pregnancy is 2% to 3%, defined as elevated TSH and normal FT_4 levels (Stagnaro-Green, 2011). The most common cause worldwide of hypothyroidism is iodine deficiency. In countries with sufficient iodine, the most common causes are autoimmune thyroiditis and iatrogenic hypothyroidism after treatment for hyperthyroidism. In the United States, the Guidelines of the American Thyroid Association (ATA) recommends 150 mcg of iodine daily during pregnancy and lactation, which is the dose in most prenatal vitamins (Alexander et al., 2017). In pregnancy, hypothyroidism has been associated with an increased risk of several complications, including:

- **a.** Preeclampsia and gestational hypertension
- **b.** Placental abruption
- **c.** Non-reassuring fetal heart rate tracing
- **d.** Preterm delivery, including very preterm delivery (before 32 weeks)
- **e.** Low birth weight
- **f.** Increased rate of cesarean section
- **g.** Postpartum hemorrhage
- **h.** Perinatal morbidity and mortality
- **i.** Neuropsychological and cognitive impairment in the child

2. Hyperthyroidism

The incidence of hyperthyroidism during pregnancy is 0.2% with overt hyperthyroidism defined as elevated FT_4 and low TSH and subclinical hyperthyroidism defined as asymptomatic low TSH and normal FT_4. Graves' disease is an autoimmune disorder with antithyroid antibodies against the TSH receptor accounting for 95% of the cases. Less common causes of hyperthyroidism also include gestational trophoblastic disease, nodular goiter, solidary toxic adenoma, viral thyroiditis, and pituitary or ovarian tumors. In pregnancy, hyperthyroidism has been associated with an increased risk of several complications, including:

- **a.** Spontaneous abortion
- **b.** Premature labor
- **c.** Low birth weight
- **d.** Stillbirth
- **e.** Preeclampsia
- **f.** Heart failure

3. Postpartum Thyroiditis

The incidence of postpartum thyroiditis is 1.1% to 21.1%, defined as an abnormal TSH level in the first 12 months postpartum in the absence of a toxic thyroid nodule or thyrotoxin receptor antibodies (Muller et al., 2001). Postpartum thyroiditis may occur after pregnancy loss (miscarriage, abortion, ectopic pregnancy) and after normal delivery.

4. Goiter

In the United States, where iodine is sufficient, true goiter during pregnancy is rare. However, in iodine-deficient regions of the world, goiter is more common during pregnancy.

B. HISTORY

1. Universal screening of asymptomatic pregnant patients for thyroid dysfunction during pregnancy is controversial and not currently recommended (ACOG, 2020). Indications for thyroid testing in pregnancy include:

a. Current thyroid therapy
b. Family history of autoimmune thyroid disease
c. Goiter
d. Morbid obesity (BMI ≥40 kg/m^2)
e. Personal history of:
   i. High-dose neck radiation
   ii. Autoimmune disease
   iii. Type 1 DM
   iv. Postpartum thyroid dysfunction
   v. Prior delivery of infant with thyroid disease
   vi. Therapy for hyperthyroidism
   vii. Decreased fertility
   viii. Recurrent miscarriage or preterm delivery
   ix. Prior thyroid surgery
   x. Age >30 years
   xi. Thyroid peroxidase (TPO) antibodies
   xii. Multiple prior pregnancies (two or more)
   xiii. Use of amiodarone, lithium, or recent administration of iodinated radiologic contrast agents
   xiv. Living in an area of moderate to severe iodine insufficiency
f. Symptoms of hypothyroidism

2. Determine if presenting signs or symptoms are present:
   a. Hypothyroidism: Fatigue, weight gain, decreased exercise capacity, constipation, dry and pale skin, brittle nails, hair loss, bradycardia, slow movement and slow speech, cold intolerance, delayed deep tendon reflexes, puffy face, tongue enlargement, periorbital edema, and hoarseness
   b. Hyperthyroidism: Failure to gain weight or weight loss with adequate food intake, thyromegaly, exophthalmos, tachycardia, elevated sleeping pulse rate, anxiety and/or nervousness, tremor, sweating, heat intolerance, proximal muscle weakness, increased bowel movements, decreased exercise tolerance, and hypertension
   c. Postpartum thyroiditis: Clinical course may vary with 25% patients present with symptoms of hyperthyroidism followed by symptoms of hypothyroidism and then recover, 43% present with hypothyroidism symptoms, and 32% present with hyperthyroidism (Stagnaro-Green, 2011). Signs and symptoms of hyperthyroidism are typically mild and consist of fatigue, weight loss, palpitations, heat intolerance, anxiety, irritability, tachycardia, and tremor. Similarly, hypothyroidism is also usually mild, leading to lack of energy, cold intolerance, constipation, sluggishness, and dry skin.

C. PHYSICAL EXAMINATION

1. Check vital signs for tachycardia, bradycardia, and hypertension.
2. Check weight for increase or decrease.
3. General appearance: Observe for diaphoresis, tremor, exophthalmos, and dry skin.
4. Inspect and palpate thyroid gland for enlargement and/or nodules.

D. LABORATORY AND DIAGNOSTIC STUDIES

1. ACOG recommends a TSH level as the first line measurement for thyroid evaluation during pregnancy. If the TSH is elevated, ACOG next recommends assessment of FT_4 (most labs now automatically reflex the FT_4 level if

the TSH is abnormal). If the TSH is decreased, ACOG recommends assessment of both FT_4 and Total T_3. However, in the presence of increased risk factors and/or signs and symptoms, other tests such as FT_3, TT_4, TBG, and TPO antibodies may be warranted. See Table 23.2 for trimester specific reference ranges.

2. In the United States, any thyroid enlargement during pregnancy is potentially abnormal requiring assessment with thyroid function tests and thyroid ultrasonography.

3. A pregnant patient with a thyroid nodule should have a TSH and ultrasound. While thyroid radionuclide scanning is contraindicated during pregnancy, a fine needle aspiration biopsy is safe during pregnancy if warranted.

E. MANAGEMENT

1. Hypothyroidism: Treat with incremental doses of levothyroxine adjusted based on the degree of TSH elevation with serum TSH measured every 4 to 6 weeks until 20 weeks gestational age and until stable. Then TSH is measured again at 24 to 28 weeks and 32 to 34 weeks gestation. TSH levels at 4 to 10 mU/L require dosing at 25 to 50 mcg/day, levels at 11 to 20 mU/L require dosing at 50 to 75 mcg/day, and levels >20 mU/L require dosing at 75 to 100 mcg/day. Treatment goal is for TSH <2.5. Patients with TSH levels between 2.5 to 4 mU/L with negative TPO antibodies are considered euthyroid, and no treatment is necessary. In patients with +TPO antibodies and TSH levels between 2.5 to 4 mU/L with a prior history of recurrent miscarriage, 50 mcg/day is advised (Ross, 2021). Antenatal testing is not recommended in pregnant individuals with medication-controlled hypothyroidism but may be considered in patients with co-existing maternal or obstetric indications. After delivery, levothyroxine dose may be decreased to pre-pregnancy dose and guided by TSH levels at 4 to 6 weeks postpartum.

2. Hyperthyroidism: Treat with incremental doses based on the degree abnormality with propylthiouracil 50 to 300 mg/day in two divided doses in the first trimester, changing to methimazole in second trimester due to risk of liver damage. Methimazole (tapazole), is not recommended in first trimester due to risk of birth defects. Methimazole is dosed at 5 to 30 mg/day in two divided doses based on the degree of TSH and FT_4 measured every 2 weeks until stable with treatment goal of FT_4 in upper one-third normal range. For pregnant individuals unable to tolerate medical treatment due to allergy or agranulocytosis, thyroidectomy during the second trimester of pregnancy may be offered after all the risks factors and potential complications have been discussed in detail. Antenatal testing should begin weekly at 32 to 34 weeks gestation in patients with poorly controlled

TABLE 23.2 TRIMESTER SPECIFIC REFERENCE RANGES FOR THYROID TESTS

TEST	NON-PREGNANT	FIRST TRIMESTER	SECOND TRIMESTER	THIRD TRIMESTER
TSH	0.3–4.3	0.1–2.5	0.2–3.0	0.3–3.0
FT_4	0.8–1.7	0.8–1.2	0.6–1.0	0.5–0.8
TT_4	5.4–11.7	6.5–10.1	7.5–10.3	6.3–9.7
FT_3	2.4–4.2	4.1–4.4	4.0–4.2	Unknown
TT_3	77.0–135.0	97.0–149.0	117.0–169.0	123.0–162.0
TBG	1.3–3.0	1.8–3.2	2.8–4.0	2.6–4.2

hyperthyroidism and fetal ultrasonography every 4 to 6 weeks after 20 weeks gestation to assess for fetal growth, hydrops, goiter, and cardiac function.

3. Postpartum Thyroiditis: Typically, the hyperthyroid phase is caused by autoimmune destruction of the thyroid resulting in the release of stored thyroid hormone; thus, antithyroid medications are not beneficial. However, peripheral beta antagonists may be used if the patient is symptomatic. It is important to differentiate postpartum thyroiditis from Grave's disease since Grave's requires antithyroid therapy. Differentiation can be done with referral for radioactive iodine uptake scan but is contraindicated during breastfeeding, and close contact with others is limited after the scan. In postpartum thyroiditis in the hypothyroid phase, patients may be treated with levothyroxine as noted prior if symptomatic and may require lifelong supplementation.

F. PATIENT EDUCATION

1. Education on symptoms of hypothyroidism include:
- **a.** Lack of energy and easily fatigued
- **b.** Feeling cold easily
- **c.** Developing coarse or thin hair
- **d.** Constipation

2. If it is not treated, hypothyroidism can weaken and slow the heart. This may leave patients feeling out of breath or tired when exercising and cause edema in the ankles. Untreated hypothyroidism can also increase blood pressure and raise cholesterol – both of which increase the risk of heart disease.

3. Treatment for hypothyroidism involves taking thyroid hormone pills every day. After taking the medication for 4 to 6 weeks, follow-up blood tests are needed to make sure the levels are adequate. The medication dose may need adjusting depending on the test results. Most people with hypothyroidism need to be on thyroid pills for the rest of their life. Levothyroxine is the medication of choice and should be taken on an empty stomach, ideally 1 hour before breakfast daily.

4. Education on common symptoms of hyperthyroidism include:
- **a.** Feeling tired or weak
- **b.** Losing weight, even when you eat normally
- **c.** Having a fast or uneven heartbeat
- **d.** Sweating a lot and having trouble dealing with hot weather
- **e.** Feeling worried
- **f.** Trembling

5. Thyroiditis after pregnancy can cause symptoms of hyperthyroidism or hypothyroidism. Sometimes people have symptoms of hyperthyroidism and then symptoms of hypothyroidism.

Common symptoms of postpartum hyperthyroidism include:
- **a.** Feeling tired or weak
- **b.** Losing weight, even when you eat normally
- **c.** Having a fast or uneven heartbeat
- **d.** Sweating a lot and having trouble dealing with hot weather
- **e.** Feeling worried
- **f.** Trembling

Common symptoms of postpartum hypothyroidism include:
- **g.** Having no energy
- **h.** Feeling cold
- **i.** Trouble having bowel movements (constipation)
- **j.** Not making enough breast milk, if breastfeeding

6. Education on nutritional sources of iodine. Good sources of iodine include dairy foods, seafood, eggs, meat, poultry, and iodized salt. It is recommended prenatal vitamins contain 150 mcg of iodine. Iodine is also important while breastfeeding for infants to receive iodine in breastmilk. Caution, too much iodine from supplements such as seaweed may be harmful.

G. CONSULTATION/REFERRAL

1. Consult with collaborating physician upon the diagnosis of hypothyroidism, hyperthyroidism, postpartum thyroiditis, and goiter in ambulatory OB settings.

2. Refer to the appropriate specialist as indicated by poorly controlled thyroid function test levels and/or worsening symptoms.

3. Referral and or co-management with maternal-fetal medicine as indicated, especially for patients with a history of irradiation for hyperthyroidism on replacement therapy.

Bibliography

Abbassi-Ghanavati, M., Greer, L. G., & Cunningham, F. G. (2009). Pregnancy and laboratory studies: A reference table for clinicians. *Obstetrics and Gynecology, 114*(6), 1326–1331. https://doi.org/10.1097/AOG.0b013e3181c2bde8

Alexander, E. K., Pearce, E. N., Brent, G. A., Brown, R. S., Chen, H., Dosiou, C., Grobman, W. A., Laurberg, P., Lazarus, J. H., Mandel, S. J., Peeters, R. P., & Sullivan, S. (2017). Guidelines of the American Thyroid Association for the diagnosis and management of thyroid disease during pregnancy and the postpartum. *Thyroid, 27*(3), 315–389. https://doi.org/10.1089/thy.2016.0457

American College of Obstetrics and Gynecologists. (2020). ACOG Practice Bulletin No. 233 thyroid disease in pregnancy. *Obstetrics & Gynecology, 135*(6), e261–e274. https://doi.org/10.1097/AOG.0000000000003893

De Groot, L., Abalovich, M., Alexander, E. K., Amino, N., Barbour, L., Cobin, R. H., Eastman, C. J., Lazarus, J. H., Luton, D., Mandel, S. J., Mestman, J., Rovet, J., & Sullivan, S. (2012). Management of thyroid dysfunction during pregnancy and postpartum: An Endocrine Society clinical practice guideline. *The Journal of Clinical Endocrinology and Metabolism, 97*(8), 2543–2565. https://doi.org/10.1210/jc.2011-2803

Leung, A. M., Pearce, E. N., & Braverman, L. E. (2009). Iodine content of prenatal vitamins in the United States. *The New England Journal of Medicine, 360*, 939–940. https://doi.org/10.1056/NEJMc0807851

Muller, A. F., Drexhage, H. A., & Berghout, A. (2001). Postpartum thyroiditis and autoimmune thyroiditis in women of childbearing age: Recent insights and consequences for antenatal and postnatal care. *Endocrine Reviews, 22*(5), 605–630. https://doi.org/10.1210/edrv.22.5.0441

Nazarpour, S., Ramezani-Tehrani, F., Simbar, M., Tohidi, M., Majd, H. A., & Azizi, F. (2017). Effects of levothyroxine treatment on pregnancy outcomes in pregnant women with autoimmune thyroid disease. *European Journal of Endocrinology, 176*, 253–265. https://doi.org/10.1530/EJE-16-0548

Negro, R., Schwartz, A., & Stagnaro-Green, A. (2016). Impact of levothyroxine in miscarriage and preterm birth delivery rates in first trimester thyroid antibody-positive women with TSH less than 2.5 mU/L. *The Journal of Clinical Endocrinology and Metabolism, 101*, 3685–3690. https://doi.org/10.1210/jc.2016-1803

Ross, D. S. (2021). Hyperthyroidism during pregnancy: Clinical manifestations, diagnosis, and causes. *UptoDate.* https://www.uptodate.com/contents/hyperthyroidism-during-pregnancy-treatment?search=hyperthyroidism%20in%20pregnancy&source=search_result&selectedTitle=1~150&usage_type=default&display_rank=1

Stagnaro-Green, A. (2004). Postpartum thyroiditis. *Best Practice & Research Clinical Endocrinology & Metabolism, 18*(2), 303–316. https://doi.org/10.1016/j.beem.2004.03.008

Stagnaro-Green, A. (2011). Overt hyperthyroidism and hypothyroidism during pregnancy. *Clinical Obstetrics and Gynecology, 54*(3), 478–487. https://doi.org/10.1097/GRF.0b013e3182272f32

24. COVID-19 During Pregnancy and Postpartum

AMY M. SEIBERT | KELLY D. ROSENBERGER

A. DEFINITIONS AND BACKGROUND

1. The severe acute respiratory syndrome coronavirus 2 (SARS-CoV-2) was first identified in China in December 2019. The disease caused by the SARS-CoV-2 virus is coronavirus disease 2019, or COVID-19. It has spread worldwide at a rapid pace and was identified as a pandemic by the World Health Organization on March 11, 2020. The body of scientific knowledge regarding this recently discovered virus is continuously evolving, and guidance may become out-of-date as new information becomes available. Practitioners are encouraged to regularly review the most updated guidance from the American College of Obstetricians and Gynecologists (ACOG), Centers for Disease Control and Prevention (CDC), and Society for Maternal-Fetal Medicine (SMFM).

2. The SARS-CoV-2 virus spreads through close person-to-person contact via inhalation of airborne droplets or direct contact with respiratory secretions on a contaminated surface. An individual who is asymptomatic can spread the disease by shedding the virus for 1 to 3 days prior to symptom onset. Once infected, individuals can remain infectious for 10 to 20 days, depending on disease severity. The incubation period is typically 5 to 6 days.

3. The virus can cause a wide range of illness severity, from asymptomatic cases or mild symptoms to more severe disease. Common symptoms of COVID-19 include fever, headache, cough, fatigue, shortness of breath, and loss of taste and smell. More severe disease can involve thromboembolism, sepsis, multiorgan system failure, and even death. Symptoms may be short-lived, or they can persist for months.

4. At the time of writing, there have been more than 46 million cases and more than 750,000 deaths from COVID-19 in the United States since January 21, 2020.

5. Because of the physiologic and immunologic changes of pregnancy, COVD-19 is more likely to cause severe illness in pregnant individuals compared to those who are not pregnant. The third trimester appears to be the most vulnerable time for severe infection. According to data released by the CDC, pregnant individuals who test positive for SARS-CoV-2 are more likely than their age-matched peers to be hospitalized, be admitted to an intensive care unit, and receive mechanical ventilation (NIH, 2021). Overall infection rates and death rates related to COVID-19 are similar in pregnant and nonpregnant individuals. Vertical transmission of COVID-19 is rare but possible.

6. Ethnic disparities in COVID-19 disease outcomes are evident. Hispanic and non-Hispanic Black populations comprise a disproportionately large percentage of COVID-19 infections, hospitalizations, and deaths in the United States. These disparities are also reflected in severe infection among pregnant individuals. Providers of obstetric care should be alert to underlying chronic conditions, including diabetes, hypertension, and obesity, as well as socioeconomic determinants of health, including housing insecurity, transportation issues, food scarcity, and shelter-in-place restrictions, making it difficult to obtain healthy foods, access to baby supplies (e.g. formula, diapers), and/or attend prenatal appointments and birthing classes. Members of the non-Hispanic Black community have the highest prevalence of obesity compared to other racial groups, which further increases the risk associated with COVID-19. Additionally, the non-Hispanic Black community has more cultural acceptance of obesity.

7. Increased incidence of depression and anxiety due to the COVID-19 pandemic have been noted. The ACOG recommends ongoing universal screening for depression during pregnancy and in the postpartum period, including during telehealth appointments.

8. Medical staff caring for patients with suspected or confirmed COVID-19 should use personal protective equipment (PPE), including N95 respirators, eye protection, gloves, and gowns. All PPE should be put on before entry into the patient's room and removed before leaving the patient's room.

B. HISTORY

1. Assess the patient for the following:
   - **a.** Fever of 100.4 °F (38 °C) or higher
   - **b.** Cough
   - **c.** Difficulty breathing or shortness of breath
   - **d.** Shaking or chills
   - **e.** Sore throat
   - **f.** Headache
   - **g.** New loss of taste or smell
   - **h.** Malaise, fatigue
   - **i.** Muscle or body aches
   - **j.** Congestion or runny nose
   - **k.** Nausea and/or vomiting
   - **l.** Diarrhea
   - **m.** Recent close exposure to someone who tested positive for COVID-19
2. Assess illness severity:
   - **a.** Increased difficulty breathing or shortness of breath
   - **b.** Difficulty completing a sentence or walking across the room without gasping for air
   - **c.** Coughing up bloody sputum
   - **d.** New pain or pressure in chest other than pain with coughing
   - **e.** Unable to keep liquids down
   - **f.** Signs of dehydration, including dizziness when standing
   - **g.** Altered mental status
3. Review history for comorbidities:
   - **a.** Diabetes, hypertension, chronic heart, liver, lung, or kidney disease, immunologic conditions, blood clotting disorders, obesity
   - **b.** Symptoms of preterm labor
   - **c.** Inability to care for self

4. Determine whether the patient received a COVID-19 vaccine. COVID-19 vaccines have been shown to be 95%, 94%, and 67% effective at preventing symptomatic illness, respectively, for the Pfizer, Moderna, and Johnson & Johnson (J&J) vaccines (Olliaro et al., 2021).

5. Assess for any signs of evolving pregnancy complications:

- **a.** Fetal movements
- **b.** Cramps
- **c.** Contractions
- **d.** Leaking fluid from vagina
- **e.** Severe headache
- **f.** Swelling

C. PHYSICAL EXAMINATION

1. Check vital signs: May have fever, tachycardia, tachypnea, and/or pulse oximetry < 95%.

2. Observe general appearance and observe lips, face, or fingertips for cyanosis.

3. Auscultate lung fields bilaterally for crackles or rales; auscultate heart for rubs, tachycardia, murmurs, or extra sounds.

4. Neurological examination: Assess the level of consciousness and for signs of meningeal irritation (e.g., nuchal rigidity and Brudzinski's and Kernig's signs).

5. Assess for fetal well-being: Check fundal height, fetal heart tones, and fetal movement.

D. LABORATORY AND DIAGNOSTIC STUDIES

1. Direct viral testing using nucleic acid amplification or antigen detection is the only specific method of diagnosis authorized by the United States Food and Drug Administration (FDA) and recommended by the CDC. Reverse transcription-polymerase chain reaction (RT-PCR) test checks respiratory secretion samples from a nasopharyngeal or oropharyngeal swab.

2. Rapid point-of-care tests may provide results within an hour. However, false negatives are common. Antibody tests have not been authorized by the FDA for diagnosing COVID-19.

3. Pulse oximetry to monitor oxygenation status

4. Complete blood count (CBC) and complete metabolic panel (CMP) if indicated by the severity of illness

- **a.** May show cytopenia, elevated triglycerides (as expected during pregnancy), ferritin, and/or serum aspartate aminotransferase (AST)
- **b.** Elevated procalcitonin level indicates a superimposed bacterial infection. Ceftriaxone plus azithromycin may be used to treat community-acquired pneumonia during pregnancy, following sputum or blood culture collection
- **c.** Laboratory findings may overlap with those found in preeclampsia or hemolysis, elevated liver enzymes, low platelet count (HELLP) syndrome; RT-PCR testing is recommended if the patient has risk factors for COVID-19

5. Chest x-ray or chest CT is not currently recommended for diagnosing COVID-19 due to lack of specificity. Imaging findings overlap with those of other viral respiratory illnesses, including influenza, H1N1, SARS, and MERS (American College of Radiology, 2020).

6. Continuous fetal monitoring if indicated by the patient's condition

E. DIFFERENTIAL DIAGNOSES

1. COVID-19
   - **a.** Mild disease: Flu-like symptoms or asymptomatic
   - **b.** Moderate disease: Dyspnea, pneumonia on imaging, fever not relieved by acetaminophen, oxygen saturation >93% on room air
   - **c.** Severe disease: Tachypnea (>30 breaths per minute), oxygen saturation <94%, increased lung involvement noted on imaging
   - **d.** Critical disease: Multi-organ dysfunction, shock, or respiratory failure
2. Upper respiratory infection, nasopharyngitis, or common cold
3. Infectious mononucleosis
4. Viral or strep pharyngitis
5. Bronchitis
6. Pneumonia
7. Influenza, type A or B
8. Preeclampsia or HELLP syndrome

F. MANAGEMENT

1. Patients with a positive COVID-19 test or suspected COVID-19 illness must self-isolate for at least 10 days following a positive test or the onset of symptoms. Additionally, symptoms must be improving, and the patient must be fever-free for at least 24 hours with no fever-reducing medication. Patients with severe illnesses that required hospitalization should follow guidance from the healthcare provider.

2. Pregnant individuals are at an increased risk for severe illness from COVID-19 and death, compared to nonpregnant people. Inform patients of potential complications, including an increased risk of preterm birth, and advise patients to contact their healthcare provider right away if symptoms worsen. If they have any difficulty in breathing or shortness of breath, new pain or pressure in the chest, are unable to tolerate liquids, have any signs of cyanosis of lips or fingertips, abnormal mental status, or uterine contractions or decreased fetal movement, they should seek immediate care at a hospital with intensive care capabilities and equipped to care for pregnant individuals. ACOG and SMFM published a helpful algorithm for assessment and care of the pregnant patient with suspected COVID-19 infection at www.acog.org/-/media/project/acog/acogorg/files/pdfs/clinical-guidance/practice-advisory/covid-19-algorithm.pdf

3. Outpatient treatment consists of comfort measures. Patients should be encouraged to rest, increase fluid intake, and self-isolate to avoid infecting others. Acetaminophen 650 mg orally every 4 hours may be used as needed for headaches, muscle aches, and to reduce fevers of 100.4 °F or more. Hyperthermia is a risk factor for adverse pregnancy outcomes. Intractable fever, or fever that is not alleviated by acetaminophen, is a sign of worsening illness and is an indication for inpatient monitoring. Information for pregnant individuals with suspected or confirmed COVID-19 is available at www.cdc.gov/coronavirus/2019-ncov/need-extra-precautions/pregnancy-breastfeeding.html.

4. According to Vaught & Halscott as published by the Society for Maternal-Fetal Medicine (2021), pregnant patients with COVID-19 disease that warrants pharmacological treatment should be admitted to the inpatient setting. Multiple pharmacological treatment options have been investigated for COVID-19. Remdesivir, azithromycin, tocilizumab, and convalescent plasma have all been used to treat severe disease in the inpatient setting and have shown varying success in decreasing the length of stay in hospital and the mortality risk. There is no known fetal toxicity risk for any of the treatments listed. While pregnant individuals have not been included in clinical trials of any pharmacological treatment for COVID-19, the SMFM and NIH recommend that any of the above treatments be offered to pregnant patients with COVID-19 who meet the criteria for compassionate use.

G. PREVENTION OF COVID-19

1. Pregnant individuals should follow the same recommendations as non-pregnant individuals for avoiding exposure to the virus.

a. Limit interactions with people who may have been exposed to or who may be infected with COVID-19.

b. Wear a mask that covers the nose and mouth completely and avoid people who are not wearing masks. ACOG and the CDC recommend masks for pregnant individuals when in public. These studies address masks and respirators during pregnancy and demonstrate no significant differences in maternal and fetal heart rates and oxygen saturation in participants wearing masks compared to those not wearing masks:

i. www.ncbi.nlm.nih.gov/pmc/articles/PMC4469179/

ii. blogs.cdc.gov/niosh-science-blog/2015/06/18/respirators-pregnancy/

iii. aricjournal.biomedcentral.com/articles/10.1186/s13756-015-0086-z

c. Practice social distancing by staying a minimum of 6 feet away from other people outside the household.

d. Wash hands frequently with soap and water.

e. Avoid activities where social distancing and hand hygiene will not be possible.

2. As of March 2021, three COVID-19 vaccines are available and have received emergency use authorization from the FDA. More vaccines are in various stages of development and trials. The initial COVID-19 vaccine trials did not include pregnant individuals; however, the FDA is observationally studying the pregnant patients who have received COVID-19 vaccines in the initial rollout before knowing they were pregnant. The COVID-19 vaccines developed by Pfizer-BioNTech, Moderna, and J&J are based on mRNA or protein subunits and contain no infectious virus. The Pfizer and Moderna vaccines are 95% and 94% effective, respectively, at preventing COVID-19 illness after the second dose (Olliaro et al., 2021).

3. The J&J vaccine is 67% effective in preventing moderate and severe disease, 85% effective overall at preventing hospitalization, and 100% at preventing death after one dose (CDC, 2021). In April 2021, the CDC and FDA recommended a temporary halt of administration of the J&J vaccine out of an abundance of caution due to rare adverse thrombosis with thrombocytopenia syndrome (TTS) in women younger than age 50. TTS is a rare condition involving blood clots and low platelets. While the CDC and FDA resumed J&J vaccination a few weeks later, the authors recommend pregnant individuals select either the Pfizer or Moderna vaccines (neither has demonstrated an increased risk of TTS) until further information becomes available.

4. In February 2021, Pfizer launched a COVID-19 vaccine trial for pregnant individuals, including 4,000 healthy participants aged 18 and older who are 24 to 34 weeks pregnant randomly assigned to receive either two doses of Pfizer/BioNTech's COVID-19 vaccine or a placebo to be given 21 days apart. The global trial will assess the vaccine's safety, immunogenicity, and tolerability, with each participant to be observed for an estimated 7 to 10 months, dependent on whether they were given a placebo or vaccine.

a. ACOG recommends that COVID-19 vaccines should not be withheld from pregnant individuals who meet the criteria for vaccination based on the Advisory Committee on Immunization Practices (ACIP)-recommended priority groups. COVID-19 vaccines should be offered to lactating individuals similar to non-lactating individuals when they meet the criteria for receipt of the vaccine based on prioritization groups outlined by the ACIP.

b. If an individual becomes pregnant after receiving the first dose of the COVID-19 vaccine series, the second dose should be administered when indicated.

c. When possible, vaccination should be timed so that patients do not receive a COVID-19 vaccine within 14 days of receipt of a routine vaccination, such as the Tdap or influenza.

d. Anti-D immunoglobin (RhoGAM) does not interfere with the immune response to vaccines and may be administered according to standard treatment protocols.

e. Common side effects of the vaccine include sore arm, redness or swelling at the injection site, headache, low-grade fever, and muscle or joint aches. Patients should be advised that side effects are a normal part of the immune reaction to the vaccine and signal the creation of antibodies to protect against COVID-19 illness.

f. Several studies have demonstrated pregnant and lactating individuals who received the Pfizer and Moderna COVID-19 vaccines pass protective antibodies on to their newborns with antibody levels much higher compared to those individuals with COVID-19 infection during pregnancy (Gray et al., 2021; Prabhu et al., 2021).

H. COMPLICATIONS

1. Pneumonia

2. Preterm delivery: Increased incidence by 60% compared to individuals without infection

3. Stillbirth: Increased incidence in pregnant individuals requiring hospitalization for COVID-19. No increased risk was noted with mild or asymptomatic disease.

4. Respiratory failure

5. Multiple organ dysfunction

6. Maternal death: Increased incidence in pregnant individuals worldwide during the pandemic

7. Preeclampsia: Increased incidence by 76% compared to individuals without infection

8. Venous thromboembolism (VTE)

I. CONSULTATION/REFERRAL

1. Consult with Maternal-Fetal Medicine specialist in cases of moderate or severe COVID-19 disease and/or obstetric complications.

2. Hospitalization is indicated for pregnant people with moderate or severe disease.

J. FOLLOW-UP

1. Advise the patient to notify a healthcare practitioner immediately if the condition worsens.

2. Within two weeks of initial diagnosis of COVID-19 for maternal/fetal well-being check

3. As recommended for ongoing prenatal care

Bibliography

American College of Obstetricians and Gynecologists. (2020). *Practice advisory: Novel coronavirus 2019 (COVID-19).* https://www.acog.org/clinical/clinical-guidance/practice-advisory/articles/2020/03/novel-coronavirus-2019

American College of Obstetricians and Gynecologists. (2021). *Practice advisory: Vaccinating pregnant and lactating patients against Covid-19.* https://www.acog.org/clinical/clinical-guidance/practice-advisory/articles/2020/12/vaccinating-pregnant-and-lactating-patients-against-covid-19

American College of Radiology. (2020). *ACR recommendations for the use of chest radiography and computed tomography (CT) for suspected Covid-19 infection.* https://www.acr.org/Advocacy-and-Economics/ACR-Position-Statements/Recommendations-for-Chest-Radiography-and-CT-for-Suspected-COVID19-Infection

Barbosa-Leiker, C., Smith, C. L., Crespi, E. J., Brooks, O., Burduli, E., Ranjo, S., Carty, C. L., Hebert, L. E., Waters, S. F., & Gartstein, M. A. (2021). Stressors, coping, and resources needed during the COVID-19 pandemic in a sample of perinatal women. *BMC Pregnancy Childbirth, 21,* 171. https://bmcpregnancychildbirth.biomedcentral.com/articles/10.1186/s12884-021-03665-0#citeas

Berghella, V., & Hughes, B. (2021). Coronavirus disease 2019 (COVID-19): Pregnancy issues and antenatal care. *UpToDate.* https://www.uptodate.com/contents/coronavirus-disease-2019-covid-19-pregnancy-issues-and-antenatal-care#!

Centers for Disease Control and Prevention. (2021a). *The advisory committee on immunizations practices' interim recommendation for use of Janssen COVID-19 Vaccine.* https://www.cdc.gov/mmwr/volumes/70/wr/mm7009e4.htm

Centers for Disease Control and Prevention. (2021b). *Pregnancy, breastfeeding, and caring for newborns.* https://www.cdc.gov/coronavirus/2019-ncov/need-extra-precautions/pregnancy-breastfeeding.html

Chmielewska, B., Barratt, I., Townsend, R., Kalafat, E., Van der Meulen, J., & Gurol-Urganci, I. (2021). Effects of the COVID-19 pandemic on maternal and perinatal outcomes: A systematic review and meta-analysis. *The Lancet, Global Health, 9*(6), e759–e772. https://www.thelancet.com/journals/langlo/article/PIIS2214-109X(21)00079-6/fulltext

Craig, A. M., Hughes, B. L., & Swamy, G. K. (2021). COVID-19 vaccines in pregnancy. *American Journal of Obstetrics & Gynecology MFM, 3*(2), 100295. https://doi.org/10.1016/j.ajogmf.2020.100295

Gray, K. J., Bordt, E. A., Atyeo, C., Deriso, E., Akinwunmi, B., Young, N., Baez, A. M., Shook, L. L., Cvrk, D., James, K., De Guzman, R. M., Brigida, S., Diouf, K., Goldfarb, I., Bebell, L. M., Yonker, L.M., Fasano, A., Elovitz, M. A., . . . Edlow, A. G. (2021). COVID-19 vaccine response in pregnant and lactating women: A cohort study. *AJOG.* https://www.ajog.org/article/S0002-9378(21)00187-3/fulltext#%20

Jering, K. S., Claggett, B. L., Cunningham, J. W., Rosenthal, N., Vardeny, O., Greene, M. F., & Solomon, S. D.. (2021). Maternal outcomes and COVID-19: Results from a large US-based cohort study of clinical characteristics and outcomes of hospitalized women giving birth with and without COVID-19. *JAMA Internal Medicine.* https://www.obgproject.com/2021/03/04/maternal-outcomes-following-childbirth-with-covid-19-results-from-a-large-us-based-population/?mc_cid=7395d163fc&mc_eid=7237b2c60f

Johns Hopkins University & Medicine. (2021). *Coronavirus resource center.* https://coronavirus.jhu.edu/us-map

Lokken, E., Huebner, E., Taylor, G., Hendrickson, S., Vanderhoeven, J., Kachikis, A., Coler, B., Walker, C. L., Sheng, J. S., Al-Haddad, B. J. S., McCartney, S. A., Kretzer, N. M., Resnick, R., Barnhart, N., Schulte, V., Bergam, B., Ma, K. K., Albright, C., Larios, V., . . . Waldorf, K. M. A. (2021). Disease severity, pregnancy outcomes and maternal deaths among pregnant patients with SARS-CoV-2 infection in Washington state. *American Journal of Obstetrics and Gynecology, 225*(1), 77.e1–77.e14. https://doi.org/10.1016/j.ajog.2020.12.1221

National Institutes of Health.(2021). COVID-19 Treatment Guidelines Panel. *Coronavirus Disease 2019 (COVID-19) Treatment Guidelines.* https://www.covid19treatmentguidelines.nih.gov/

Mahendra, V., & Murugan, S. (2020). Pregnant patients and COVID-19. In H. Prabhakar, I. Kapoor, and C. Mahajan (Eds.), *Clinical synopsis of COVID-19* (pp. 185–201). Springer. https://doi.org/10.1007/978-981-15-8681-1_11

Olliaro, P., Torreele, E., & Vaillant, M. (2021). COVID-19 vaccine efficacy and effectiveness—the elephant (not) in the room. *Lancet, 2*(7), e279–e280. https://www.thelancet.com/journals/lanmic/article/PIIS2666-5247(21)00069-0/fulltext

Onwuzurike, C., Diouf, K., Meadows, A., & Nour, N. (2020). Racial and ethnic disparities in severity of COVID-19 disease in pregnancy in the United States. *International Journal of Gynecology and Obstetrics, 151*(2), 293–295. https://doi.org/10.1002/ijgo.13333

Prabhu, M., Murphy, E. A., Sukhu, A. C., Yee, J., Singh, S., Eng, D., Zhao, Z., Riley, L. E., & Yang, Y. J. (2021). Antibody response to coronavirus disease 2019 (COVID-19) messenger RNA vaccination in pregnant women and transplacental passage into cord blood. *Obstetrics & Gynecology*, *138*(2), 278–280. https://doi.org/10.1097/AOG.0000000000004438

Salem, D., Katranji, F., & Bakdash, T. (2021). COVID-19 infection in pregnant women: Review of maternal and fetal outcomes. *International Journal of Gynecology and Obstetrics*, *152*(1), 291–298. https://doi.org/10.1002/ijgo.13533

Schwartz, D. A. (2020). The effects of pregnancy on women with COVID-19: Maternal and infant outcomes. *Clinical Infectious Diseases*, *71*(16), 2042–2044. https://doi.org/10.1093/cid/ciaa559

Vaught, J., & Halscott, T. (2021). Management considerations for pregnant patients with COVID-19. *Society for Maternal Fetal Medicine*. https://s3.amazonaws.com/cdn.smfm.org/media/2668/SMFM_COVID_Management_of_COVID_pos_preg_patients_1-7-21_(final).pdf?mc_cid=69ebd86ca6&mc_eid=7237b2c60f

Villar, J., Ariff, S., Gunier, R. B., Thiruvengadam, R., Rauch, S., Kholin, A., Roggero, P., Prefumo, F., do Vale, M. S., Cardona-Perez, J. A., Maiz, N., Cetin, I., Savasi, V., Deruelle, P., Easter, S. R., Sichitiu, J., Conti, C. P. S., Ernawati, E., Mhatre, M., . . . Papageorghiou, A. T. (2021). Maternal and neonatal morbidity and mortality among pregnant women with and without COVID-19 infection. *JAMA Pediatrics*. https://jamanetwork.com/journals/jamapediatrics/fullarticle/2779182?guestAccessKey=fed2ea98-6893-42aa-87e4-9664222f3842&utm_source=For_The_Media&utm_medium=referral&utm_campaign=ftm_links&utm_content=tfl&utm_term=042221

Appendices

A. Patient Resources and Instructions

KELLY D. ROSENBERGER | NANCY J. CIBULKA | MARY LEE BARRON

CHAPTER 1

INTERNET/WEB RESOURCES

American College of Obstetricians and Gynecologists. (2019). ACOG Committee Opinion No. 762: Prepregnancy Counseling. *Obstetrics & Gynecology,* 133(1), e78–e89. doi: 10.1097/AOG.0000000000003013

ACOG Patient Resources: www.acog.org/womens-health/faqs/good-health-before-pregnancy-prepregnancy-care

Before, Between and Beyond Pregnancy. beforeandbeyond.org/

Centers for Disease Control and Prevention: www.cdc.gov/preconception/planning.html

www.cdc.gov.ezp.slu.edu/ncbddd/preconception

Every Woman California: everywomancalifornia.org/

March of Dimes: www.marchofdimes.org/pregnancy/before-pregnancy.aspx

CHAPTER 2

GENETICS RESOURCES FOR PARENTS

National Institutes of Health, U.S. National Library of Medicine. Genetics home reference. medlineplus.gov/genetics/. This is a consumer-friendly guide to understanding more than 1,300 syndromes and genetic conditions.

American College of Obstetricians and Gynecologists. (2016, September). FAQ 164 Prenatal genetic diagnostic tests; FAQ 165 Prenatal genetic screening tests. www.acog.org/womens-health/faqs/prenatal-genetic-diagnostic-tests

Cystic Fibrosis Foundation. (n.d.). Retrieved from www.cff.org

March of Dimes. Cystic fibrosis and pregnancy. www.marchofdimes.org/complications/cystic-fibrosis-and-pregnancy.aspx

March of Dimes. Your family health history. www.marchofdimes.org/pregnancy/your-family-health-history.aspx

Mayo Clinic. Sickle cell anemia. www.mayoclinic.org/diseases-conditions/sickle-cell-anemia/symptoms-causes/syc-20355876

U.S. Department of Health and Human Services, National Institutes of Health, & National Heart, Lung, and Blood Institute. Thalassemias. www.nhlbi.nih.gov/health-topics/thalassemias

U.S. Department of Health and Human Services, National Institutes of Health, National Heart, Lung, and Blood Institute. Sickle cell disease. www.nhlbi.nih.gov/health-topics/sickle-cell-disease

U.S. Department of Health & Human Services. National Human Genome Research Institute Family Health Histories for patients and families. www.genome.gov/Health/Family-Health-History/Patients-Families

CDC. Family health history. www.cdc.gov/genomics/famhistory/knowing_not_enough.htm?CDC_AA_refVal=https%3A%2F%2Fwww.cdc.gov%2Ffeatures%2Ffamilyhealthhistory%2Findex.html

U.S. National Library of Medicine. PubMed Health. (2021). Sickle cell disease. www.ncbi.nlm.nih.gov/books/NBK482384/

U.S. National Library of Medicine. PubMed Health. (2021). Thalassemia. www.ncbi.nlm.nih.gov/books/NBK545151/

U.S. National Library of Medicine. PubMed Health. (2020). Cystic fibrosis (CF). www.ncbi.nlm.nih.gov/books/NBK493206/

Support Groups and Additional Information

Cystic fibrosis: cysticfibrosis.com/

Families of SMA: www.curesma.org/living-with-sma/

National Fragile X Foundation: fragilex.org/

National Heart, Lung, and Blood Institute: www.nhlbi.nih.gov/

National Tay-Sachs and Allied Diseases Association: rarediseases.org/organizations/national-tay-sachs-and-allied-diseases-association-inc/

Sickle Cell Disease Association of America: www.sicklecelldisease.org/

RESOURCES FOR HEALTHCARE PROFESSIONALS

Resources for Teratogenic Exposures in Pregnancy

American Academy of Pediatrics (AAP). www.aap.org/en-us/professional-resources/Pages/Professional-Resources.aspx

American College of Obstetricians and Gynecologists (ACOG). www.acog.org/

Food and Drug Administration (FDA). www.fda.gov/

March of Dimes. www.marchofdimes.org/pregnancy/over-the-counter-medicine-supplements-and-herbal-products.aspx

www.marchofdimes.org/pregnancy/alcohol-during-pregnancy.aspx

National Birth Defects Prevention Network. www.nbdpn.org/

National Birth Defects Prevention Study (Centers for Disease Control and Prevention): www.nbdps.org/National Institutes of Health (NIH). www.nichd.nih.gov/health/topics/pregnancy/conditioninfo

National Women's Health Information Center (U.S. Department of Health and Human Services [DHHS]). www.womenshealth.gov/

Organization of Teratology Information Specialists (OTIS). MotherToBaby: mothertobaby.org/about-otis/

REPROTOX (a subscription is required to access information). reprotox.org/

Teratogen Information System (TERIS) and Shephard's Catalog of Teratogenic Agents (a subscription is required to access some but not all information). deohs.washington.edu/teris/health-care-providers

Society for Birth Defects Research & Prevention (formerly known as The Teratology Society). birthdefectsresearch.org/

Genetics Textbooks and Compendia

Beery, T. A., Workman, M. L., & Eggert, J. A. (2018). *Genetics and genomics in nursing and health care* (2nd ed.). F. A. Davis.

Briggs, E. G., Freeman, R. K., Roger, K., Towers, C. V., & Forinash, A. B. (2017). *Drugs in pregnancy and lactation: A reference guide to fetal and neonatal risk* (11th ed.). Wolters Kluwer.

Shepard, T. H., Lemire, R. J., & Polifa, J. (2020). *Catalog of teratogenic agents.* Now online and currently distributed internationally by three publishers: IBM/Watson (Micromedex), RightAnswer.com and ToxPlanet. An electronic version of the catalog is also distributed by the University of Washington as a standalone product in conjunction with the TERIS database.

Tonkin, E., Calzone, K., Jenkins, J., Lea, D., & Prows, C. (2011). Genomic education resources for nursing faculty. *Journal of Nursing Scholarship, 43*, 330–340.

U.S. National Center for Biotechnology Information, National Institutes of Health, & National Library of Medicine. GeneTests. (2017). *Home page for GeneTests, GeneReviews, Laboratory and Clinic directories and educational material.* www.ncbi.nlm.nih.gov/sites/GeneTests

CHAPTER 3

NUTRITION IN PREGNANCY

2020–2025 Dietary Guidelines. www.dietaryguidelines.gov/resources/2020-2025-dietary-guidelines-online-materialsAmerican. Dietetic Association Resources for Women. www.eatright.org/for-women

Maternal Intake of Seafood and Omega-3 Fatty Acids. www.uptodate.com/contents/fish-consumption-and-marine-omega-3-fatty-acid-supplementation-in-pregnancy

U.S. Department of Agriculture Interactive Dietary Reference Intake and Estimated Energy Requirement Calculator. www.nal.usda.gov/fnic/interactiveDRI

CHAPTER 5

Resources for Healthcare Providers:

Al-Zidan, R. H. (2021). *Drugs in pregnancy: A handbook for pharmacists and physicians.* Apple Academic Press, Inc.

CHAPTER 6

PATIENT INSTRUCTIONS FOR FETAL ACTIVITY RECORD (OR KICK COUNTS)

Frequent fetal activity indicates a healthy baby. Monitor your baby's movements twice each day (morning and evening). Bring the record to each appointment.

1. Lie down on your side in a relaxing environment with no distractions. Continue to rest until you are aware of 10 baby movements.
2. If your baby moves 10 times in 1 hour or less, place a check under "Morning" or "Evening" in the following activity record.
3. If you are not aware of 10 movements in *1 hour or less*, repeat the same procedure for the next hour.
4. If you feel 10 movements during the second hour, you can be reassured that your baby is doing well. Continue monitoring *twice each day*.
5. If you do not feel 10 movements during the second hour, *contact your provider* or follow the instructions that your provider has previously given you.

DATE	MORNING	EVENING

Provider's name and phone number and any special instructions should be listed here.

CHAPTER 7

RESOURCES FOR SUCCESSFUL AND SAFE BREASTFEEDING

American Academy of Pediatrics. www.aap.org

American College of Nurse-Midwives. www.midwife.org

American College of Obstetricians and Gynecologists. www.acog.org/womens-health/infographics/breastfeeding-your-baby-breastfeeding-positions

Association of Women's Health, Obstetric and Neonatal Nurses (AWHONN). Healthy Mom & Baby at www.health4mom.org/category/healthy-moms/breastfeeding/

—www.thebump.com/topics/parenting-breastfeeding online community of mothers and nursing professionals

Centers for Disease Control and Prevention. www.cdc.gov/breastfeeding/index.htm

La Leche League (LLL) Breastfeeding Helpline 877-452-5324. www.llli.org/breastfeeding-info/

www.facebook.com/pg/LaLecheLeagueUSA/events/.

Maternal health and nutrition during breastfeeding (Beyond the basics). www.uptodate.com/contents/maternal-health-and-nutrition-during-breast-feeding-beyond-the-basics?search=patient-information-maternal-health-and-nutrition-during-breastfeeding-beyond-the-basics&source=search_result&selectedTitle=1~150&usage_type=default&display_rank=1

Womenshealth.gov offers a free online publication: Your Guide to Breastfeeding at www.womenshealth.gov/breastfeedingfact sheets on a variety of important topics (800)-994-9662.

Medications and Breastfeeding

LactMed, National Library of Medicine, National Institutes of Health.

www.nlm.nih.gov/toxnet/index.html https://www.nlm.nih.gov/toxnet/Accessing_LactMed_Content_from_NCBI_Bookshelf.htmlDatabase includes alternate drugs to consider.

CHAPTER 8

RESOURCES ON POSTPARTUM DEPRESSION FOR PATIENTS

ACOG Patient Page, Postpartum Depression (FAQs) at www.acog.org/womens-health/faqs/postpartum-depression

eMedicine's Depression Center includes information on Postpartum Depression at www.emedicinehealth.com/depression/center.htm

March of Dimes Postpartum Depression Information at www.marchofdimes.org/pregnancy/postpartum-depression.aspx

National Institute of Mental Health, National Institutes of Health, Department of Health and Human Services Phone: 866 615 6464 or 866 415 8051 (TTY) or 1-800-662-HELP (4357)

www.nimh.nih.gov/health/topics/depression/

Postpartum Education for Parents Phone: 805-564-3888

Postpartum Support International Phone: 855-631001 or 6314222255

National Suicide Prevention Lifeline Phone: 800-273TALK (8255) or online chat

Substance Abuse and Mental Health Services Administration Publications, U.S. Department of Health and Human Services Phone: 877-726-4727

WomensHealth.Gov (800–994–9662). Depression during and after pregnancy fact sheet at www.womenshealth.gov/publications/our-publications/fact-sheet/depression-pregnancy.html

CHAPTER 9

PATIENT AND PROVIDER RESOURCES FOR DENTAL CARE AND ORAL HEALTH DURING PREGNANCY

American Academy of Pediatrics. www.aap.org

American Academy of Periodontology. www.perio.org

American College of Obstetricians and Gynecologists. www.acog.org

American Dental Association. www.ada.org

California Dental Association. www.cdafoundation.org/education/perinatal-oral-health

Institute of Medicine. (2011). *Advancing oral health in America*. www.hrsa.gov/publichealth/clinical/oralhealth/advancingoralhealth.pdf

www.hrsa.gov/sites/default/files/publichealth/clinical/oralhealth/advancingoralhealth.pdf

Share with Women patient education handout from the American College of Nurse Midwives, onlinelibrary.wiley.com/page/journal/15422011/homepage/share-with-women

WebMd Oral Health Center, www.webmd.com/oral-health/dental-care-pregnancy

CHAPTER 11

PATIENT INFORMATION FOR RESPIRATORY ILLNESS IN PREGNANCY

American Academy of Allergy, Asthma, and Immunology. www.aaaai.org

American Lung Association. www.lungusa.org

Asthma topics. www.cdc.gov/asthma/default.htm

Centers for Disease Control and Prevention. www.cdc.gov

Homecare for the flu. www.cdc.gov/flu/takingcare.htm

Mayo Clinic medical information and tools for healthy living. www.mayoclinic.org/patient-care-and-health-information

National Heart, Lung, and Blood Institute. www.nhlbi.nih.gov

The National Library of Medicine. www.nlm.nih.gov/medlineplus/healthtopics.html

Pregnant women and influenza. www.cdc.gov/flu/protect/vaccine/pregnant.htm

Seasonal influenza. www.cdc.gov/flu

Upper respiratory tract infection: Adult treatment guidelines. www.cdc.gov/getsmart/campaign-materials/treatment-guidelines.html

UptoDate for Patients and Caregivers (free Beyond the Basics content). www.uptodate.com/home/uptodate-subscription-options-patients

CHAPTER 18

PATIENT RESOURCES ON PREECLAMPSIA

American College of Obstetricians and Gynecologists (ACOG). *For patients: Preeclampsia and high blood pressure during pregnancy FAQs.* www.acog.org/womens-health/faqs/preeclampsia-and-high-blood-pressure-during-pregnancy?utm_source=redirect&utm_medium=web&utm_campaign=otn

Up to Date Patient education: Preeclampsia (Beyond the basics). www.uptodate.com/contents/preeclampsia-beyond-the-basics?search=patient-information-preeclampsia-beyond-the-basics&source=search_result&selectedTitle=1~150&usage_type=default&display_rank=1

March of Dimes. (2021). *Pregnancy complications: Preeclampsia.* www.marchofdimes.org/complications/preeclampsia.aspx

Mayo Clinic. (2014). *Preeclampsia.* www.mayoclinic.org/diseases-conditions/preeclampsia/symptoms-causes/syc-20355745

National Heart Lung and Blood Institute. (n.d.). *High blood pressure in pregnancy.* www.nhlbi.nih.gov/health-topics/high-blood-pressure

Preeclampsia Foundation. www.preeclampsia.org/

Grow by WebMD. (2021). *Preeclampsia.* www.webmd.com/baby/preeclampsia-eclampsia#1

CHAPTER 19

PATIENT RESOURCES FOR UP-TO-DATE INFORMATION ABOUT PRETERM LABOR AND PRETERM BIRTH PREVENTION

American College of Obstetricians and Gynecologists Patient Page, www.acog.org/patients

Centers for Disease Control and Prevention. (2021). *Pregnancy.* www.cdc.gov/pregnancy/index.html

Centers for Disease Control and Prevention, Division of Reproductive Health. (2015). *Preterm birth.* www.cdc.gov/reproductivehealth/maternalinfanthealth/pretermbirth.htm

Funai, E. F. (2021). *Patient education: Preterm labor (Beyond the basics).* www.uptodate.com/contents/preterm-labor-beyond-the-basics?source=search_result&search=preterm+labor&selectedTitle=1%7E5

March of Dimes. (2021). *Fighting premature birth.* www.marchofdimes.org/mission/prematurity-campaign.aspx

March of Dimes. (2021). *Preterm labor and premature birth.* www.marchofdimes.org/preterm-labor-and-premature-baby.aspx

Mayo Clinic Staff. (2021). *Preterm labor.* www.mayoclinic.org/diseases-conditions/preterm-labor/symptoms-causes/syc-20376842

U.S. National Library of Medicine. National Institutes of Health. (2021). *Premature babies: Medline plus* (The National Library of Medicine provides links to the latest research on prematurity). medlineplus.gov/prematurebabies.html

Grow by WebMD. (2021). *Premature labor and birth – The basics explained*. www.webmd.com/baby/understanding-preterm-labor-birth-basics#1

CHAPTER 20

PATIENT RESOURCES ON HIV PREVENTION AND PREGNANCY

Resources and topics from the Centers for Disease Control and Prevention are available at www.cdc.gov/hiv and include the following:

- AIDS.gov
- Federal resources on HIV/AIDS
- AIDSInfo
- Information on treatment and clinical trials
- Black Women's Health Imperative. bwhi.org/
- The Black Women's Health Imperative seeks to improve the health of Black women by providing wellness education and services, health information, and advocacy
- Get tested: HIV Testing Resources,
- Locate an HIV and sexually transmitted infection testing location near you.
- HIV/AIDS Fact Sheets
- HIV Basics
- HIV by Group (including pregnancy)Information and resources for women and HIV
- HIV Risk and Prevention
- HIV Risk Reduction Tool at hivrisk.cdc.gov/
- HIV Research· HIV in the Workplace
- WomensHealth.gov Sponsored by the Department of Health and Human Services Office on Women's Health; empowering women to live healthier lives www.womenshealth.gov/

CDC at www.cdc.gov supports the dissemination of effective HIV behavioral interventions for women, such as the following:

Sistering, Informing, Healing, Living, and Empowering (SIHLE) is a group-level intervention aimed at reducing risk behaviors among sexually active Black teenagers aged 14 to 18 years.

Sister to Sister is a brief, one-on-one, skills-based behavioral intervention for sexually active African American women aged 18 to 45 years to reduce sexual risk behaviors and prevent HIV and other sexually transmitted infections.

Women Involved in Life Learning from Other Women (WILLOW) is a social-skills building and educational intervention for adult heterosexual women, aged 18 to 50 years, living with HIV infection.

CHAPTER 21

RESOURCES FOR ZIKA INFORMATION AND PREVENTION IN PREGNANCY

American College of Obstetricians and Gynecologists: Zika virus and pregnancy at www.acog.org/womens-health/infographics/zika-virus-and-pregnancy

Zika prevention information at www.cdc.gov/zika/prevention/index.html
Latest Zika travel notices at wwwnc.cdc.gov/travel/page/zika-information
Zika virus information at www.cdc.gov/zika/
Zika and pregnancy at www.cdc.gov/zika/pregnancy/index.html

CHAPTER 22

PROFESSIONAL DEVELOPMENT COURSES ON DISASTER PREPAREDNESS FOR HEALTHCARE PROVIDERS

Disaster Preparedness and Response by Nurses is a two-contact-hour web-based course originally funded by Sigma Theta Tau International and the Red Cross. It is available for a nominal fee at www.nursingce.com/ceu-courses/disaster-planning

Funded by Congress, the Centers for Disease Control and Prevention sponsors disaster preparedness training for 14 Preparedness and Emergency Response Learning Centers (PERLC) throughout the United States to meet the educational needs of the public health work force. Core competency-based training is provided to states, local, and tribal public health authorities through short single-module courses and longer series. Learn more at www.cdc.gov/phpr/perlc.htm and emergency.cdc.gov/coca/trainingresources.asp

National Nurse Emergency Preparedness Initiative (NNEPI) course, Nurses on the Front Line: Preparing for Emergencies and Disasters, is an interactive web-based course available at nnepi.gwnursing.org/

RESOURCES ON DISASTER PREPAREDNESS FOR PARENTS AND PROFESSIONALS

American Academy of Pediatricians. www.aap.org

American Congress of Nurse-Midwives, Emergency preparedness for childbirth.

www.midwife.org/ACNM/files/ccLibraryFiles/Filename/000000000731/Emergency%20Preparedness%20for%20Childbirth.pdf

American College of Obstetricians and Gynecologists. www.acog.org and www.acog.org/clinical/clinical-guidance/committee-opinion/articles/2010/06/preparing-for-disasters-perspectives-on-women

American Red Cross. www.redcross.org

Association of Women's Health, Obstetrics, and Neonatal Nursing. www.awhonn.org

Centers for Disease Control and Prevention. www.cdc.gov

For specific information about natural disasters or weather emergencies, see e emergency.cdc.gov/disasters

Federal Emergency Management Agency (FEMA), www.fema.gov or www.ready.gov provides detailed information for making a plan at www.fema.gov/pdf/areyouready/areyouready_full.pdf

La Leche League. www.llli.org

March of Dimes. www.marchofdimes.com

U.S. Department of Health and Human Services Office on Women's Health. www.womenshealth.gov

Women and Infants Service Package, National Working Group for Women and Infant Needs in Emergencies, White Ribbon Alliance. www.ennonline.net/attachments/836/wisp-final-07-27-07-usa.pdf

Several apps are available for emergency alert, family safety, first aid, pet care, blood donation, shelter, and more. Get more information at www.fema.gov/about/news-multimedia/mobile-app-text-messages and www.redcross.org/get-help/how-to-prepare-for-emergencies/mobile-apps.html

The National Health Security Preparedness Index Report can be found at www.tfah.org/wp-content/uploads/2021/03/TFAH_ReadyOrNot2021_Fnl.pdf

CHAPTER 23

RESOURCES FOR THYROID DISORDERS IN PREGNANCY AND POSTPARTUM

Society Guideline Link – Hypothyroidism. www-uptodate-com.proxy.cc.uic.edu/contents/society-guideline-links-hypothyroidism?search=thyroid%20diseases%20and%20pregnancy&topicRef=16609&source=see_link

Information for Patients: Patient Education: Congenital hypothyroidism. www-uptodate-com.proxy.cc.uic.edu/contents/congenital-hypothyroidism-the-basics?search=thyroid%20diseases%20and%20pregnancy&topicRef=16609&source=see_link

Society Guideline Link – Hyperthyroidism. www-uptodate-com.proxy.cc.uic.edu/contents/society-guideline-links-hyperthyroidism?search=thyroid%20diseases%20and%20pregnancy&topicRef=7884&source=see_link

Information for Patients - Patient education: Hyperthyroidism (overactive thyroid) and pregnancy. www-uptodate-com.proxy.cc.uic.edu/contents/hyperthyroidism-overactive-thyroid-and-pregnancy-the-basics?search=thyroid%20diseases%20and%20pregnancy&topicRef=7884&source=see_link

Society Guideline Links: Thyroid disease in pregnancy. www-uptodate-com.proxy.cc.uic.edu/contents/society-guideline-links-thyroid-disease-in-pregnancy?search=thyroid%20diseases%20and%20pregnancy&topicRef=7831&source=see_link

Information for Patients - Patient education: Thyroiditis after pregnancy. www-uptodate-com.proxy.cc.uic.edu/contents/thyroiditis-after-pregnancy-the-basics?search=thyroid%20diseases%20and%20pregnancy&topicRef=7831&source=see_link

CHAPTER 24

COVID-19 RESOURCES

Experts are learning more every day about the new coronavirus that causes COVID-19. The American College of Obstetricians and Gynecologists (ACOG), the Centers for Disease Control (CDC), Society for Maternal-Fetal Medicine (SMFM), American College of Nurse Midwives (ACNM), and the Association of Women's Health, Obstetric and Neonatal Nurses (AWHONN) are following the situation closely. The following resources are updated as new information becomes available for pregnant and breastfeeding individuals.

American College of Obstetricians and Gynecologists. *Coronavirus, pregnancy, and breastfeeding: A message for patients.* www.acog.org/womens-health/faqs/coronavirus-covid-19-pregnancy-and-breastfeeding

Centers for Disease Control and Prevention. www.cdc.gov/coronavirus/2019-ncov/index.html

Centers for Disease Control and Prevention. *Information for healthcare workers.* www.cdc.gov/coronavirus/2019-nCoV/hcp/index.html

Centers for Disease Control and Prevention. *Information for clinic preparedness.* www.cdc.gov/coronavirus/2019-ncov/hcp/clinic-preparedness.html

Centers for Disease Control and Prevention. *Information for managing COVID-19 patients.* www.cdc.gov/coronavirus/2019-ncov/hcp/clinical-guidance-management-patients.html

Centers for Disease Control and Prevention. *Information for COVID-19 vaccination.* www.cdc.gov/vaccines/covid-19/index.html

Centers for Disease Control and Prevention. *Use of cloth face coverings to help slow the spread of COVID-19.* www.cdc.gov/coronavirus/2019-ncov/prevent-getting-sick/diy-cloth-face-coverings.html

Centers for Disease Control and Prevention. *Public health recommendations for vaccinated persons.* www.cdc.gov/vaccines/covid-19/info-by-product/clinical-considerations.html

Centers for Disease Control and Prevention. *Travel guidance.* www.cdc.gov/coronavirus/2019-ncov/travelers/index.html

Centers for Disease Control and Prevention. *COVID-19 Travel recommendations by destination.* www.cdc.gov/coronavirus/2019-ncov/travelers/map-and-travel-notices.html

Centers for Disease Control and Prevention. Coping with stress for healthcare workers. www.cdc.gov/coronavirus/2019-ncov/hcp/mental-health-healthcare.html

Society for Maternal Fetal Medicine. *Patient education: COVID-19 vaccines and pregnancy.* www.highriskpregnancyinfo.org/covid-19

The Path to Zero: Key Metrics for COVID Suppression. globalepidemics.org/key-metrics-for-covid-suppression/

U.S. Department of State – Bureau of Consular Affairs. *COVID-19 traveler information.* travel.state.gov/content/travel/en/traveladvisories/ea/covid-19-information.html

B. Screening Tools

MARY LEE BARRON | KELLY D. ROSENBERGER

I. SUBSTANCE USE

A. SUBSTANCE USE RISK PROFILE—PREGNANCY SCALE

1. Have you ever smoked marijuana?
2. In the month before you knew you were pregnant, how many beers, how much wine, or how much liquor did you drink?
3. Have you ever felt that you needed to cut down on your drug or alcohol use?

Scoring: Answering yes to one question = moderate risk; answering yes to two or three questions = high risk of having a positive screen for alcohol or illicit drug use.

B. CAGE-AID

Have you ever felt that you needed to cut down on your drug or alcohol use? Have people annoyed you by criticizing your drinking or drug use? Have you felt bad or guilty about your drinking or drug use? Have you ever had a drink or used drugs in the morning to steady your nerves or to get rid of a hangover (eye-opener)?

Scoring: Item responses on the CAGE questions are scored 0 for "no" and 1 for "yes" answers, with a higher score being an indication of drug or alcohol problems. A total score of two or greater is considered clinically significant.

The American College of Obstetricians and Gynecologists offers information on Marijuana and Pregnancy at www.acog.org/womens-health/faqs/marijuana-and-pregnancy

II. TOBACCO USE

A. 5 As

1. *Ask*: Ask the patient to choose a statement that best describes smoking status.
2. *Advise*: Ask permission to share the health message about smoking during pregnancy.
3. *Assess*: Readiness to change.
4. *Assist*: Briefly explore problem-solving methods and skills for smoking cessation.
5. *Arrange*: Let the patient know that you will be following up on each visit; assess smoking status at subsequent prenatal visits; affirm efforts to quit (U.S. Preventive Services Task Force, 2021).

III. DEPRESSION

A. TWO-QUESTION BRIEF

1. Over the past 2 weeks, have you felt down, depressed, or hopeless?
2. Over the past 2 weeks, have you felt little interest in doing things?

B. ANTENATAL EXPOSURE TO DEPRESSION RESOURCE

The Massachusetts General Hospital Center for Women's Mental Health at Harvard University offers information at womensmentalhealth.org/posts/depression-fathers-increases-risk-adolescent-depression/

C. EDINBURGH POSTNATAL DEPRESSION SCALE

The Edinburgh Postnatal Depression Scale is available at med.stanford.edu/content/dam/sm/ppc/documents/DBP/EDPS_text_added.pdf

A score of 10 or greater indicates the likelihood of depression but not its severity.

D. American College of Obstetricians and Gynecologists offers screening information at resources and overview of depression tools for screening

www.acog.org/womens-health/faqs/depression-during-pregnancy

IV. INTIMATE PARTNER VIOLENCE

A. The hurt, insult, threaten, and scream (HITS) Instrument

Both English and Spanish versions of the four-item HITS instrument have sensitivity and specificity greater than 85%. HITS consists of the following four screening questions:

"How often does your partner...

1. Hurt: Physically hurt you (e.g., push, slap, hit, kick, punch)?
2. Insult: Insult or talk down to you?
3. Threaten: Threaten you with harm?
4. Scream: Scream or curse at you?"

Patients responded to each of these items with a 5-point frequency format: never, rarely, sometimes, fairly often, and frequently.

Score values could range from a minimum of 4 to a maximum of 20 (Sherin, Sinacore, Li, Zitter, & Shakil, 1998).

A HITS cut-off score of 11 or greater indicates a woman who is victimized.

B. THE ONGOING VIOLENCE ASSESSMENT TOOL

This four-item tool has a specificity of 83% to 85% and a sensitivity of 86% to 93% when used in an emergency department and on varied populations of men and women.

1. At the present time, does your partner threaten you with a weapon?
2. At the present time, does your partner beat you so badly that you must seek medical help?
3. At the present time, does your partner act like he or she would like to kill you?
4. My partner has no respect for my feelings (never, rarely, occasionally, often, always) (Weiss, Ernst, Cham, & Nick, 2003).

C. ONGOING ABUSE SCREEN OR ABUSE ASSESSMENT SCREEN (FIVE ITEMS)

1. Are you presently emotionally or physically abused by your partner or someone important to you?

2. Are you presently being hit, slapped, kicked, or otherwise physically hurt by your partner or someone important to you?
3. Are you presently being forced to have sexual activities?
4. Are you afraid of your partner or any one of the following (circle if applicable): husband/wife; ex-husband/ex-wife; boyfriend/girlfriend; stranger?
5. (If pregnant) Have you been hit, slapped, kicked, or otherwise physically hurt by your partner or someone important to you during pregnancy (Weiss et al., 2003)?
6. Scoring procedures: If any questions on the screen are answered affirmatively, the ongoing abuse screen is considered positive for ongoing abuse.

D. THE HUMILIATION, AFRAID, RAPE, KICK (HARK) INSTRUMENT

1. Humiliation: Within the past year, have you been humiliated or emotionally abused in other ways by your partner or your ex-partner?
2. Afraid: Within the past year, have you been afraid of your partner or ex-partner?
3. Rape: Within the past year, have you been raped or forced to have any kind of sexual activity by your partner or ex-partner?
4. Kick: Within the past year, have you been kicked, hit, slapped, or otherwise physically hurt by your partner or ex-partner?

One point is given for every yes answer; a score of greater than 1 is positive for intimate partner violence (IPV) (Sohal, Eldridge, & Feder, 2007).

E. THE WOMAN ABUSE SCREENING TOOL

1. In general, how would you describe your relationship?
   a lot of tension some tension no tension
2. Do you and your partner work out arguments with
   great difficulty some difficulty no difficulty
3. Do arguments ever result in you feeling put down or bad about yourself?
   often sometimes never
4. Do arguments ever result in hitting, kicking, or pushing?
   often sometimes never
5. Do you ever feel frightened by what your partner says or does?
   often sometimes never
6. Has your partner ever abused you physically?
   often sometimes never
7. Has your partner ever abused you emotionally?
   often sometimes never
8. Has your partner ever abused you sexually?
   often sometimes never

To score this instrument, the responses are assigned a number. For the first question, "a lot of tension" gets a score of 1 and the other two get a 0. For the second question, "great difficulty" gets a score of 1 and the other two get 0. For the remaining questions, "often" gets a score of 1, "sometimes" gets a score of 2, and "never" gets a score of 3 (Brown, Lent, Brett, Sas, & Pederson, 1996). The items are summed to calculate the overall score. The interpretation is based on clinical judgment as no fixed positive scoring is assigned.

F. HAWAII RISK INDICATORS SCREENING TOOL

Based on the medical record or interview, score items as "true," "false," or "unknown."

1. Unmarried
2. Partner employed
3. Inadequate income

4. Unstable housing
5. No phone
6. Education less than 12 years
7. Inadequate emergency contacts
8. History of substance use
9. Inadequate prenatal care
10. History of abortions
11. History of psychiatric care
12. Abortion unsuccessfully sought or attempted
13. Adoption sought or attempted
14. Marital or family problems
15. History of depression

Positive screen: true score on item numbers 1, 9, or 12; two or more true scores; seven or more unknown (Duggan et al., 2000).

V. SCREENING FOR FOOD SECURITY (DOES THE HOUSEHOLD HAVE ENOUGH FOOD?)

INSTRUCTIONS: Select the appropriate answers depending on the number of persons and number of adults in the household.

Provider: I'm going to read you several statements that people have made about their food situation. For these statements, please tell me whether the statement was *often* true, *sometimes* true, or *never* true for (you/your household) in the past 12 months—that is, since last (name of current month).

1. The first statement is, "The food that (I/we) bought just didn't last, and (I/we) didn't have money to get more." Was that often, sometimes, or never true for (you/your household) in the past 12 months?

[]Often true
[]Sometimes true
[]Never true
[]Don't know (DK) or refused

2. "(I/we) couldn't afford to eat balanced meals." Was that often, sometimes, or never true for (you/your household) in the past 12 months?

[]Often true
[]Sometimes true
[]Never true
[]DK or refused

3. In the past 12 months, since last (name of current month), did (you/you or other adults in your household) ever cut the size of your meals or skip meals because there wasn't enough money for food?

[]Yes
[]No (Skip 3a)
[]DK (Skip 3a)

3a. [IF YES ABOVE, ASK] How often did this happen—almost every month, some months but not every month, or in only 1 or 2 months?

[]Almost every month
[]Some months, but not every month
[]Only 1 or 2 months
[]DK

4. In the past 12 months, did you ever eat less than you felt you should because there wasn't enough money for food?

[]Yes
[]No
[]DK

5. In the past 12 months, were you very hungry but didn't eat because there wasn't enough money for food?

[]Yes
[]No
[]DK

USER NOTES: Coding Responses and Assessing Households' Food Security Status:

Responses of "often" or "sometimes" on questions 1 and 2 and "yes" on 2, 3, and 4 are coded as affirmative (yes). Responses of "almost every month" and "some months but not every month" on 3a are coded as affirmative (yes). The sum of affirmative responses to the six questions in the module is the household's raw score on the scale.

Food security status is assigned as follows:

1. Raw score 0 to 1—High or marginal food security (raw score 1 may be considered marginal food security, but a large proportion of households that would be measured as having marginal food security using the household or adult scale will have a raw score of zero on the six-item scale).
2. Raw score 2 to 4—Low food security
3. Raw score 5 to 6—Very low food security

BIBLIOGRAPHY

American College of Obstetricians and Gynecologists Committee Opinion no. 757. (2018). Screening for perinatal depression. *Obstetrics & Gynecology, 132*(5), e208–e212. https://doi.org/10.1097/AOG.0000000000002927

Brown, J. B., Lent, B., Brett, P., Sas, G., & Pederson, L. (1996). Development of the woman abuse screening tool for use in family practice. *Family Medicine, 28*, 422–428.

Duggan, A., Windham, A., McFarlane, E., Fuddy, L., Rohde, C., Buchbinder, S., & Sia, C. (2000). Hawaii's Healthy Start program of home visiting for at-risk families: Evaluation of family identification, family engagement, and service delivery. *Pediatrics, 105*, 250–259.

Ewing, J. A. (1984). Detecting alcoholism: The CAGE questionnaire. *JAMA, 252*, 1905–1907. https://doi.org/10.1001/jama.1984.03350140051025

Sherin, K. M., Sinacore, J. M., Li, X. Q., Zitter, R. E., & Shakil, A. (1998). HITS: A short domestic violence screening tool for use in a family practice setting. *Family Medicine, 30*(7), 508–512.

Sohal, H., Eldridge, S., & Feder, G. (2007). The sensitivity and specificity of four questions (HARK) to identify intimate partner violence: A diagnostic accuracy study in general practice. *BMC Family Practice*. https://doi.org/10.1186/1471-2296-8-49 *8*,49

U.S. Preventive Services Task Force. (2021). *Tobacco smoking cessation in adults, including pregnant persons: Interventions.* https://www.uspreventiveservicestaskforce.org/uspstf/recommendation/tobacco-use-in-adults-and-pregnant-women-counseling-and-interventions

USDA Food Security Survey. (2012). *U.S. household. food security survey module: Six-item short form.* Economic Research Service, USDA. https://www.ers.usda.gov/media/8282/short2012.pdf

Weiss, S., Ernst, A., Cham, E., & Nick, T. (2003). Development of a screen for ongoing intimate partner violence. *Violence and Victims, 18*(2), 131–141. https://doi.org/10.1891/vivi.2003.18.2.131

C. Common Approach to HIV Testing in Pregnancy for Barnes-Jewish Hospital: A Consensus of the HIV Perinatal Working Group of Washington University School of Medicine

NANCY J. CIBULKA | KELLY D. ROSENBERGER

The goal of routine HIV testing in pregnancy is to prevent perinatal transmission of HIV without patients feeling judged or stigmatized. Testing can occur using an opt-out counseling approach, but it is inappropriate to test a patient for HIV without her knowledge. The decision to decline testing should be respected.

A. FIRST PRENATAL VISIT

1. All patients will be offered HIV testing at the first prenatal visit in an opt-out fashion. This test will be a standard HIV fourth-generation antibody test, sent to the lab. Opt-out language should be used: "An HIV test will be performed as a part of routine prenatal care for all patients. Is that okay?" Patients who decline will again be offered testing later in the pregnancy.

2. Patients who decline will be asked why they decline in an attempt to get 100% compliance with testing and dispel any myths or concerns related to the test. All patients will be encouraged to accept the test without judgment and informed that the pediatrician will want the result to care for the baby. The reason for declining the test should be documented.

3. Patients can be counseled that if the HIV test is positive, knowing the diagnosis and treating appropriately can decrease transmission to the newborn from about 25% to less than 2%.

4. Positive results will be confirmed with additional testing.

5. A patient who has confirmed HIV infection will be informed about the results and counseled by the primary physician or nurse practitioner. The patient will be linked to care for adult and pediatric infectious disease (ID) clinics. Maternal-fetal medicine/obstetrics consult will be obtained.

B. 34- TO 36-WEEK VISIT

1. A third-trimester standard HIV-1 and HIV-2 fourth-generation antibody test will be offered in an opt-out fashion for all patients around 34 to 36 weeks. This test will also be done in an opt-out fashion with the patient being informed that this is a part of routine prenatal care. The wishes of patients who decline this screening will be respected, and the patient will be asked the reason for declining the test, which should be documented. If a patient declines, they should be asked whether there are any risks for HIV transmission during the pregnancy, including a new sexual partner, multiple sexual partners, a sexually transmitted infection during the pregnancy, intravenous (IV) drug use, occupational blood exposure, living in area with high HIV prevalence, or having a HIV infected partner. If any of these are positive, then the testing should be strongly encouraged.

2. Patients can be counseled that if the HIV test is positive, knowing the diagnosis and treating appropriately can decrease transmission to the newborn.

C. ADMISSION TO PREGNANCY ASSESSMENT CENTER OR LABOR AND DELIVERY

1. Patients with no prenatal care or who are presenting at more than 36 weeks should be assessed to see whether HIV testing is appropriate.

2. Rapid HIV testing using OraQuick enzyme immune assay (EIA) is available as a point-of-care test in the hospital. This testing will be performed using a rapid testing method on whole blood (preferred) or saliva as a point-of-care test in the pregnancy assessment center.

3. All available prenatal records should be reviewed before approaching patients about HIV testing, including recent hospital and laboratory visits.

4. Patients who have had both first-trimester and third-trimester negative HIV tests should not be offered repeat rapid testing unless very high risk (i.e., partner with HIV or recent IV drug use).

5. Patients who do not have prenatal records available should be asked whether they had HIV testing during the pregnancy and if a third-trimester test was done.

6. Patients who have not had HIV testing at any time during the pregnancy should receive an OraQuick point-of-care test using an opt-out counseling approach.

7. Patients who have a first-trimester negative HIV test and no third-trimester test should be offered OraQuick opt-out testing based on any positive risk factors such as:

- **a.** Recent IV drug use or sex with IV drug user
- **b.** A sexually transmitted infection within the last year
- **c.** A positive answer to the question, "Have you had a new sexual partner or more than one partner during your pregnancy?"

D. TEST RESULTS

1. Patients with positive OraQuick testing should have Western blot testing done as soon as possible.

2. For patients in the third trimester, an infectious disease consult should be called immediately for follow-up of any positive or indeterminant test results.

3. Patients with a positive HIV-1 or HIV-2 antibody test should have HIV ribonucleic acid viral load testing performed rapidly (especially in the third trimester).

4. For patients in the third trimester, an infectious disease consult should be called immediately for follow-up of any positive or indeterminant tests. Pediatricians should also be notified of patients expected to deliver during this hospitalization.

5. Situations may arise when it is necessary to counsel patients and start zidovudine (also known as ZDV or AZT) based on an unconfirmed OraQuick test. This should be discussed with the patient privately, and AZT should be recommended and started until follow-up testing confirms or refutes the diagnosis or the patient delivers. Breastfeeding should not be performed until the diagnosis is clearly negative. An infectious disease consult should be obtained to assist in test interpretation and counseling. Pediatricians should be notified as well to allow time for discussion about a treatment plan for the infant.

Reprinted with permission from the HIV Perinatal Working Group of Washington University School of Medicine.

D. Federal Employment Laws on Work Break

MARY LEE BARRON | KELLY D. ROSENBERGER

1. Bathroom Breaks

There is no federal law that directly addresses bathroom breaks; however, the Occupational Safety and Health Administration determined that an employer may not impose unreasonable restrictions on employees' use of the [toilet] facilities. In other words, there are no strict rules regarding time limits or pay for bathroom breaks, but workers should have access to bathrooms and be able to use them when needed.

2. Health Breaks

Title I of the Americans with Disabilities Act (ADA) is designed to prevent discrimination in the workplace against individuals with disabilities. Under the ADA, an employer must make reasonable accommodation for special needs. This includes breaks for individuals with diabetes to have snacks and check their blood levels. The ADA does not provide a list of other health breaks, instead preferring the details to be worked out between employer and worker or, if necessary, in court.

3. Meal Period

If an employee is relieved of work duties during a meal break, the period is considered to be unpaid time. Federal law requires the employer to pay for the meal period if the employee is not completely relieved of his work duties. Paid meal periods count toward the employee's 40-hour workweek.

4. Nursing Break

The Patient Protection and Affordable Care Act was enacted on March 23, 2010, with a provision for nursing mothers. The provision requires employers to make reasonable efforts to extend breaks and a private location to a nursing mother for the purpose of expressing breast milk for her child. The provision extends this right to the mother for up to 1 year after the child's birth.

5. Rest Break

Authorized rest breaks are generally scheduled for 20 minutes or less. Federal law views such breaks as paid time. As paid time, the period counts toward the time needed to complete a 40-hour workweek. Employees are paid an overtime premium for hours worked in excess of 40 hours for the week.

6. Sleep Breaks

Employees who work for more than 24 consecutive hours may need breaks to sleep. Federal employment laws do not mandate that employers provide sleeping breaks in these circumstances. However, if the worker arranges such a break with the employer, the employer does not need to pay for the break. According to the Fair Labor Standards Act (FLSA), sleeping breaks are not hours worked. To qualify as a sleeping break, the period must be between 5 and 8 hours.

Read more: Federal Employment Laws on Breaks at www.ehow.com/about_5208554_federal-employment-laws-breaks.html#ixzz257pp7AhK

www.dol.gov/general/topic/workhours/breaks

PREGNANCY DISCRIMINATION

Pregnancy discrimination involves treating a woman (an applicant or employee) unfavorably because of pregnancy, childbirth, or a medical condition related to pregnancy or childbirth (see www.eeoc.gov/pregnancy-discrimination).

PREGNANCY DISCRIMINATION AND WORK SITUATIONS

"The Pregnancy Discrimination Act (PDA) forbids discrimination based on pregnancy when it comes to any aspect of employment, including hiring, firing, pay, job assignments, promotions, layoff, training, fringe benefits such as leave and health insurance, and any other term or condition of employment."

PREGNANCY DISCRIMINATION AND TEMPORARY DISABILITY

If a woman is temporarily unable to perform her job because of a medical condition related to pregnancy or childbirth, the employer or other covered entity must treat her in the same way as it treats any other temporarily disabled employee. For example, the employer may have to provide light duty, alternative assignments, disability leave, or unpaid leave to pregnant employees if it does so for other temporarily disabled employees.

In addition, impairments resulting from pregnancy (e.g., gestational diabetes or preeclampsia, a condition characterized by pregnancy-induced hypertension and protein in the urine) may be disabilities under the ADA. An employer may have to provide a reasonable accommodation (such as leave or modifications that enable an employee to perform her job) for a disability related to pregnancy, absent undue hardship (significant difficulty or expense). The ADA Amendments Act of 2008 makes it much easier to show that a medical condition is a covered disability. For more information about the ADA, see www.eeoc.gov/laws/types/disability.cfm

For information about the ADA Amendments Act, see www.eeoc.gov/laws/types/disability_regulations.cfm and www.eeoc.gov/regulations-related-disability-discrimination

PREGNANCY DISCRIMINATION AND HARASSMENT

It is unlawful to harass a woman because of pregnancy, childbirth, or a medical condition related to pregnancy or childbirth. Harassment is illegal when it is so frequent or severe that it creates a hostile or offensive work environment or when it results in an adverse employment decision (such as the victim being fired or demoted). The harasser can be the victim's supervisor, a supervisor in another area, a coworker, or someone who is not an employee of the employer, such as a client or customer.

PREGNANCY, MATERNITY, AND PARENTAL LEAVE

Under the PDA, an employer who allows temporarily disabled employees to take disability leave or leave without pay must allow an employee who is temporarily disabled because of pregnancy to do the same.

An employer may not single out pregnancy-related conditions for special procedures to determine an employee's ability to work. However, if an employer requires employees to submit a doctor's statement concerning their ability to work before granting leave or paying sick benefits, the employer may require employees affected by pregnancy-related conditions to submit such statements.

Furthermore, under the Family and Medical Leave Act (FMLA) of 1993, a new parent (including foster and adoptive parents) may be eligible for 12 weeks of leave (unpaid or paid if the employee has earned or accrued it) that may be used for care of the new child. To be eligible, the employee must have worked for the employer for 12 months before taking the leave and the employer must have a specified number of employees (see www.dol.gov/whd/regs/compliance/whdfs28.htm)

PREGNANCY AND WORKPLACE LAWS

Pregnant employees may have additional rights under the FMLA, which is enforced by the U.S. Department of Labor. Nursing mothers may also have the right to express milk in the workplace under a provision of the FLSA enforced by the U.S. Department of Labor's Wage and Hour Division (see www.dol.gov/whd/regs/compliance/whdfs73.htm)

For more information about the FMLA or break time for nursing mothers, go to www.dol.gov/agencies/whd or call 202-693-0051 or 1-866-487-9243 (voice), 202-693-7755 (TTY); website: www.dol.gov/general/topic/workhours/fmla

E. Telehealth Resources and Best Practice Guides

KELLY D. ROSENBERGER

The COVID-19 public health emergency has significantly changed the way healthcare services may be delivered for pregnant and postpartum individuals offering more opportunities for telehealth. It is now easier for NPs to offer and get reimbursed for telehealth services. Telehealth can also make healthcare services safer, more private, and more convenient for patients to access care from their homes.

Telehealth can break down barriers, especially for patients living in rural and/or remote communities. It connects patients and providers to a wider network, regardless of location, making it easier to connect patients with specialists, unique treatments, providers, and patient communities who speak their native language or come from a similar cultural background. Telehealth also offers more privacy than face-to-face care, often making patients more willing to seek healthcare treatment. The benefits of telehealth for pregnant individuals have also been explored in rural settings, where access to care is often limited or nonexistent. Many rural hospitals have closed their maternity wards because of cost or other factors. The reduction in maternity facilities has resulted in significant gaps in care for pregnant individuals across the country. With telehealth, patients in rural locations can be treated by providers outside of their immediate vicinity. This allows for a wider network of provider options and facilitates a connection to maternal-fetal medicine specialists if necessary. Patients can access care immediately instead of having to travel long distances to the clinic or wait for an appointment that may not occur for days or even weeks.

Providing healthcare services via telehealth takes planning. It requires new ways of delivering care, different workflow and procedures, as well as a new business model. It is important to understand the pros and cons for NPS and the patients served to decide if providing telehealth services is right for a NP practice.

In the United States, >85% of pregnant individuals are considered low risk. For these patients, telehealth can be used to augment traditional care. Telehealth interventions can also replace some in-person appointments that primarily exist to confirm that both the pregnant individual and fetus are healthy (a conclusion that can often be reached at home). With telehealth, pregnant individuals can decrease the amount of in-person doctor's visits during the prenatal period while still maintaining a high quality of care and patient satisfaction. Integrating new telehealth services for low-risk pregnant individuals is an innovative option to ensure access to prenatal and postpartum care during the COVID-19 pandemic.

With telehealth, a pregnant individual is able to monitor weight and track both blood pressure and fetal heart rate in the comfort of one's own home. If experiencing abnormal or confusing results, the patient simply reaches out to the NP. This allows for a constant stream of communication between patient and NP throughout the prenatal period and limits unnecessary utilization of costly medical resources, such as obstetric providers, clinic time, and nursing support.

There is research to support that telehealth is a good option for pregnant individuals. A study out of the Mayo Clinic evaluated the efficacy of self-monitoring (weight, fundal height, blood pressure, fetal heart rate), text-based communication between care team and patient, and an online community (a forum moderated by a nurse where cohorts of pregnant individuals could consult with one another and their providers). The study found many benefits of the telehealth model, including: increased sense of control and reassurance, lower cost of care, increased access for high-acuity patients, supportive partnerships between care team and pregnant individual, increased patient satisfaction, increased patient engagement and continuity of care, less time away from work, facilities savings, and increased provider engagement and satisfaction. The study concluded that telehealth aided in anticipating the needs of patients and provided access to care in a way that better accommodates the lives of patients.

NPs need to decide what telehealth services will be provided and should define the current service gaps and the problems needing solutions. ACOG has urged state officials to adopt evidence-based policies, including telehealth and remote patient monitoring, that prioritize access to high-quality care, including affordable durable medical equipment (DME) for risk-appropriate pregnant and postpartum individuals. Increasing the availability of DME for pregnant and postpartum women will improve access to comprehensive obstetric telehealth services, ease burdens on hospitals and other healthcare facilities, and reduce the risk of exposure for patients and health care professionals.

NPs need to understand the local State Medicaid agencies' DME benefit coverage so that prescriptions for at-home blood pressure cuffs, pulse oximeters, scales, blood glucose monitors, and fetal heart rate monitors may be provided. ACOG guidance indicates that blood pressure, glucose, and weight monitoring are essential components of comprehensive obstetric care, and state making the availability of at-home monitoring equipment is essential for improving access to telehealth services for pregnant and postpartum individuals. States can eliminate coverage barriers and other inequities for DME, with the following measures: guarantee coverage without cost-sharing, limit the use of utilization management techniques, and implement payment parity for telehealth visits. NPs also need to understand low-income patients, those who live in rural areas, and patients who do not have access to a tablet or smartphone may not be able to access audio-video telehealth services. The Centers for Medicare and Medicaid Services has implemented payment parity for Medicare audio-only visits.

There are many resources available for both patients and healthcare providers, and the American Association of Nurse Practitioners® (AANP) has listed some telehealth resources at: www.aanp.org/practice/practice-management/technology/telehealth

Here are other telehealth resources:

Centers for Medicare and Medicaid Services (CMS) General Provider Telehealth and Telemedicine Toolkit. www.cms.gov/files/document/general-telemedicine-toolkit.pdf

CMS Telehealth Video. www.youtube.com/watch?v=Bsp5tIFnYHk

Medicaid Telehealth Overview. www.medicaid.gov/medicaid/benefits/downloads/medicaid-telehealth-services.pdf

Medicare Telehealth Waiver FAQs. edit.cms.gov/files/document/medicare-telehealth-frequently-asked-questions-faqs-31720.pdf

www.cms.gov/About-CMS/Agency-Information/OMH/equity-initiatives/c2c/consumer-resources/telehealth-resources

BIBLIOGRAPHY

American College of Obstetricians and Gynecologists. (2020). Implementing telehealth in practice. *Obstetrics & Gynecology, 135*(2). https://doi.org/10.1097/AOG.0000000000003671 https://journals.lww.com/greenjournal/Fulltext/2020/02000/Implementing_Telehealth_in_Practice.44.aspx

Reynolds, R. M. (2020). Telehealth in pregnancy. *The Lancet Diabetes & Endocrinology, 8*(6), 459–461. https://doi.org/10.1016/S2213-8587(20)30158-3

Snyder, E. F., & Kerns, L. (2021). Telehealth billing for nurse practitioners during COVID-19: Policy updates. *The Journal for Nurse Practitioners, 17(3)*, 258–263. https://doi.org/10.1016/j.nurpra.2020.11.015

Weigel, G., Frederiksen, B., & Ranji, U. (2020). *Telemedicine and pregnancy care. Women's Health Policy Brief.* https://www.kff.org/womens-health-policy/issue-brief/telemedicine-and-pregnancy-care/

F. LGBTQIA+ Resources

KELLY D. ROSENBERGER

There are many resources available for both patients and healthcare providers related to LGBTQIA+ health. The Centers for Disease Control and Prevention website offers a variety of links with general information, data resources, and LGBTQAI+ health-related organizations and coalitions at www.cdc.gov/lgbthealth/links.htm. Many people in the LGBTQIA+ community are choosing or desiring to become parents. The various pathways to parenthood for LGBTQIA+ individuals may be complex and include several challenges such as barriers to healthcare, transgender hormonal procedures and surgeries that may impact the ability to conceive as well as other fertility issues. More information regarding LGBTQIA+ and pregnancy can be found at www.babymed.com/gay-and-lesbian-pregnancy/lgbt-gay-lesbian-bisexual-transgender-pregnancy-and-parenting#.

Creating a gender-inclusive, accurate, and affirming clinical environment is important and the language used can be powerful. NPs should address each patient based on the patient's own self-reported identity, pronouns, and terms without assuming gender or how someone identifies. By just asking, NPs can create a clinical environment that is inclusive and affirming of various identities, experiences, and perspectives. While there is no one-size-fits-all terminology, Table F-1 provides a guide to using more inclusive "umbrella terms" when providing healthcare.

TABLE F-1 INCLUSIVE TERMS

INSTEAD OF...	USE...
Maternal/Paternal	Parental
Mother/Mom	Parent/Birthing-Parent
Pregnant Women Pregnant Woman	Pregnant People Pregnant Individual
Father/ Dad	Parent
Breastfeeding	Lactation
Women's Health	Reproductive Health
Breast Pump	Lactation Device
Female/Male Reproductive Organs	Internal/External Reproductive Organs
Feminine Products	Menstrual Products
Transsexual	Transgender
Sex Change Operation	Gender Affirming Surgery
Preferred Pronouns	Pronouns

Source: BMC Pregnancy and Childbirth (bmcpregnancychildbirth.biomedcentral.com); LGBTQ Parenting Network (lgbtqpn.ca); Trans Student Educational Resources (transstudent.org)

Additional Resources may be found at:

The Gay, Lesbian, Bisexual, and Transgender Health Access Project's Community Standards of Practice for the Provision of Quality Health Care Services to Lesbian, Gay, Bisexual, and Transgender Clients is a framework that addresses personnel, client's rights, intake and assessment, service planning and delivery, confidentiality, and community outreach and health promotion. Available at www.glbthealth.org/ CommunityStandardsofPractice.htm.

The National Coalition for LGBT Health has many resources, including Guiding Principles for LGBT Inclusion in Healthcare. These principles highlight key health issues facing lesbian, gay, bisexual, and transgender individuals and communities to ensure health equity. Available at lgbthealth.webolutionary.com/sites/default/files/ Guiding%20Principles.pdf.

The Joint Commission's Advancing Effective Communication, Cultural Competence, and Patient- and Family-Centered Care: A Roadmap for Hospitals (Oak Brook, IL: Joint Commission Resources, 2010) contains leadership Resource Guide recommendations and suggested frameworks, issues, and practice examples. Available at www.jointcommission.org/assets/1/6/A RoadmapforHospitalsfinalversion727.pdf.

The C-CAT is an organizational performance assessment toolkit from the Ethical Force Program® at the American Medical Association (AMA) designed to assist organizations in meeting the needs of a diverse patient population. Emphasizing the importance of patient-centered communication, the C-CAT provides a broad-based set of scores about an organization's communication climate and can help healthcare organizations assess how effectively they communicate. More information is available at www.ama-assn.org/ama/pub/physician-resources/medical-ethics/the-ethical-force-program/patient-centered-communication/organizational-assessment-resources. page.

The National Prevention Council, created through the Affordable Care Act and chaired by the U.S. Surgeon General, has developed the National Prevention Strategy: America's Plan for Better Health and Wellness. This 2011 publication includes references to the need for additional information about health issues within the LGBT subpopulations. Available at www.healthcare.gov/center/councils/nphpphc/strategy/report.pdf.

The U.S. Agency for Healthcare Research and Quality's Health Care Innovations Exchange includes an "Innovation Profile" about a comprehensive set of strategies developed by the University of California, San Francisco (UCSF) Medical Center. These communication protocols and inclusive policies, along with ongoing training, led to more equitable, culturally competent care for LGBT patients. Available at www.innovations.ahrq.gov/ content.aspx?id=2737.

The Gay and Lesbian Medical Association (GLMA) Guidelines for Care of Lesbian, Gay, Bisexual, and Transgender Patients provides guidance for assessing provider's practices, offices, policies, and staff training in regard to LGBT inclusivity and recommended actions to improve the access to quality care for the LGBT population. Available at www.glma.org/_data/n_0001/resources/live/GLMA%20guidelines%202006%20FINAL.pdf. GLMA's Web site contains many other resources and more information at www.glma.org.

Healthy People 2020, from the U.S. Department of Health and Human Services, is the government's 10-year agenda for improving the health of all Americans. One objective is to improve the health, safety, and well-being of LGBT individuals. A section specific to LGBT health is available at www.healthypeople.gov/2020/ topicsobjectives2020/overview.aspx?topicid=25.

The Centers for Disease Control and Prevention (CDC) Web site includes a page on LGBT health that offers links to more detailed information for each subpopulation. Available at www.cdc.gov/lgbthealth/index.htm.

The Fenway Institute Web site contains information and numerous resources available at www.fenwayhealth.org

A Provider's Handbook on Culturally Competent Care: Lesbian, Gay, Bisexual and Transgendered Population, produced by Kaiser Permanente National Diversity Council for Kaiser Permanente, offers guidance on providing culturally competent care to LGBT populations. Available at www.audacityofpride.com/ audacity_of_pride/Medical_resources_files/KP%20LGBT%20handbook.pdf.

The American Medical Association's GLBT Advisory Committee Web page contains several resources, including a video on how to take a sexual health history, creating an LGBT–friendly practice, effectively communicating with LGBT patients, and understanding LGBT health issues. Available at www.ama-assn.org/ama/pub/about-ama/our-people/member-groups-sections/glbt-advisory-committee/glbt-resources.page.

Index